Palgrave Studies In Play, Performance, Learning, and Development

Series Editor

Lois Holzman
East Side Institute for Group
and Short Term Psychotherapy
New York, New York, USA

This series showcases research, theory and practice linking play and performance to learning and development across the life span. Bringing the concerns of play theorists and performance practitioners together with those of educational and developmental psychologists and counsellors coincides with the increasing professional and public recognition that changing times require a reconceptualization of what it means to develop, to learn and to teach. In particular, outside of school and informal learning, the arts, and creativity are coming to be understood as essential in order to address school failure and isolation. Drawing upon existing expertise with in and across disciplinary and geographical borders and theoretical perspectives, the series features collaborative projects and theoretical crossovers in the work of theatre artists, youth workers and scholars in educational, developmental, clinical and community psychology, social work and medicine—providing real world evidence of play and theatrical-type performance as powerful catalysts for social-emotional-cognitive growth and successful learning.

Advisory Board: Patch Adams, Founder, Gesundheit Institute, USA; Natalia Gajdamaschko, Simon Fraser University, Canada; Kenneth Gergen, Professor, Swarthmore College, USA and Tilburg University, the Netherlands; Artin Gonçu, Professor, University of Illinois at Chicago, USA; James Johnson, Professor, Pennsylvania State University, USA; Fernanda Liberali, Professor, Pontific Catholic University of São Paulo, Brazil; Yuji Moro, Professor, University of Tsukuba, Japan; Alex Sutherland, Professor, Rhodes University, South Africa; Jill Vialet, Founder and CEO, Playworks, USA.

More information about this series at
http://www.springer.com/series/14603

Peter Smagorinsky
Editor

Creativity and Community among Autism-Spectrum Youth

Creating Positive Social Updrafts through Play and Performance

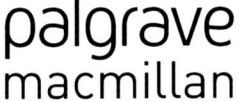

Editor
Peter Smagorinsky
The University of Georgia
Athens, Georgia, USA

Palgrave Studies In Play, Performance, Learning, and Development
ISBN 978-1-137-54796-5   ISBN 978-1-137-54797-2 (eBook)
DOI 10.1057/978-1-137-54797-2

Library of Congress Control Number: 2016958219

© The Editor(s) (if applicable) and The Author(s) 2016
This work is subject to copyright. All rights are solely and exclusively licensed by the Publisher, whether the whole or part of the material is concerned, specifically the rights of translation, reprinting, reuse of illustrations, recitation, broadcasting, reproduction on microfilms or in any other physical way, and transmission or information storage and retrieval, electronic adaptation, computer software, or by similar or dissimilar methodology now known or hereafter developed.
The use of general descriptive names, registered names, trademarks, service marks, etc. in this publication does not imply, even in the absence of a specific statement, that such names are exempt from the relevant protective laws and regulations and therefore free for general use.
The publisher, the authors and the editors are safe to assume that the advice and information in this book are believed to be true and accurate at the date of publication. Neither the publisher nor the authors or the editors give a warranty, express or implied, with respect to the material contained herein or for any errors or omissions that may have been made.

Cover illustration: © SPUTNIK / Alamy Stock Photo

Printed on acid-free paper

This Palgrave Macmillan imprint is published by Springer Nature
The registered company is Nature America Inc.
The registered company address is: 1 New York Plaza, New York, NY 10004, U.S.A.

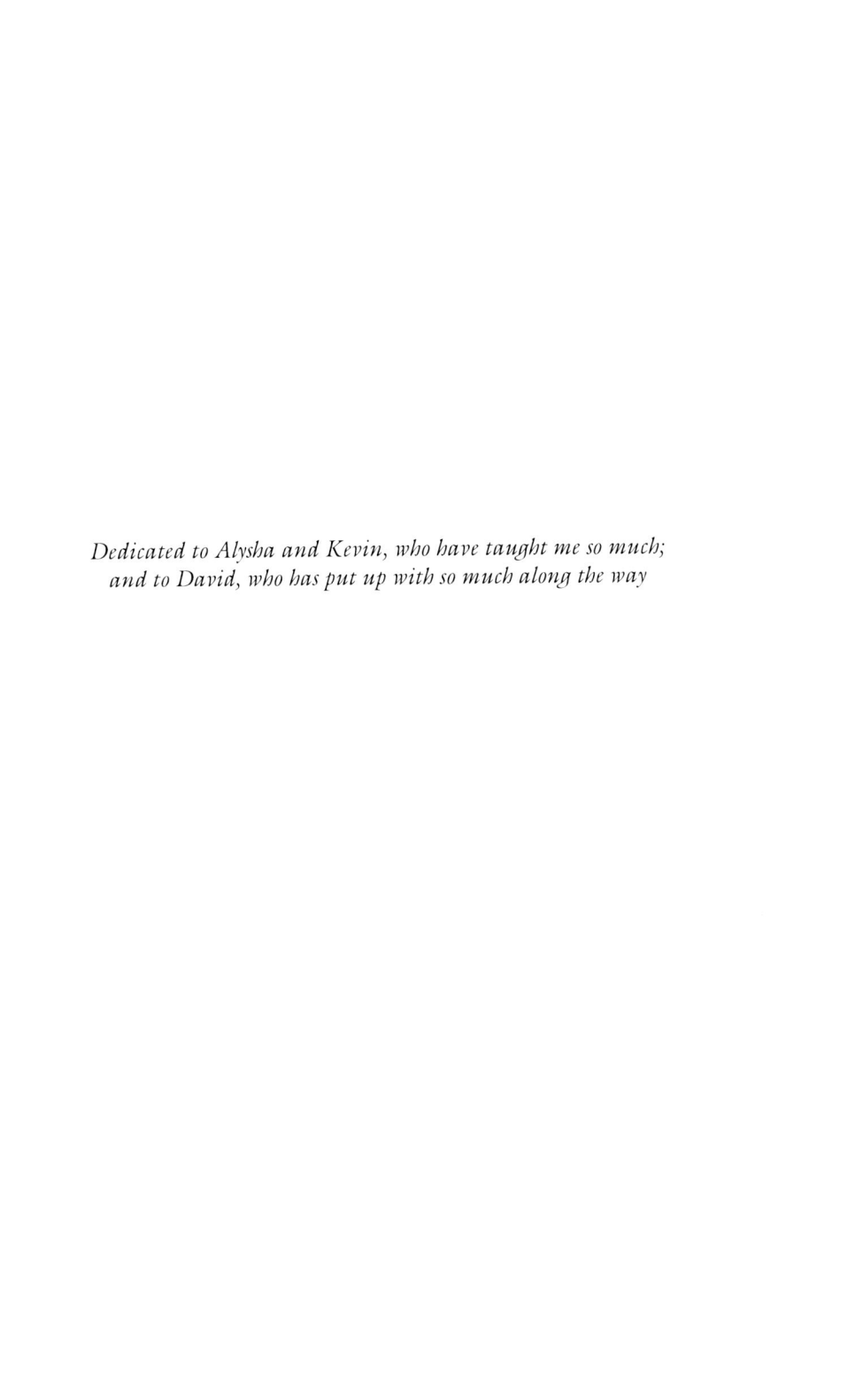

*Dedicated to Alysha and Kevin, who have taught me so much;
and to David, who has put up with so much along the way*

SERIES EDITOR FOREWORD

I am delighted to launch this series, "Studies in Play, Performance, Learning and Development" with such an eclectic and creative book as *Creating Positive Social Updrafts through Play and Performance: Fostering Creativity and Community among Autism-Spectrum Youth*. Peter Smagorinsky has done a wonderful job creating a themed volume in which scholars and practitioners speak passionately and informatively about some of the most cutting-edge work being done by, with, and for young people diagnosed on the autism spectrum. These authors, aided immeasurably by the mental health, play/performance, and Vygotskian framework presented in Smagorinsky's chapters, give readers the gift of their relationships with the people with whom they work and play. There is no dead prose within the pages of this book!

In the beginning, I envisioned the series as an opportunity to bring together some things that too often remain apart: (1) theory, research, and practical intervention related to (2) what we know—and still need to discover—about the human activities of playing and performing with (3) what we know—and need to still discover—about human learning and development. And while the cross fertilization of the "play and performance" folks with the "learning and development" people is underway, the scholars and practitioners engaged in this kind of work are spread out in many fields—from education; developmental, social, and organizational psychology; psychotherapy; and counseling to drama and the performing arts, performance studies, and applied and educational theater.

For two decades, I have had the privilege of meeting, learning from, and partnering with hundreds of people like the contributors to *Creating*

Positive Social Updrafts in the USA and globally. What I hear again and again is a desire to expand their own voices and reach, so that they may continue to innovate and discover more about the kinds of activities that help individuals, groups—indeed, humanity—go beyond the present conditions. My thanks to Smagorinsky and his contributors for their leadership in this effort.

New York, NY, USA   Lois Holzman

Foreword

This is an important and timely book. Notions of diversity and inclusion have too often tended to draw upon outdated and deeply troubled social hierarchies of racial categories. This definition of diversity, while seeking to right longstanding social ills that have perpetuated racial and social inequities, has, more often than not, left out many people whose difference is not visible.

The understanding that diversity is something visible is as outdated as it is a deeply troubled and troubling practice. It leads to methods of identifying diversity by a quick glance at people's faces or quantifying it by determining numbers of people needed from specific groups in order to be representative of their ratio in the entire population. This notion of diversity tends to tokenize people of color, on the one hand, while overlooking people whose differences are not visible, on the other hand. White people and people of mixed race, for instance, who have different orientations toward sexuality and gender, different ways of learning, and different ways of behaving, remain unseen when viewed from this narrow definition of diversity. In these pages, definitions of diversity and practices of inclusion are expanded through finely crafted chapters that show autism-spectrum youths learning through play and performance.

An accomplished scholar of learning and literacy, Peter Smagorinsky is uniquely positioned to speak to the topic of fostering creativity and community among autism-spectrum learners. In the first three chapters, he critiques the willful ignorance of peoples whose class and race positions afford them the luxury of disinterestedness and disregard for the lives and perseverance of autism-spectrum youths. The remaining chapters of the book assemble a well-versed range of professionals who offer several entry points to and in-depth perspectives on working with autism-spectrum youth and their families. They speak of methods for learning and teaching that draw upon social therapies, inclusive theater, exploring expression through Shakespeare, pretend play, collaborative online anime spaces, performance pedagogies, and poetry in order to illustrate how these learning spaces can cultivate social updrafts of mutually sustaining learning relationships.

Throughout, readers learn about the myth of mental illness, a myth that individualizes a disorder—treating it as pathology and disability that manifests itself in the symptoms of diseased thinking and maladapted behavior— as though mental illness is a sickness that needs to be treated by finding just the right cure for that person. The writers gathered here offer instead an understanding of the trials and affordances of different epistemologies and approaches to interacting with the world. In doing so, the authors challenge the conception of neurodiversity as a deficit, a biological deficiency, or an individual lack of ability. Each in this collection begins with the assumption that the onus to change is not on the autism-spectrum youths themselves, but on all students, teachers, parents, professors, and administrators alike who work and learn with these children and youths.

This book offers concrete descriptions of playful social learning moments that help create positive social updrafts. This book allows readers to see diversity in a broader way, to conceptualize integration and inclusion as playful, inviting, and creative sets of shared practices that open up new spaces for learning through the mutually sustaining and reciprocal relationships. This book helps to envision fresh ways for dwelling in the borders of differences, visible or not.

Associate Dean of Academic Affairs,
Diversity and Inclusion
College of Social Sciences and Humanities
Northeastern University
617-373-3349

Ellen Cushman

Acknowledgements

This book was a long time in the making. Thanks to Lois Holzman for inviting me to develop it and for her endless patience in allowing it to stumble, take detours, and finally take shape through our many discussions and written exchanges. Nick Walker was also generous in helping me with certain difficult phrasings in characterizing autistic people. Thanks as well to the contributors who have helped me illustrate the construct of positive social updraft with their programs and research. Finally, I appreciate the help of the friendly folks at Palgrave Macmillan for supporting this project and helping to bring it home.

Contents

Part I Theoretical Framework ... 1

1 Introduction ... 3
Peter Smagorinsky

2 Toward a Social Understanding of Mental Health ... 33
Peter Smagorinsky

3 Adaptation as Reciprocal Dynamic ... 51
Peter Smagorinsky

Part II Deliberately Crafted Activity Settings ... 77

4 Social Therapy and Family Play ... 79
Christine LaCerva

5 Shakespeare and Autism: Reenvisioning Expression, Communication, and Inclusive Communities ... 105
Robin Post

6   We Don't Want to Fit in: A Reflection
    on the Revolutionary Inclusive Theater Practices
    of The Miracle Project and Actionplay for Adolescents
    on the Autism Spectrum   129
    Aaron Feinstein

7   The DisAbility Project: A Model for Autism-Specific
    Creativity and Civic Engagement Within the Broader
    Context of Difference   153
    *Joan Lipkin, Marcy Epstein, Paula Heller,
    and Peter Smagorinsky*

8   Curious Incidents: Pretend Play,
    Presence, and Performance Pedagogies
    in Encounters with Autism   187
    Nicola Shaughnessy

Part III   Mainstream Activity Niches   217

9   The Collaborative Online Anime
    Community as Positive Social Updraft   219
    Leslie S. Cook and Peter Smagorinsky

10 Composing Poetry and a Writer's Identity:
    Positive Social Updrafts in a Community of Writers   243
    Christine M. Dawson

11 An Autistic Life, Animated Through the
    World of Disney: A Loving Autoethnography   269
    Peter Smagorinsky

Contributors   293

Index   297

List of Figures

Fig. 5.1	The HHM circle	108
Fig. 5.2	The Doyoyoying game	110
Fig. 5.3	Teaching Caliban his name	112
Fig. 5.4	Actors model the games	117
Fig. 5.5	Actor modeling emotional expression	125
Fig. 7.1	Survey	172
Fig. 8.1	The alien puppet	188
Fig. 10.1	Three drafts of "Yosemite Still Life"	256

PART I

Theoretical Framework

CHAPTER 1

Introduction

Peter Smagorinsky

As a person with autism I want to emphasize the importance of developing the child's talents. Skills are often uneven in autism, and a child may be good at one thing and poor at another. I had talents in drawing, and these talents later developed into a career in designing cattle handling systems for major beef companies. Too often there is too much emphasis on the deficits and not enough emphasis on the talents. Abilities in children with autism will vary greatly, and many individuals will function at a lower level than me. However, developing talents and improving skills will benefit all. If a child becomes fixated on trains, then use the great motivation of that fixation to motivate learning other skills. For example use a book about trains to teaching reading, use calculating the speed of a train to teach math, and encourage an interest in history by studying the history of the railroads. ~Temple Grandin (Adams et al. 2012)

In forests and tide pools, the value of biological diversity is resilience: the ability to withstand shifting conditions and resist attacks from predators. In a world changing faster than ever, honoring and nurturing neurodiversity is civilization's best chance to thrive in an uncertain future. ~Steve Silberman (2013)

Both of the quotes with which I open this chapter speak about the potential of autistic[1] people to live lives that are personally fulfilling and that

P. Smagorinsky (✉)
Department of Language and Literacy Education, The University of Georgia, USA

contribute to the well-being of society. Unfortunately, however, those on the spectrum tend to be viewed negatively as weird, sick, disabled, disordered, abnormal, and laden with deficits. This book is an effort both to shift the public conception of autistic people toward an understanding of assets and possibility, and to illustrate how the people who surround those on the spectrum may adapt their beliefs and conduct to enable autistic people lead lives that are satisfying and fulfilling.

In this book we take a perspective grounded in Vygotsky's (1987) notion of culturally mediated human development, one that is focused on potential and concerned with fostering it through social processes. In considering questions of development, I always summon a question I heard James Wertsch pose at a conference: *Development toward what?* Given my agreement with Wertsch's (1985) summation of L.S. Vygotsky's historical-cultural-social perspective on psychology, I extend that question to include attention to critical related factors: *Development through what mediational channels, development through which mediational tools, development in light of whose priorities and value systems, and development toward what social and cultural endpoints?*

The contributors to this volume assert that autism is less a static condition than a set of traits that provide the basis for the development of personality through participation in significant cultural activities. This perspective on human difference is available through Vygotsky's (1993) writing in the field known as *defectology*, a term whose unfortunate name I unpack in Chap. 2. This field falls within the general purview of Vygotsky's individual, social, cultural, and historical developmental psychology and is concerned with people of physical and cognitive difference—primarily the deaf, blind, and cognitively impaired children of the early Soviet Union (see Chap. 2). We have adapted a Vygotskian perspective to consider twenty-first-century treatment of those who are classified with what are commonly known as autism spectrum *disorders* (ASD) (see Smagorinsky 2011a, 2012a, b, 2014a, b; Cook and Smagorinsky 2014), a pathology-oriented characterization that we contest in this volume.

According to the Centers for Disease Control and Prevention (2015), "Autism spectrum *disorder* (ASD) is a group of developmental *disabilities* that can cause significant social, communication and behavioral challenges" (n. p.; emphasis added). This statement reveals the pathological way in which autism is defined, even by those who consider themselves sympathetic to the autistic population. The National Institute of Neurological Disorders and Stroke (2016) further states, "The severity of

ASD can vary greatly and is based on the degree to which social communication, insistence of sameness of activities and surroundings, and repetitive patterns of behavior affect the daily functioning of the individual" (n. p.). Greater symptomatic degrees of this "neurological disorder" are treated as indications of "severity," again suggesting that the greater the presence of traits, the more diseased one is considered. Autism, in the view of the general public and the services through which they are informed, is thus widely viewed as an abnormality and disablement of severe consequences.

The authors of this volume take a very different perspective not only in their rejection of this pathological perspective but also in their focus of attention in promoting greater well-being. They are especially attentive to the need for *adaptations in the social environment of human development* (see Chap. 3), rather than solely focusing on individuals who are considered anomalous; and the role of *play and performance* within these social channels to allow groups to construct boundaries and means of self-regulation sensitive to the needs of the whole group.

This emphasis on participation in cultural activity runs counter to the asocial manner in which autism is often conceived. The authors of the chapters in the book demonstrate how autism-spectrum children and youth may be taken up in a *positive social updraft* through which their actions may be channeled in ways that affirm their worth and status within social groups. As the Silberman (2013) quote that begins this chapter suggests, the point is twofold: to address the developmental needs of those on the spectrum, and to enrich the whole of society with the qualities available from those who have long been considered pathetic and abnormal and are best treated with isolation and neglect.

The authors in this volume document the poverty of the perspective that views the human race as hierarchical and human development as measurable through prescriptive notions of normality, a scale that inevitably finds autism-spectrum children and youth (and adults) to be defective. Rather, the contributors work from the premise that human life, although socially channeled toward a common motive within broad societies, includes unlimited endpoints and accompanying pathways for individuals and their social groups to travel. Throughout history, society has provided general value systems and outcomes through which both personal and collective actions are mediated. Individuals within societies are typically socially pressured to take on the identity afforded by those cultural streams, from the leverage of national policies for general populations such as youth in school to more micro-level forces such that left-handed people must adapt to living a right-handed life.[2]

People in the USA and other competitive Western societies are raised within a set of tensions that value conformity to rules on the one hand, and individualism on the other. Human development within such tensions can be subject to a great deal of dissonance, especially for those whose individualism provides a poor fit with societal convention. Such people tend to be treated as oddballs and weirdos, scorned as deficient for their different orientations and ways of engaging with the world.

In this volume, the authors attend especially to autistic people, particularly children and adolescents, whose differences typically lead to their rejection and dismissal by the general population as being of lesser social value. Their differences might be rooted in neurological makeup that produces classifications of deficiency and disorder, might follow practices of a nondominant culture, may be a consequence of external trauma, may have origins in physical or cognitive points of difference that impinge on what are considered typical ways of being, or might proceed from other circumstances. In contrast, the contributors describe how social contexts may be found, constructed, or adapted so that children and youth on the autism spectrum may be treated as contributing members to the greater social order, even as they do so through different means of engagement.

An Alternative to the Standard, Individualistic View of Human Development

The contributors to this volume are particularly concerned about the ways in which social groups, especially those that are dominant, tend to construct environments that limit the types of people who may participate in their activities with confidence and positive reinforcement. We share Vygotsky's (1993) assumption that if problems follow from a person developing in a manner contrary to what is anticipated by others, *these problems are social* rather than deficiencies of the individual.

There is a tendency to locate the individualistic perspective on what is called "mental health"—a term I trouble later in this chapter—as the special province of Western societies. Yet societies from outside the Western purview share this perspective as well. Lee (1997) states that

> Most Asian Americans attempt to deal with their psychological problems without seeking professional services. Many tend to rely on the family in dealing with their problems. Traditional families often treat mental disorders by urging the disturbed family members to change their behavior. They believe that self-control, will power, avoidance of unpleasant thoughts,

keeping busy, and trying not to think too much about problems can help individuals to deal with their troubles. Each family member, including the extended family members, may offer his or her recommended treatment. When the troubled person and his or her family are not able to resolve the problem, they often turn to resources available in their community, such as elders, spiritual healers, ministers, monks, herbalists, fortune tellers, or physicians. Many come to mental health professionals as the last resort, while others are forced to receive counseling by the courts, hospitals, schools, and other social services agencies. (n.p.)

Although there is attention to changes within the family, the onus, as in Western approaches, is on individual self-control, or perhaps on individualized treatments such as acupuncture. Within this perspective, the individual is *disturbed, disordered*, or *troubled*—a view that fits well within the Western view, and in need of repair. This perspective is common among diagnosticians and is pervasive among the general public, becoming near axiomatic in the ways in which people who exhibit anomalous tendencies are socially and medically constructed in U S society and beyond.

In this volume the authors question this emphasis on the individual as the locus of responsibility for difference, shifting attention instead to the environment. Paradoxically perhaps, we assume that although all human conduct and development are socially mediated so that cultures have definable contours and processes, those outcomes and processes are not deterministic, and a dominant culture's ideal destinations or means of arriving at them do not suit all. Further, especially in large nations composed of people of many cultural orientations, multiple pathways and outcomes must be available such that the notion of standardization to a norm becomes too preposterous a condition to impose on multifarious people and subgroups. In our conception, cultural variation includes the cultures that involve people who carry classifications regarding their "mental health" in that their goals, practices, and social standards typically have a particular character that requires adaptive thinking and action on the part of its participants and, from our perspective, on the part of those who surround them.

Typically, however, societies develop beliefs about propriety that lead the majority to view neurodivergent people as having deficiencies that should be corrected. The solution to deafness is to repair the problem with a cochlear implant; the solution for people considered to be mentally ill is to provide the individual with therapy and medication; the solution to being left-handed is to require right-handed performance; and so on. As I know from my own experiences with systemic anxiety, Asperger's traits, and obsessive-compulsiveness, medication can provide relief from anxiety and other conditions that make social life a challenge. Yet such interventions are designed to change the individual's neurological functioning and thus address only a part of what makes life difficult. Similarly, therapy tends to address the individual's feelings of distress. What it does not contribute to is a *change in the social setting* in which the individual is considered to be abnormal, or sick, or disordered, or any number of other pejorative deficit conceptions.

In contrast, many on the autism spectrum *don't want to be normal*. One person on the Asperger's spectrum has characterized the *neurotypical* population—those of "typical" neurological functioning, that is, those who have a style of neurocognitive functioning that falls within the dominant societal standards of "normality"—as follows: "Neurotypical syndrome is a neurobiological disorder characterized by preoccupation with social concerns, delusions of superiority, and obsession with conformity" (quoted by Blume 1998). This preoccupation with following social norms and conventions, to many on the spectrum, is a useless waste of time, and not to be emulated or striven for. Not only is neurotypicality not to be desired, it is considered by those on the spectrum to be debilitating in its own way, focused on appearances and concerned with fitting into other people's notions of how to engage with the world.

The Medical Model, and Difference as a Disease of the Individual

The authors in this volume distance themselves from the *medical model* of treatment of human difference (Laing 1971), which is focused on the physical origins and symptoms of difference and attempts to repair them, as a medical doctor might address bodily maladies from warts to kidney failure. This emphasis on individual difference as a form of disease has been called the *pathology paradigm*, which involves, according to Walker (2013), the following assumptions:

1. There is one "right," "normal," or "healthy" way for human brains and human minds to be configured and to function (or one relatively narrow "normal" range into which the configuration and functioning of human brains and minds ought to fall).
2. If your neurological configuration and functioning (and, as a result, your ways of thinking and behaving) diverge substantially from the dominant standard of "normal," then there is Something Wrong With You. (n. p.)

Neurological variation in the medical model is considered largely as a *disorder*, treatable primarily by medicinal or at times surgical intervention for the patient who is inevitably described as *suffering* from the point of difference. Contributors to this volume do acknowledge the role of interventions that attend to the physical source of difference, such as an antidepressant that employs serotonin reuptake inhibitors. We see, however, such solutions as partial and aimed symptomatically, rather than at the broader culture that defines difference as deficiency and in need of repair.

The medical model tends to be cure-oriented and focused on the sick individual. These remedies are viewed as ways to normalize the condition according to societal mores. This approach is vulnerable to a tendency noted by Hjörne and Säljö (2004) in which professionals encountering a complex social situation categorize people in ways that solve *their own* problems of diagnosis but not those of the people purportedly being served, a problem that Daniels (2006) argues inhibits assistance more than it helps. In this sense, categorizing serves as a sociocultural process and not necessarily a medical diagnosis of firm reliability, a process controlled by the diagnosticians at times to the detriment of the autistic person.

In contrast, the authors are interested in human development in social, cultural, and historical settings. An emphasis on socially situated development shifts the emphasis from cure to participation in meaningful cultural activities through which differences cease to be prohibitive in enabling engagement. Rather than relying on the repair of a deficit, this approach attends to what Vygotsky (1993) calls "roundabout" means of mediating social engagement, such as the blind person's use of a white cane to navigate unfamiliar spaces and traffic patterns. The goal is not to provide sight to the blind, but to provide people lacking sight with other ways of processing and maneuvering about their surroundings so as to participate more fully in cultural activity.

Concurrently, and of paramount importance, the goal is to *alter how people view and accommodate the blindness in others*. Although physical limitations such as the inability to see are not the focus of this volume, the general principle of seeking alternative mediational means for participation in general cultural activity remains central to our approach to considering how social groups may treat neurodivergent people inclusively.

Walker (2013) characterizes this alternative perspective as the *neurodiversity paradigm* (cf. Silberman 2015), one that involves the following assumptions:

1. Neurodiversity—the diversity of brains and minds—is a natural, healthy, and valuable form of human diversity.
2. There is no "normal" or "right" style of human brain or human mind, any more than there is one "normal" or "right" ethnicity, gender, or culture.
3. The social dynamics that manifest in regard to neurodiversity are similar to the social dynamics that manifest in regard to other forms of human diversity (e.g., diversity of race, culture, gender, or sexual orientation). These dynamics include the dynamics of social power relations—the dynamics of social inequality, privilege, and oppression—as well as the dynamics by which diversity, when embraced, acts as a source of creative potential within a group or society. (n. p.)

The term "neurodiversity," coined by autistic Australian sociologist Judy Singer in the 1990s as part of a broader effort among people on the spectrum to assert their humanity in the face of the debilitating assumptions that surround them, was popularized by Harvey Blume (1998), who wrote in *The Atlantic* magazine, "Neurodiversity may be every bit as crucial for the human race as biodiversity is for life in general. Who can say what form of wiring will prove best at any given moment? Cybernetics and computer culture, for example, may favor a somewhat autistic cast of mind" (n. p.). Still regarded by mainstream researchers as "controversial," this perspective takes the position that neurological differences should be recognized and respected, as would other types of diversity in the human makeup. This rejection of the medical model and its accompanying pathology paradigm, and this acceptance of a modified version of the neurodiversity paradigm, are central values articulated by the contributors to this collection.

Is Mental Health Strictly Mental?

One area I've struggled to articulate throughout my effort to understand life on the autism spectrum is the conception of what it means to be mentally healthy or ill. My conversations with my series editor Lois Holzman during the production of this volume have been helpful in my developing an understanding, if not expertise, in this area. In essence, she has helped me recognize the difficulties that I, along with many others, have had with making a break with the medical model of mental health. On one hand, I've rejected it in accepting the Vygotskian notion that having an anomalous mental orientation is primarily a social problem rather than a problem of the individual; on the other hand, I have simultaneously struggled to distance myself from terminology and related concepts to which I've been exposed for my whole life of over six decades. As with any effort to surpass an inadequate paradigm, mine still feels the influence of extant, well-established ideas, ideas that I feel deep in my bones. The production of this book represents an intentional, determined effort to break with the perceptions of difference that have surrounded me for over 60 years.

I will begin with the common term "mental illness." Mental illness is characterized on the website of one of the nation's most vigorous and respectable advocacy groups, the National Alliance on Mental Illness (NAMI) (1996–2011), as follows:

> Mental illnesses are medical conditions that disrupt a person's thinking, feeling, mood, ability to relate to others and daily functioning. Just as diabetes is a disorder of the pancreas, mental illnesses are medical conditions that often result in a diminished capacity for coping with the ordinary demands of life.... Without treatment the consequences of mental illness for the individual and society are staggering: unnecessary disability, unemployment, substance abuse, homelessness, inappropriate incarceration, suicide and wasted lives. The economic cost of untreated mental illness is more than 100 billion dollars each year in the United States.

NAMI's definition of mental illness follows the medical model of diagnosis inscribed in the manual published by the American Psychiatric Association (1994) for responding to mental health issues. Although I am grateful for all of the sincere work undertaken by NAMI, I see their phrasing as falling within the deficit view of mental health difference, as indicated by their use of the word "disorder" and "diminished."

Their analogy of repairing a defective pancreas has its appeal, suggesting that science and medicine can repair what nature couldn't get right the first time around. I have been saved by medicine and science before, and am not against Western medicine or the rational science that provides its foundation. If it weren't for medical interventions, I'd be writing this chapter from the grave.

However, I find the extrapolation from malfunctioning organs to atypical mental frames of mind to be misapplied. A defective human vital organ that is left untreated leads to death as a consequence of biological malfunctioning. A pancreatic impairment is amenable to treatment that provides the body with what the defective pancreas does not by means of insulin replacements. Doctors can even transplant a new pancreas to replace the faulty organ. Treating a disabled pancreas thus focuses directly on the pancreas itself such that its functions are either replicated artificially or replaced by a substitute. No one needs to reconceive the pancreas, or the person whose pancreas fails to produce insulin properly, in order for this intervention to work.

What is commonly thought of as mental health, however, is not analogous to physical illness in this fashion. Although such consequences as suicide may be attributed to severe depression (Fenton 2000), depression itself is not deadly in the manner of a pancreatic dysfunction, and doctors cannot transplant neurological components from one body to another (at least, not during the era of this book's production). Medications are available to alter the manner in which the nervous system works and thus temper disturbing thoughts and feelings; I take one such drug myself for chronic anxiety and obsessive-compulsiveness (see Smagorinsky 2011a) and am grateful for its availability and its calming effect on my otherwise über-intense demeanor. My drug is known as "the detachment drug" for its ability to help users become less maniacally obsessed with all that's wrong with life. Those obsessions used to make my life very challenging and at times quite miserable for me and for those who surrounded me.

My reliance on that daily pill, however, or my need for additional medications to suppress panic attacks when I board airplanes or speak in public, does not mean that I accept the full range of assumptions that the medical community makes about mental makeups that depart from the evolutionary norm. The analogy between mental health and physical illness contributes to the idea that people who are different are the only ones with a responsibility to change themselves. Although attention to stigma is included in the perspective articulated by research and doctors, it is termed as a means of understanding the treatment of *individuals'* nonstandard neurological functioning, rather than *changes in the environment* such that neurodivergence[3] is not stigmatized pathologically, with or without medical intervention.

I have thus far focused on where the issue is located—in the "sick" individual or the insensitive environment—a conundrum regarding which I have a fairly clear answer, one that should be evident to the reader by now. But there are greater complexities that merit attention. By characterizing the various states of mind as involving *mental* health or illness, the issues are not confined only to the affected individual; they are located in "the mind," a construct that in common thought is a function of the brain. Mental illness is thus thought generally to be a problem within an individual's head, as "He's sick in the head," "She's a head case," "He went mental," and other phrasings imply.

However, those working within the Vygotskian tradition tend to embrace Wertsch's (1991) extension of Vygotsky's notion of tool mediation to include the axiom that *the mind extends beyond the skin*. Mind is not only a full-body experience, one that melds cognition, affect, neurology, trauma, diet, and much else; it is a distributed phenomenon, linked inextricably to whatever mediational tools, including engagement with people and their social environments, that people use both to process and represent their worlds and in turn act on them. In other words, "mental health" and "mental illness" mischaracterize neurodivergence by locating it as a problem in the head, and nowhere else.

Problems follow aplenty from conceptualizing the mind as encased within the skull, and from considering "mental health" to be primarily a property of dysfunctional neurologically motivated cognition that can be straightened out with proper interventions, at times of a very behaviorist sort (see Feinstein, this volume). This tendency to treat the mind as a compartmentalized portion of the individual body is consistent with much available through the medical model of "mental health" treatment, as is viewing atypical makeups as solely the province of a discrete neurological system. It follows from such assumptions that the best, and perhaps only, way to "treat" difference is to medicate the neurological system to normalize it and, in turn, moderate whatever mental activity produces anomalous ways of being in the world.

In advancing this perspective, I am not claiming that one's neurological system is irrelevant; my own body would disagree. I am asserting, however, that the neurological system is among many factors in the overall construction of a disposition and way of engaging with one's surroundings, one that is affected by the social environment and its treatment of difference. This broadened perspective, one that assumes neuroplasticity rather than static hard-wiring, opens the door for approaches to difference that include efforts beyond individual medication and therapy.

The neurological system is known as the body's information processor, without which a human (or other creature that includes one) could not function. It includes two major subsystems: the central nervous system, including the brain and spinal cord with its many nerve fibers that produce electronic impulses; and the peripheral nervous system, which includes cranial and spinal nerves that reach the rest of the body. The peripheral nervous system includes the somatic nervous system (consciously controlled muscle movements) and the autonomic nervous system (involuntary activities such as breathing), which in turn includes the sympathetic system (cell and organ functions activated by threat) and the parasympathetic system (which inhibits cell and organ function and slows the body down following a response to threat). This whole system is not autonomous, but may be affected by a variety of external factors: diet, attacks on the immune system, stress, and exposure to heavy metals.

As this account indicates, there's a lot more to how one is neurologically organized than what is strictly "mental." Further, the mind's functioning is also a consequence of how the environment supports an individual's or a group's engagement with the social surroundings. With an extension to the role of social life in how difference is constructed and acted on by others, both relationally and in the sign and tool systems that structure social life, the neurodiversity paradigm might better be called the *socially mediated neurodiversity paradigm*.

What is then called "mental health" is quite deceptive, and as many rhetoricians and discourse analysts have asserted, the discursive environment of human activity provides a principal means of structuring belief systems and accompanying social practices. Neurodivergence does not follow solely from the "hard-wiring" of the neurological system. Some, and perhaps many, sources of difference are neurological in orientation, such as a bipolar personality, described by NAMI (n.d.) as "a brain *disorder* that causes unusual shifts in mood, energy, activity levels, and the ability to carry out daily tasks" (n. p.; emphasis added). Some mental health challenges follow from environmental factors such as the events that result in trauma, such as when depression follows from the death of a loved one (Depression and Bipolar Support Alliance n.d.). Yet other classifications are contested, such as instances of overdiagnosis and overmedication of people to address what are considered aberrations in their behavior. In such instances the DSM provides diagnosticians with pathologizing views of patients and thus mental illness classifications (Frances 2010). The tendency to over-classify children and youth of minoritized racial groups as having abnormal makeups is especially pernicious and corresponds with dominant culture expectations for how they are perceived (Lee and Neuharth-Pritchett 2008).

The authors in this volume contest this deficit perspective, instead viewing neurodiverse populations as having potential, a premise that sees their current state developmentally and amenable to socially mediated formation into productive lives of fulfillment. The possibilities available through such a perspective tend to be social and activity-oriented, foregrounding present activity with a future orientation in how one participates with others in social performances, often undertaken with a playful, experimental frame of mind through which new boundaries are explored and constructed to channel activity productively. (See http://www.madinamerica.com/ for ongoing discussion of this perspective in relation to socially mediated neurodivergence.)

This recognition leads me to a final observation in this section: The public's conception of people of neurodivergent makeups tends to rest on the extremes. On the one hand, there are savants, the sort of character played by Dustin Hoffman in the film *Rain Man* (Levinson 1988), whose autism produces a narrow form of genius that can be channeled into productive activity (although the film's ultimate destination, the gaming tables of Las Vegas, might be considered a dubious use for these abilities). On the other hand, there are people whose frustrations lead them to violent outbursts; these are the sort of people for whom President Obama included a provision in his proposed gun laws to address mental health (National Conference of State Legislatures 2016). For the vast majority between the savants and the threats, however, attention has been limited. This population in the middle provides the focus for this volume.

An Environmental Approach

The shift in attention to the social environment of human development requires one to consider how settings can be altered to allow more human types to be regarded in supportive, appreciative ways, rather than to herd all people through the same developmental chute. Such an adaptation on the part of those in the environment, rather than requiring change only of the individual, has been difficult to achieve. Institutions have become more accommodating in the last few decades, for example, providing such features as wheelchair-accessible ramps and, when affordable, such services as sign interpreters. By and large, however, the onus for adjusting to being different has been placed on the individual of atypical makeup rather than on the surrounding community. The problem of adaptation (see Chap. 3) is thus thrust on the person with the fewest resources to acclimate, while those whose lives are least compromised by difference have minimal responsibility for altering their thinking and conduct. If the stress of adapting individually to one's surroundings can itself produce additional risks for those already considered "at risk" in society (Lee 2008), then shifting attention from the individual to the surroundings would lessen the sense of disaffiliation and alienation often experienced by people exhibiting difference.

Because the neurodivergent population is viewed as deficient, they are subject to what Vygotsky (1993) calls the *secondary disability*. Vygotsky undertook studies of people impaired by continual war in Eastern Europe during World War I and the ensuing Russian Revolution and Civil War. In his sadly neglected oeuvre on "defectology,[4]" Vygotsky (1993) outlines his conclusions on how to account for those people who lack critical physical and mental capabilities such as sight or full-bodied movement.

According to Vygotsky (1993), people do not know that they are different until they are treated as such, often accompanied by the judgmental extremes of scorn and pity. In his conception, their points of difference are not the source of their troubles. Rather, the problem is created by those who treat them as if they have lower social value, producing a *secondary disability* of feelings of inferiority, a malady that is far more harmful to them than the initial source of difference itself. Vygotsky (1993) asserted that "the social aspect formerly diagnosed as secondary and derivative, in fact, turns out to be primary and major. One must boldly look at this problem as a social problem" (p. 112). The authors in this volume take this bold approach in their consideration of how to provide satisfying channels of activity through which autistic people may lead satisfying lives in which their strengths, rather than their points of variance, are foregrounded to serve as assets that are affirmed through social engagement in worthwhile cultural activities.

Positive Social Updraft

Vygotsky's (1993) work in defectology emphasizes, "Full social esteem is the ultimate aim of education inasmuch as all the processes of overcompensation are directed at achieving social status" (p. 57). The solution for anomalous people, he argued, is for other people to contribute to feelings of value by including those who are different in cultural practice such that they have opportunities to participate in ways that take advantage of their assets. In prior work I have used the metaphor of "positive social updraft" to characterize the social channels through which neurodivergent people might be swept up into broader cultural streams such that they feel valued, appreciated, and empowered, and such that they direct their energies toward constructing social futures of promise and potential (Cook and Smagorinsky 2014; Smagorinsky 2013; Walker and Smagorinsky 2013).

I adopted the metaphor of *updraft* from the process of wind currents, such as those that are swept up through a chimney. These currents both have an upward motion themselves and catch other elements in their draft, carrying them upward in their flow. A wind draft is also evident among racers who follow other competitors in order to be drawn along in the air currents they create in their wake. A social updraft provides cultural mediational means that propel people socially "upward" and thus allow people of atypical makeups to become fully involved in significant cultural activity that brings them a feeling of belonging and appreciation.

I have used this metaphor in a variety of contexts. In some cases I have argued that school-based and extracurricular programs such as music, theater, and art can provide the social updraft for youth who are disaffected from established institutions, particularly school. Supporting such programs, I have argued, can help youth whose points of difference—race, immigration status, area of residency, social class, sexual identity, neurodivergence, and many others—often lead to feelings of alienation. Involvement in such programmatic opportunities can provide them with a socially sanctioned activity in which their worth becomes validated, leading to a greater likelihood that they may become more productively involved in other areas of society and its activities.

Such channels illustrate the construct of a *positive social updraft*: an activity system that enables full involvement in worthwhile cultural action, particularly among those who are considered to be social or cultural outsiders who might otherwise be limited in opportunities for legitimate social participation. Although the term "positive" is relative in interpretation, on the whole it refers to socially constructive practices that lead to the achievement of cultural ends. Some cultural practices and the larger purposes toward which they are put, even though they may lead to personal validation, could be considered other than positive for the broader society, for example, physically violent gang activity on one extreme and interpersonally violent social cliques on the other (see Miller et al. 2013). The authors in this volume assume that a positive social updraft contributes to a constructive orientation to social life, broadly speaking. It changes the dynamics of those in the surroundings whose adaptations require of them both a greater empathy toward others and a more astute recognition that their own norms may be prejudicial toward people who follow different orders.

Attention to the social environment of development shifts the focus from considering difference as repairable deficit to providing neurodivergent people with a sense of belonging and affirmation, assisted by increased self-regulation that enables them to learn and develop within cultural contours. It shifts the language of disorder to a conception of difference as different order. It reconceives deficits as potential strengths through a process in which social judgments that produce secondary disabilities give way to enabling environments that allow new strengths and assets to emerge through social activity. Rather than curing people's differences so that they fit in with extant societal ways and means, this perspective seeks to *change the surroundings* to accommodate a broader range of stances, perspectives, and manners. Social dysphoria becomes, if not always euphoria, at least a position farther toward that end of the affective continuum.

THE ROLE OF PLAY AND PERFORMANCE IN SOCIALLY CHANNELED DEVELOPMENT

I have focused thus far on the traits of environments through which positive social updraft may become available to people of difference and in turn contribute to their learning, development, and reciprocal affirmation. The inclusion of playful, performative dimensions in these contexts enables high-level engagement both with others and with their personal developmental needs. "Performance" is often conceived of as being formal, with the goal of producing a great aesthetic effect on audiences. Indeed, Vygotsky's (1971) early work on the theater was dedicated to understanding those formal features of art (including theater) that produced particular, "intelligent" emotional responses in audiences (Smagorinsky 2011b). Yet performance, argues Goffman (1959), is central to everyday life's dramaturgical engagement, a position taken by Vygotsky (1933) when his attention shifted from artistic products to matters of human development.

Yaroshevsky (1989) reports that Vygotsky jotted the following notes in a 1929 notebook: "Dynamics of the individual=drama....The individual as a participant in a drama....Psychology is humanised" (Yaroshevsky, p. 217). The performative aspects of social life were, according to Yaroshevsky, of great interest to Vygotsky, in part because of his great passion for theater. But formal drama was less important in his conception of psychology than everyday social performance that involves each person as "a character of the drama of life on the social stage" (Yaroshevsky, p. 219). This drama takes place among people in everyday interactions, with drama emerging through relational exchanges. Dramatic tensions, he argued, are also present within the individual, indicating that the development of personality is a consequence of the internal and external dramatic conflicts a person experiences in everyday life, the sort of dialectic tension that was central to his Marxist orientation to psychology. To Vygotsky, the development of personality is fundamentally dramatic and the phenomenon of art is at its heart psychological, suggesting the necessity of both in the development of consciousness.

Performance in everyday drama involves what Vygotsky termed "play": experimentation at the borders of convention such that rules are tested and socialization is enabled through activity at the boundaries of propriety. Play involves imaginatively taking on roles and trying out personas that are related to "the child's needs, inclinations, incentives, and motives to act" (Vygotsky 2002/1933, n. p.) in relation to unsatisfied desires, with the ultimate goal of adapting external rules to self-regulatory ways of thinking. Vygotsky sums up the process by saying, "At the end of play development, rules emerge; and the more rigid they are, the greater the demands on the child's application, the greater the regulation of the child's activity, the more tense and acute play becomes" (n. p.). The road to this self-regulatory state of consciousness is paved with imaginative play through which boundaries begin to shape thinking, speech, and action into coherent sets of social practices.

Here's an example borrowed from Chap. 9 of this volume: To produce anime art, one must follow conventions of the genre if one is to be taken seriously and accorded social status and respect; and in so doing, one must work at the limits of one's abilities and conception of appropriate content. How one arrives at producing the form, and what role one takes in larger group productions, involves experimental play that seeks to work at the borders of one's potential and the limits of social and textual genres, and to do so through dramatic engagement with one's own ambivalence and the response of others. Through such playful engagement, learners may test their understandings and perhaps serendipitously discover new juxtapositions that produce new hybrid ways of being (John-Steiner and Meehan 2000). This conception of play and performance is fundamentally consistent with Vygotsky's (1987/1934) understanding of the activity involved in an individual's growth in social, cultural, and historical settings.

Although artistic and other performative products are valued in the work undertaken by this volume's contributors and their participants, even more critical are the developmental processes involved in playful exploration of the boundaries of both formal genres and personal possibilities within social activities. This experimentation with social rules and assumptions is enabled, through performance, to allow people to act "a head taller" and thus use playful activity to serve a developmental role (Vygotsky 1978; cf. Holzman 2009). Playful experimentation with social boundaries is available when constraints become amenable to the suspension of disbelief in the limitations' reification, and when possibilities for new growth follow. This process in turn contributes to the construction of new social contexts that potentially alter one's social profile and lead to different ways of seeing and being seen and considered to have potential for moving life forward as a fully accepted participant in community life. Such pathways are afforded within the positive social updraft of productive, imagination-infused joint activity.

Overview of the Chapters

This book is designed to collect the perspectives of scholars and practitioners whose research has considered the role of social environments in human development, with a particular emphasis on constructing inclusive and accommodative settings that minimize the *secondary disability* of inferior feelings among people of socially mediated neurodivergence by optimizing the developmental value of play and performance. Some of these environments are deliberately constructed for therapeutic purposes, such as the settings provided by psychologists for those seeking treatment. Others are socially available and entered without provocation, such as the online anime community that is presumably open to any participant. What the authors share is a belief that social groups, more than individuals, are responsible for adaptations that affirm autistic people and support their healthy emotional growth, and that opportunities for imaginative play and performance become available through which these adaptations become possible. We hope that this volume provides both an argument on behalf of this approach and a series of illustrations that others may adapt to provide more accommodating environments for the world's great and varied neurodivergence.

Part 1: Theoretical Framework

Following this introductory chapter, I explore the topic of neurodiversity in "Toward a Social Understanding of Neurodiversity." I open with a review of a set of concerns about the ease with which society elides attention to neurodiversity through a series of related phenomena: the problem of *privileged irresponsibility*, through which people with societal assets overlook the problems of people in need; the construct of *epistemological ignorance*, in which those with privilege feel no need to know or understand the needs of those they have *othered* and no obligation to help them persevere; the *benign neglect* that allows such conduct to become normalized in everyday life; and the ways in which their treatment as inferior beings becomes appropriated by those subjected to neglect. With these concepts established, I expand on Vygotsky's (1993) conception of defectology in order to provide the foundation for subsequent chapters' illustration of the positive social updraft available through specific means of collective activity. As noted throughout this introduction, cognitive, neurological, and physical differences are often pathologized by others as problems of the individual and not the responsibility of the social group. This chapter contests that orientation and proposes, based on Vygotsky's formulation, a *social understanding of what is commonly known as mental health* that is less oriented to individual illness and more centered on adaptations made by the broader society to accommodate and support a neurodiverse population.

"Adaptation as Reciprocal Dynamic" centers on the role of adaptation in addressing human variation. I review Darwin's (1859) outline of evolutionary adaptation and consider various efforts to apply his concepts to human society (e.g., Spencer 1857). Adaptation tends to be considered to be the task of individuals and particular species, yet the phenomenon of co-adaptation was central to Darwin's explanation of evolution. This chapter, like the first, helps to set the stage for the remainder of the chapters, which rely on the constructs presented to illustrate mediational settings in which imaginative play may contribute to adaptations by both autistic people and by those who surround them to produce affirmational relationships and a positive social updraft.

Part 2: Deliberately Crafted Activity Settings

In this section, contributors describe therapeutic and performative settings deliberately designed to provide autism-spectrum children and youth with a positive social updraft through which their roles benefit both the group and themselves. Christine LaCerva begins by exploring the methodology of multi-family social therapy groups of adults and children that she has developed as part of a broader social therapeutic approach created by Fred Newman and Lois Holzman. The focus of this work is on the human capacity to play and perform (including to play and perform conversation) and its implications for emotional growth and development. In contrast to traditional play therapy that focuses on the individual child or family, LaCerva illustrates the work of therapy groups designed to facilitate children and the adults working and playing together to create their collective emotional and social development, with this chapter focusing on youth on the autism spectrum. The chapter includes examples from practice as well as a delineation of the theoretical and methodological underpinnings of the performative psychology, *social therapy*. Designed as a playground for emotional and social growth, social therapy groups interrupt psychology's fascination with the individual self and shift attention to the group. It helps therapists and patients alike restrain the knee-jerk impulse to dig into the psyche of the individual or analyze the dynamics of the family unit. In its place is an activity theoretical approach of organizing environments that facilitate both adults and children working together to create new ensemble performances of their relational lives.

Joan Lipkin, Marcy Epstein, Paula Heller, and I next describe The DisAbility Project, which uses formal drama as a means to counter dominant perspectives on "disability," which project director Lipkin conceives of in terms of abilities that go unnoticed in a culture of disability. This chapter is unique in this collection in that autism-spectrum children and youth are not the sole focus of the program; they are among the difference classifications served by this project. The DisAbility Project involves the performance by professional performers of a series of 8 to 12 scripts written to amplify aspects of life with what are commonly known as disabilities. The acting troupe always includes performers who are considered by the broader society to be handicapped in some way. The scripts are not strictly performed, however. Rather, they serve as the stimulus for involving the audience in discussions of difference, with performances interrupted, interludes between skits serving as opportunities to explore the themes featured, and brief activities before and after performances designed to invite personal reflection on beliefs about the self and others. The performances themselves serve as a context for allowing a positive social updraft. The expectation is that when the audience disperses, they will be moved to create new enabling environments for atypical people in their lives. Although autism-spectrum people are but one of many differently enabled people served by this ensemble, the lessons of the project are consistent with the autism-specific activities described throughout the volume.

Aaron Feinstein, working from a theatrical background, writes about the use of performance in creating ways for youth on the autism spectrum to expand their social confidence through the performance of their individual affinities in his program's collaborative after-school improvisational performance-based workshops. The Actionplay model for working with youth is based in the work of the pioneering developmental psychologist Stanley Greenspan, whose DIR/Floortime™ model created an individualized, relationship-based, developmental approach to helping youth on the autism spectrum grow in their social and cognitive development. Greenspan coined the term "follow the child's lead" in building developmentally appropriate social, familial, and educational environments for children on the autism spectrum. The child's "lead" applies to the unique affinities and interests of many children on the autism spectrum that are often viewed as distractions or extinguishable behaviors in academic environments. Many of these affinities may offer insights into the unique sensory processing differences of youth on the autism spectrum, as well as providing opportunities for greater social connectivity and relatedness. Because of the use of compliance-based models in education, many children on the autism spectrum lose confidence in social and academic environments, which can be detrimental to their social and developmental growth. Actionplay provides an accepting and inclusive group-based social approach to creating performances that respect the unique differences and affinities of the individual on the autism spectrum, and creates opportunities for shared social experiences in the creation of original works of art, film, and theatrical performance.

Robin Post next provides insights available through the Hunter Heartbeat Method (HMM) for creating dramatic possibilities for autistic youth. Through this project, autistic children transform the complexities of Shakespeare's poetry and storytelling into a sequence of games that are specifically tailored to address the communicative and social challenges faced by children on the autism spectrum. This chapter describes how the HMM builds safe communities where communication is explored through the physical, vocal, and emotional life of Shakespeare's characters and expressed through the rhythm of life that is Shakespeare's iambic pentameter. The chapter also describes how the pedagogical principles of structure, play, praise, and empowerment underpin the HMM and create communities where children on the spectrum and teaching artists alike are encouraged to share and express their humanity.

Nicola Shaughnessy concludes Part 2 with an account of her "Imagining Autism: Drama, Performance and Intermediality as Interventions for Autism" program, which uses play and performance to address the three main traits of autism: those related to language and communication, social interaction and emotional regulation, and flexibility in thought or social imagination. The play afforded by this program relies on *guided improvisation* in the context of an environment that is both organized and free, allowing autistic children and youth to improvise within a structured environment. By involving the participants in a form of pretend play, the program allows for exploratory engagement through which interactional capabilities are developed, ideally such that they can be reemployed in what she refers to as "naturalistic" social settings. By creating an immersive social environment, one in which participants are aware of the artifice of the elements, Imagining Autism seeks to create the conditions for learning within the performative world of theater, in turn providing a positive social updraft through which they can undertake development toward a valued social future in a setting in which their differences are not viewed as deficits.

Part 3: Mainstream Activity Niches

The next three chapters feature youth development in the context of existing social settings, entered informally and with minimal adult guidance, and at times in the face of adult resistance. With Leslie S. Cook, I present a case study of a young woman diagnosed with a set of related conditions, including chronic depression, Asperger's syndrome, Tourette's syndrome, obsessive-compulsiveness, and an oppositional defiant makeup. Through her involvement in the online anime community, she found an affirmational social setting in which her differences were constructed as strengths and, in contrast to her experiences with the material world and the social lives of her peer group at school, she was recognized as a key contributor to the artistic and narrative worlds available online. In contrast to her parents' concerns that excessive computer time would delay her social development, her online involvement provided her with her primary peer cohort and means of social support. Her intensive involvement in a narrow field of interest enabled her Asperger's and obsessive-compulsive tendencies to serve as assets in her exploration of highly focused topics and projects requiring attention, thus serving her developmental needs well. Within the parameters of the anime genre, her work involved the production of both art and collaborative narrative composing in the medium of "fan fiction," in which popular fictional series are subjected to new treatments by groups of fans producing new stories based on the characters. The chapter considers the inappropriateness of forcing people with dispositions favoring concentrated work into broader interests that amplify their anxiety—much as society forces left-handers to abandon their natural tendencies and requires right-handedness so that they appear to fit in better, regardless of the psychological damage done behind the physical screen.

Christine M. Dawson next describes her research with Scott, a youth on the autism spectrum who became involved in poetic communities of practice. She followed his online poetry writing experiences for six months, during which he composed poems primarily through his participation in an online poetry short course/workshop. Dawson is especially interested in how Scott defined himself and how he used writing as a mediational tool toward self-definition, and how these self-definitions shaped what he did as a poet. He described himself deliberately, at that time, as a "poet-memoirist" and as an "advanced student of writing," which served to empower him in tangible ways and shape how he participated in his writing practices (e.g., how he chose to interpret assignments and feedback, and how he engaged with revision). He deliberately did not identify as an "autistic poet" and resisted that definition and identification of himself as disabled, thus fighting back against the possibility of a secondary disability through his assertion of his qualities as a poet. Dawson explores Scott's composing practices in this online space, analyzing how he used his writing to define himself in his own terms through the poetry he created through this social medium.

In the final chapter I examine the story told by journalist Ron Suskind (2014) in his family memoir *Life Animated: A Story of Sidekicks, Heroes, and Autism*. Suskind narrates his family's experiences with their autistic son, Owen, who suddenly shuts down as a toddler and eventually animates his life by means of engaging with characters from Disney films. By ventriloquizing through the voices, experiences, and perspectives of various characters, Owen comes to understand his role in life as a "sidekick," an archetypal character occurring in most Disney films who assists the film's hero on his or her journey. Rather than discouraging Owen's obsession with Disney, the family joins in his viewings and performances of characters, allowing him to grow into means of using dialogue to communicate and express himself. This highly local family setting then extended to other areas of life, including Disney animators themselves, who became available through the Pulitzer-winning Suskind's many professional connections. The chapter thus considers how the cultivation of activity within a seemingly remote and narrow medium, and the performance of characters' personas within these channels, enabled the emergence of a personality that could easily have been shut down and muted by forcing Owen to act like a normal kid or to tone down his obsession with Disney films.

Conclusion

Taken together, this volume both theorizes the social context of human development and provides examples of how social contexts may be both created and found that allow autistic children and youth to find their place in a world that is not well designed for their needs. These social contexts must be malleable and adaptable, rather than rigid such that the only adaptations must come from those who are ill-equipped to make them. By considering these formal and informal contexts and what they enable for autism-spectrum children and youth, readers may reconsider their own approach to difference and consider those on the autism spectrum with greater understanding and be willing to change their attitudes, conduct, and configurations of space to accommodate more sympathetically the order followed by people from outside the typical range of neurological functioning. If that task is taken up more broadly by families, communities, and societies, life will become more gratifying for people who have historically felt at odds with their surroundings because of the assumption of deficiency accorded them by people who do not understand their needs and who are unwilling to accommodate them. As suggested by neurodiversity's origin in the notion of biodiversity's salutary benefits for the environment, this perspective and accompanying actions will also make the social world a richer, more dynamic place for all who inhabit it.

Notes

1. In my original phrasing here, I wrote "those who live with autism." In responding to an early draft, Nick Walker wrote what follows. I include his response to share my own struggles with my own discursive construction of neurodiversity as I try to shift paradigms through the production of this book. Nick wrote: "We don't 'live with autism,' we're autistic. Autism isn't separate from who we are; it's not a roommate, a pet, or a disease. Language that seeks to portray

autism as something separate from the autistic person's self is a hallmark of the pathology paradigm. Such language does actual harm to autistic people, especially children, because it encourages the mentality that autism could be 'removed' from a person if the right 'treatment' could be found."

2. According to Wikipedia's entry on *Bias against left-handed people*: "Western countries also attempt to convert left-handed children due to cultural, societal and religious biases. Schools tend to urge children to use their right hands, sometimes against the wishes of the child's parents. In America until corporal punishment was outlawed in schools it was not uncommon for students to be physically punished for writing with their left hands (Binns 2006): 'I was educated in the USA in Catholic school in the 60s. My left hand was beaten until it was swollen, so I would use my right right [sic] hand' ... 'I had a teacher who would smack my left hand with a yardstick every time she caught me writing with my left hand' ... 'My fourth grade teacher [...] would force me to use my right hand to perform all of my school work. If she caught me using my left hand, I was hit in the head with a dictionary. It turned out that she believed left handers were connected with Satan'"(Holder 1996–2005).

3. I originally wrote "neurodiversity," but Nick Walker helped me rephrase with the following note: "The term here is 'neurodivergence,' rather than 'neurodiversity.' 'Neurodivergent' means 'not neurotypical,' and 'neurodivergence' is 'divergence from neurotypical norms.' 'Neurodiversity' does NOT mean 'being non-neurotypical'—all humans, including the neurotypical ones, are part of the spectrum of human neurodiversity, just as White people are part of the spectrum of human racial diversity. See http://neurocosmopolitanism.com/neurodiversity-some-basic-terms-definitions/"

4. This term, or at least its translation into English, suggests a deficit perspective, as do other terms (e.g., *abnormal psychology*) associated with it. This term, according to McCagg and Siegelbaum (1989), was introduced to Russians in 1912 by V. P. Kashenko without present-day connotations, and it remains in service today in spite of its implications of defectiveness. Vygotsky's approach, however, belies these connotations in his continual assertion that although social acceptance produces the self-esteem that enables wholehearted participation in cultural practice, those who must do so through roundabout means are not of a lower disorder.

References

Adams, J. B., Edelson, S. M., Grandin, T., Rimland, B., & Johnson, J. (2012). *Advice for parents of young autistic children.* San Diego: Autism Research Institute. Retrieved November 10, 2015, from http://www.autism.com/understanding_advice

American Psychiatric Association (1994). *Diagnostic and statistical manual of mental disorders* (4th ed.). Washington, DC: American Psychiatric Association.

Binns, C. (2006). What makes a lefty: Myths and mysteries persist. *Live Science.* Retrieved October 6, 2014, from http://www.livescience.com/655-lefty-myths-mysteries-persist.html

Blume, H. (1998).Neurodiversity: On the neurological underpinnings of geekdom.*The Atlantic.* Retrieved January 18, 2016, from http://www.theatlantic.com/magazine/archive/1998/09/neurodiversity/305909/

Centers for Disease Control and Prevention. (2015). *Autism spectrum disorders (ASD).* Atlanta: Centers for Disease Control and Prevention. Retrieved February 9, 2016, from http://www.cdc.gov/ncbddd/autism/index.html

Cook, L. S., & Smagorinsky, P. (2014). Constructing positive social updrafts for extranormative personalities. *Learning, Culture and Social Interaction, 3*(4), 296–308.Retrieved August 4, 2015, from http://www.petersmagorinsky.net/About/PDF/LCSI/LCSI_2014.pdf

Daniels, H. (2006). The dangers of corruption in special needs education. *British Journal of Special Education, 33*(1), 4–9.

Darwin, C. (1859). *On the origin of species by means of natural selection, or the preservation of favoured races in the struggle for life.* London: John Murray. Retrieved August 4, 2015, from http://www.literature.org/authors/darwin-charles/the-origin-of-species/

Depression and Bipolar Support Alliance. (n.d.). *Coping with unexpected events: Depression and trauma.* Chicago: Author. Retrieved October 20, 2015, from http://www.dbsalliance.org/site/PageServer?pagename=education_brochures_coping_unexpected_events

Fenton, W. S. (2000). Depression, suicide, and suicide prevention in schizophrenia. *Suicide and Life-Threatening Behavior, 30,* 34–49.

Frances, A. J. (2010). Psychiatric fads and overdiagnosis: Normality is an endangered species. *Psychology Today online.* Retrieved October 20, 2015, from https://www.psychologytoday.com/blog/dsm5-in-distress/201006/psychiatric-fads-and-overdiagnosis

Goffman, E. (1959). *The presentation of self in everyday life.* New York: Anchor Books.

Hjörne, E., & Säljö, R. (2004). "There is something about Julia." Symptoms, categories, and the process of invoking ADHD in the Swedish School: A case study. *Journal of Language, Identity, and Education, 3*(1), 1–24.

Holder, M. K. (1996–2005). *Gauche! Lefthanders in society.* Retrieved October 6, 2014, from http://www.indiana.edu/~primate/lspeak2.html#educators

Holzman, L. (2009). *Vygotsky at work and play.* New York: Routledge.

John-Steiner, V. P., & Meehan, T. M. (2000). Creativity and collaboration in knowledge construction. In C. D. Lee & P. Smagorinsky (Eds.), *Vygotskian perspectives on literacy development: Constructing meaning through collaborative inquiry* (pp. 31–50). New York: Cambridge University Press.

Laing, R. D. (1971). *The politics of the family and other essays.* New York: Routledge.

Lee, C. D. (2008). The centrality of culture to the scientific study of learning and development: How an ecological framework in education research facilitates civic responsibility. *Educational Researcher, 37*(5), 267–279.

Lee, E. (1997). *Working with Asian Americans: A guide for clinicians.* New York: Guilford.

Lee, K., & Neuharth-Pritchett, S. (2008). Attention deficit/hyperactivity disorder across cultures: Development and disability in contexts. *Early Childhood Development and Care, 178*(4), 339–346.

Levinson, B. (1988). *Rain Man.* Beverly Hills: United Artists.

McCagg, W. O., & Siegelbaum, L. H. (1989). *The disabled in the Soviet Union past and present, theory and practice.* Pittsburgh:University of Pittsburgh Press. Retrieved November 3, 2015, from http://digital.library.pitt.edu/cgi-bin/t/text/text-idx?c=pittpress;cc=pittpress;view=toc;idno=31735057895033

Miller, s. j., Burns, L. D., & Johnson, T. S. (Eds.). (2013). *Generation BULLIED 2.0: Prevention and intervention strategies for our most vulnerable students.* New York: Peter Lang.

National Alliance on Mental Illness. (1996–2011). *What is mental illness: Mental illness facts.* Arlington: Author. Retrieved July 20, 2011, from http://www.nami.org/template.cfm?section=about_mental_illness

National Alliance on Mental Illness. (n.d.). *What is bipolar disorder?* Arlington: Author. Retrieved October 20, 2015, from http://www.nimh.nih.gov/health/publications/bipolar-disorder-in-adults/index.shtml

National Conference of State Legislatures. (2016). *President Obama's 2015 executive actions on gun control.* Washington, DC: National Conference of State Legislatures. Retrieved January 18, 2016, from http://www.ncsl.org/research/civil-and-criminal-justice/summary-president-obama-gun-proposals.aspx

National Institute of Neurological Disorders and Stroke. (2016). *Autism spectrum disorder fact sheet.* Bethesda: National Institute of Neurological Disorders and Stroke. Retrieved February 9, 2016, from http://www.ninds.nih.gov/disorders/autism/detail_autism.htm

Silberman, S. (2013). Neurodiversity rewires conventional thinking about brains. *Wired.* Retrieved January 18, 2016, from http://www.wired.com/2013/04/neurodiversity/

Silberman, S. (2015). *NeuroTribes: The legacy of autism and the future of neurodiversity*. New York: Avery.

Smagorinsky, P. (2011a). Confessions of a mad professor: An autoethnographic consideration of neuroatypicality, extranormativity, and education. *Teachers College Record, 113*, 1701–1732. Retrieved August 4, 2015, from http://www.petersmagorinsky.net/About/PDF/TCR/TCR2011.pdf

Smagorinsky, P. (2011b). Vygotsky's stage theory: The psychology of art and the actor under the direction of perezhivanie. *Mind, Culture, and Activity,18*,319–341. Retrieved August 4, 2015, from http://www.petersmagorinsky.net/About/PDF/MCA/MCA2011.pdf

Smagorinsky, P. (2012a). Vygotsky, "defectology," and the inclusion of people of difference in the broader cultural stream. *Journal of Language and Literacy Education, 8*(1), 1–25. Retrieved August 4, 2015, from http://jolle.coe.uga.edu/wp-content/uploads/2012/05/Vygotsky-and-Defectology.pdf

Smagorinsky, P. (2012b). "Every individual has his own insanity": Applying Vygotsky's work on defectology to the question of mental health as an issue of inclusion. *Learning, Culture and Social Interaction,1*(1), 67–77. Retrieved August 4, 2015, from http://www.petersmagorinsky.net/About/PDF/LCSI/LCSI_2012.pdf

Smagorinsky, P. (2013). My View: Hear the music–STEM studies aren't the only path to a better future. *CNN Schools of Thought*. Retrieved August 4, 2015, from http://schoolsofthought.blogs.cnn.com/2013/01/22/hfr-my-view-hear-the-music-stem-studies-arent-the-only-path-to-a-better-future/

Smagorinsky, P. (2014a). Who's normal here? An atypical's perspective on mental health and educational inclusion. *English Journal, 103*(5), 15–23. Retrieved August 4, 2015, from http://www.petersmagorinsky.net/About/PDF/EJ/EJ2014.pdf

Smagorinsky, P. (2014b). Taking the diss out of disability. *Teachers College Record*. Available at http://www.tcrecord.org/Content.asp?ContentID=17771

Spencer, H. (1857). Progress: Its law and causes. *The Westminster Review, 67*, 445–447, 451, 454–456, 464–65. Retrieved August 4, 2015, fromhttp://www.fordham.edu/halsall/mod/spencer-darwin.asp

Suskind, R. (2014). *Life animated: A story of sidekicks, heroes, and autism*. New York: Kingswell.

Vygotsky, L. S. (1971/1925). *The psychology of art* (trans: Scripta Technica, Inc.). Cambridge, MA: MIT Press.

Vygotsky, L. S. (1978). *Mind in society: The development of higher psychological processes* (M. Cole, V. John-Steiner, S. Scribner, & E. Souberman, Eds.). Cambridge, MA: Harvard University Press.

Vygotsky, L. S. (1987/1934). Thinking and speech. In L. S. Vygotsky, *Collected works* (Vol. 1, pp. 39–285) (R. Rieber & A. Carton, Eds.; trans: Minick, N.). New York: Plenum.

Vygotsky, L. S. (1993). *The collected works of L. S. Vygotsky. Volume 2: The fundamentals of defectology (abnormal psychology and learning disabilities)* (R. W. Rieber & A. S. Carton, Eds.; trans: Knox, J. E. & Stevens, C.B.). New York: Plenum.

Vygotsky, L. S. (2002/1933). *Play and its role in the mental development of the child.* (trans: Mulholland, C.). Retrieved October 7, 2014, from https://www.marxists.org/archive/vygotsky/works/1933/play.htm

Walker, N. (2013). Throw away the master's tools: Liberating ourselves from the pathology paradigm. *Neurocosmopolitanism: Nick Walker's notes on neurodiversity, autism, and cognitive liberty.* Retrieved January 17, 2016, from http://neurocosmopolitanism.com/throw-away-the-masters-tools-liberating-ourselves-from-the-pathology-paradigm/

Walker, M., & Smagorinsky, P. (2013). The power of school music programs: Students come for the music and stay for the math. *Atlanta Journal-Constitution.* Retrieved August 4, 2015, from http://blogs.ajc.com/get-schooled-blog/2013/01/01/the-power-of-school-music-programs-students-come-for-the-music-and-stay-for-the-math/?cxntfid=blogs_get_schooled_blog

Wertsch, J. V. (1985). *Vygotsky and the social formation of mind.* Cambridge: Harvard University Press.

Wertsch, J. V. (1991). *Voices of the mind: A sociocultural approach to mediated action.* Cambridge: Harvard University Press.

Yaroshevsky, M. (1989). *Lev Vygotsky* (trans: Syrovatin, S.). Moscow: Progress Publishers.

CHAPTER 2

Toward a Social Understanding of Mental Health

Peter Smagorinsky

My goal in this chapter is to contest the deficit views of people who are discursively constructed as being mentally ill or disordered. In the following sections I review related work on how difference becomes pathologized, and draw on Vygotsky's (1993) work in the field of *defectology*—an unfortunately named effort to integrate blind, deaf, and people otherwise lacking common physical traits into society's streams of activity[1]—to provide a *social understanding of mental health*. This effort is undertaken in order to outline a social view of anomalous mental health makeups that is less oriented to individual illness (see Chap. 1) and more centered on adaptations made by the broader society to accommodate and support a wider range of mental health profiles (see Chap. 3).

PRIVILEGED IRRESPONSIBILITY, THE BANALITY OF EVIL, AND BENIGN NEGLECT

Virtually every society has some history of oppressive social structures. This chapter is about neither race nor gender, but I see parallels between the issues articulated currently in South Africa to account for artifacts of

P. Smagorinsky (✉)
Department of Language and Literacy Education, The University of Georgia, USA

apartheid and the manner in which people of anomalous mental frameworks for engaging with the world are treated by those whose neurological makeup more closely follows the evolutionary norm.

Bozalek's (2014) account of *privileged irresponsibility*, invoked to consider differential treatment and opportunity for women and Blacks in South Africa, is instructive in extrapolating from well-known forms of oppression to those that are less visible or discussed, including those that concern neurodivergence. Drawing on Tronto's (1993) formulation, Bozalek argues that the needs of the privileged are more likely to be considered important and met than those of the marginalized, With the result that people with little political power or status are overlooked and neglected. More recently, Tronto (2013) has offered the construct of *epistemological ignorance* in which those with privilege feel no need to know or understand the needs of the oppressed and thus have little sense of obligation to provide them with appropriate attention, support, and care. As a consequence, the lives of those on the margins or in subjugated social positions are vulnerable to the phenomenon of *dualism*,[2] in which the life circumstances of social outsiders are constructed and represented as inferior to those of people from the dominant culture.

Dualism involves three processes that reify established social positioning. Through *inferiorization*, marginalized social groups are viewed as being in deficit to the norms, and thus to the inherent worth, of the dominant group. Inferiorization in turn produces *interiorization*, the manner in which oppressed people internalize the negative constructions to which they are continually exposed. The ultimate consequence is *othering*, the separation of society into dominant groups ("us") and subordinate groups ("them"), with the latter presumed to be essentially deficient and irreparable and thus a nuisance to society's good, unless they can bring themselves through individual acts of determination up to the standards of the dominant culture. We hear of this quality in the modern call for "grit" (Tough 2013)—that toughness and initiative that allow those at the bottom to lift themselves up to the top without disturbing the system or changing its structure.

Those who are *othered* become available for exploitation, particularly in terms of providing labor that benefits those who comprise society's dominant culture. South African examples include Blacks who are discouraged from even pursuing high-status and well-compensated work, and women whose life trajectories are steered toward low-paying service professions such as teaching and nursing. Bozalek's (2014) examples could almost as easily have been culled from modern-day USA as well (Thomas 2014) as from other nations with colonial histories and undoubtedly from nations with any hierarchical social structure.

The phenomenon of privileged irresponsibility maps onto the notion of *banality of evil* (Arendt 1963), as conceived in response to the trial of Nazi death camp architect Adolph Eichmann in Jerusalem. The construct refers to the manner in which the horrific treatment of other human beings may become normalized to the point that ordinary citizens come to accept evil and atrocities as part of daily life. These offenses are supported and enabled by their very banal and mundane character. By accepting appalling acts as ordinary within society's normative functioning, even those who do not commit barbarous actions themselves are participants in evil.

Arendt's (1963) attention centered on Nazi culture's inhumane treatment of Jews, an act that became normalized for Nazi-era Germans, yet by current standards it is almost universally considered barbaric and criminal. My own attention to neurodiversity centers on normalized deficit views toward autistic people and the banality of the evil of ignoring their circumstances and possibilities. I must acknowledge that prior to my own acceptance of my own place on the Asperger's syndrome spectrum, I was complicit in the evil of disregarding the needs of people considered mentally ill in all of the ways that I critique in this essay (see Smagorinsky 2011a).

My growing understanding of neurodiversity is informed by the scholarship on privileged irresponsibility and the banality of evil, although I recognize that this issue generally lacks the dimension that treats lower-status people as labor mules who make life easier for the privileged. People discursively and conceptually characterized as mentally ill are pathologized in ways that relieve the rest of society of the need to care about them, viewing their condition as a problem for doctors and not themselves. The pathologized often interiorize a belief in their own inferiority for being different; and they are othered such that their problems are not those of society. Rather, the banality of their circumstances leads them to be the concern of only themselves and the small number of people who know and care about them, or who treat them as invalids—a term that could refer both to their status as sickly and to their lack of social validity.

Those politicians and taxpayers who allow care to be underfunded, often leading to despicable conditions for those outside the evolutionary norm that in turn exacerbate their state of mind, contribute to their wretched conditions by ignoring them and considering them to be a problem outside their own life's purview. The banality of this neglect leads to the societal evil of their circumstances being solely the problem of the people considered to be inferior and to have little potential to make positive contributions to society.

With neurological anomaly being the problem of those who are othered by the dominant social group, neurologically atypical people are treated with *benign neglect*. This term was proposed by US Senator Daniel Patrick Moynihan (1970) to muffle the explosive racial uproar taking place during Richard M. Nixon's presidency. Moynihan wrote a 1969 memo, exposed the following year, in which he recommended to the president, "The time may have come when the issue of race could benefit from a period of 'benign neglect.' The subject has been too much talked about. The forum has been too much taken over to hysterics, paranoids, and boodlers on all sides. We need a period in which Negro progress continues and racial rhetoric fades." The term has come to reference any approach to a social problem in which those in power ignore it rather than address it head-on, in hopes that it eventually resolves itself. Such privileged irresponsibility allows people in dominant social positions to accept the banality of evil social conditions. This perspective might provide comfort to those among society's dominant upper tier, yet it is virtually guaranteed to exacerbate the conditions that affect those for whom being different presents continual challenges and obstacles, many of which are social in construction.

Vygotsky and Defectology

I next draw on Vygotsky's (1993) defectological writing to provide a perspective on neurodiversity that helps to address the problems of privileged irresponsibility, the banality of evil, and the benign neglect of social problems to provide a different perspective, one that is less pathologically oriented and more concerned with effecting changes in the people surrounding those who exhibit anomalous ways of being. This social view is derived from Vygotsky's interest in socially situated human development, broadly speaking. His attention to the social, cultural, and historical basis of human development included his work in the area of *defectology*, a field centered on the treatment and education of the many people deafened, blinded, maimed, and otherwise physically and mentally traumatized by Eastern Europe's continual warfare from 1914 to 1924, culminating with the formation of the Soviet Union (for an extended review of these circumstances, see Smagorinsky 2012a).

In prior work (Smagorinsky 2011a, 2012a, b, 2014) I have adapted Vygotsky's defectological writing to what I have, prior to this volume, called "mental health" in the US context. I propose extrapolating his views on people of cognitive and physical difference to take a more socially oriented approach to neurodivergence. To do so I draw on bodies of work dedicated to inclusive approaches to social difference and power differentials in colonial societies and apply them to the issue of autism, which is often subject to the same problems of pathologization and deficit characterizations to which the more familiar areas of race and gender are prone.

Vygotsky's views of the biologically different are constructed so that individual people's potential may be better realized through greater understanding of their circumstances and through adaptations by the people around them, rather than through their characterization as fundamentally sick and deficient people who are outside the need for "us" to change "our" lives so that "they" may better prosper. The term "defectology" mischaracterizes Vygotsky's (1993) approach to differences from the evolutionary norm, which he did not consider to be defective or prohibitive in enabling a full immersion in societal life. Rather than focusing on atypical people themselves, Vygotsky shifted attention to the *settings of human development* and their role in supporting and accommodating them. Vygotsky's view of the "defect" is encapsulated in his assertion that "blindness is not merely a defect, a minus, a weakness, but in some sense is also the source of manifestations of abilities, a plus, a strength (however strange or paradoxical this may seem!)" (p. 97). He argued that departures from the evolutionary norm simply call for alternative or "roundabout" means of mediation. Vygotsky's approach was thus positive and forward-looking and dedicated to cultivating potential, resisting the societal tendency to take a "philanthropic, invalid-oriented point of view" toward difference (p. 75).

Given his rejection of difference as a sign of disorder and defectiveness, Vygotsky (1993) rejected deficit views (Kotik-Friedgut and Friedgut 2008), instead situating his attention to difference in his broader developmental approach. The potential for more optimistic, future-oriented, and possibility-centered settings for development is available, he argued. Educators in particular should focus not on difference, but on one's "physical and psychological reaction to the handicap" (p. 32). Although he uses the term "handicap"—at least in translation—his overall conception of difference was one of potential rather than impediment. This attention to language and its implications is critical to my efforts to reconceive anomalous neurological functioning as less a pathological condition to be repaired and more a different orientation to the world that may produce a unique perspective. Adopting this view can be challenging given that those with bipolar, obsessive-compulsive, depressive, and other atypical personality makeups can appear to lack what others have in terms of personal stability and social functioning. People with extreme orientations away from the norm can seem socially threatening and at times appear dangerous to others, although the risks that they present might be moderated if they themselves were treated differently.

With the goal of discursively constructing anomalous ways of being more positively, I have used two terms, "extranormal" and "neuro-atypical," to account for those whose makeup stands outside the norm—not in deficit, but in relation to different orientations to the social and natural worlds (Smagorinsky 2011a). I use the term "extranormal" and its derivatives because terms such as "non-normal" assume that there is indeed a social norm, suggesting that those of different makeup are in deficit to the majority. Extranormal provides a more inclusive term that suggests additional possibilities for those having a profile outside the typical range.

"Neuro-atypical" is derived from *neurotypical*, the term that many diagnosed with Asperger's syndrome use for people not considered to be on the autism spectrum. Neurotypicals, to those whose makeups fall within the Asperger's syndrome spectrum, do not necessarily possess enviable qualities. Rather, from this perspective, neurotypicals are unfortunately obsessed with conforming to social rules. They occupy time, attention, and energy that could be put to better use and often put on false fronts that mask their genuine beliefs and opinions. Neuro-atypical simply characterizes difference as another way of being, one that is neither abnormal nor disordered but capable of producing perspectives and insights not available to those within what the majority consider to be the typical range.

Vygotsky's Views on Feelings of Inadequacy

Vygotsky (1993) argued that the feelings of inadequacy that often accompany cognitive or physical difference usually have one of two very different effects on those affected. Most often, the secondary disability follows from a sense of stigma that leads to long-term feelings of inferiority that may produce what Vygotsky termed *moral insanity*: the manner in which people are catalyzed into violent reactions against those who treat them as deficient. More positively, feelings of inadequacy can produce generative action. I next relate these two consequences of feelings of inadequacy to issues of neurodiversity.

Stigma and Secondary Disabilities

To Vygotsky (1993), feelings of inferiority that follow from being othered—to use Tronto's (1993) terms rather than Vygotsky's—serve as a secondary disability to the primary disability (to use a flawed term) of being physically or neurologically anomalous. Shifting attention from the pathologized individual to the social milieu, he argued that the place to begin is with the environment, not the individual. He emphasized the need for an inclusive view of difference such that all people, regardless of their differences, could find alternative pathways of development that result in full participation and appreciation in society's broader activities. Without a supportive environment, those who do not fit the diagnostic norm experience the secondary disability of feelings of inferiority. This condition corresponds to the process of *interiorization* in which people of difference appropriate negative judgments from their incessant social presence and accept the belief that difference and deficit are coterminous.

Vygotsky (1993) notes that people do not consider themselves as different until treated by others as such. His key insight is that the people surrounding neuro-typicals construct a potentially disabling environment of pity, rejection, scorn, and other negative means of reinforcement that lead to the inevitable conclusion that one is indeed inferior—a process of inferiorization, to use Tronto's (1993) term. Vygotsky was concerned with how people feel as a result of how they are treated. He emphasized self-esteem, which in his view follows from being treated in a manner that validates one's life as full and capable of contributing to society through productive labor. "Full social esteem," he insisted, "is the ultimate aim of education inasmuch as all the processes of overcompensation are directed at achieving social status"[3] (p. 57). Any conception that separated the intellect from affect, he argued, overlooks the fact that "thought and affect are parts of the same, single whole, and that whole is human consciousness" (p. 236).

This attention to the role of affect in overall human development is realized in what my colleagues and I have called *meta-experience*: the manner in which experience is experienced so as to frame new experiences (Smagorinsky 2011b; Smagorinsky and Daigle 2012; Smagorinsky et al.

2010). Those who are treated as defective bring their accompanying feelings of inferiority and deficiency to new experiences. These feelings in turn frame new experiences, reinforcing the belief that one is inadequate and disordered, a process corresponding to Tronto's (1993) related notions of inferiorization and interiorization. Addressing these feelings by normalizing difference, Vygotsky (1993) believed, is critical to enabling one to develop the higher mental functions characteristic of general cultural ways of engaging with the world. Vygotsky emphasized that "the changing relationship between affect and intellect is the very essence of the entire psychological development of a child" (p. 239). This change does not come about through individual acts of will, but rather through changes in how atypical people are constructed and treated by those who surround them.

Neurodivergent people realize their feelings of inferiority in diverse ways, often such that they become further pathologized. Vygotsky (1993) refers to one such response as *moral insanity*, which in his parlance refers to the way in which those who are ill-treated lash out at those who consider them pitiful and inferior. He asserts that this condition is entirely situational and relational; change the setting, he argues, and the retaliatory conduct will cease. As is typical of Vygotsky's conception, he views the problem as a social problem, rather than an incurable malady of the individual in isolation. Striking back against the oppressor, to borrow Bozalek's (2014) formulation for the relationship between dominant and marginalized people, rarely is viewed in such sympathetic terms. Rather, retaliation is simply taken as further evidence of a deficient or disordered mind, one that the individual must get repaired before reentering the social groups that are comprised of people who feel no obligation themselves to change or accommodate.

Inadequacy as a Stimulus for Generative Action

Vygotsky (1993) also found that one's response to feelings of inadequacy may produce generative action to circumvent the source of the feelings—the point of physical or neurological difference—through adaptation (see Chap. 3). This transformation requires a focused volitional effort that is socially reinforced. Vygotsky (1993) viewed compensatory development to be an instance of a generative response to difference. This adaptive, intentional initiative to respond to the environment involves working toward the satisfaction of social goals. Neuro-atypical people often seek to find social niches in which to find acceptance, thus providing the impetus to develop roundabout means of navigating society to compensate for the absence of conventional psychological or physical tools.

Unfortunately, this second notion of adaptation prevails in society. That is, rather than relying on the majority of people to adapt their thinking and behavior to allow for people of difference to find acceptance, they individualize difference and place the full burden of adaptation on the person with the fewest resources for achieving the outcome of social acceptance. Undoubtedly, some blend of the two adaptive behaviors would be of greatest benefit: People of difference would be motivated to achieve the social goal of acceptance and thus seek means of working toward it by roundabout means, and the majority would provide channels of activity through which such immersion would become possible. When irresponsible privilege negates this second option and leads to benign neglect of the needs of others, thus producing the indifference that characterizes the banality of evil, the full responsibility falls upon the neurodivergent population, those who have appropriated strong feelings of inferiority from the negative (scornful) and superficially positive (charitable) treatment by others and thus doubt their worth or feelings of healthy acceptance and social competence.

Integrating People of Difference with the Broader Cultural Stream

Vygotsky (1993) argued that society's goal ought to be to promote its culture's higher mental functions—those ways of thinking that represent cultural knowledge that form the basis of social life, rather than simple biological maturation—in all citizens, regardless of how that development is mediated. He did not focus his attention on the source of difference itself, taking instead the position that the goal of all human development is the fostering of higher mental processes. Vygotsky's (1987/1934) outline of higher mental functions influenced his view of educating society's atypical population. "The greatest possibilities for the development of the abnormal child," he wrote, "most likely lie in the higher, rather than the lower, functions" (p. 198). By this he meant that rather than attending to the biological (lower) points of difference, society should promote the development of frameworks for thinking appropriated through cultural practice: the higher mental functions. These ways of thinking are available through participation in life in the social group, suggesting that pathologizing individuals and sequestering them from society will only exacerbate, rather than address and remedy, the social problems that follow from difference.

Vygotsky's (1993) vision was geared toward the ultimate developmental goal of achieving socialization and social status. Toward that end he employed a multifaceted approach. For anomalous people, collaborative action in everyday social activity helps to foster alternative pathways toward conventional ends. Just as important, however, are adaptations undertaken by the collaborator, who must cease to view the evolutionarily different child as a deficient or disordered member of "the other," lower-order social group: "the task is not so much the education of blind children as it is the reeducation of the sighted. The latter must change their attitude toward blindness and toward the blind. The reeducation of the sighted poses a social pedagogical task of enormous importance" (p. 86). This reeducation, he concluded, requires those in the social mainstream to "overcome the very notion of a handicap" (p. 93).

Vygotsky's (1993) thus formulated an inclusive view toward those of biological difference. He continually emphasized the importance of fitting in societally, of being included and accepted, in the midst of critical biological and developmental difference. It is instructive to return to his fundamental postulation that human development involves two near-concurrent lines, one biological and one cultural. The biological line is the one that appears prevalent in conceptions of difference that rely on individualistic and pathological judgments of deficit. The biological line is "hard-wired" in the process of conception. Although some reconstituting is possible—a person can be provided a prosthetic leg in the absence of a biological one; Lasik surgery can convert opaque vision to serviceable vision in many patients—for the most part, people live with the biological affordances with which they are born.

Vygotsky's developmental approach led him to take a greater interest in the cultural line of development, which begins at birth[4] and is mediated by adult projections of a social future and the actions and practices that promote that outcome (Cole 1996). That cultural line of development, one promoted through social engagement, is the one, I further argue, that is just as appropriate for neurodivergence as it was to the physical points of difference that motivated Vygotsky's (1993) investigations in the field of defectology.

Illustration of Positive Social Updraft

In accordance with this volume's titular attention to *positive social updraft* (Cook and Smagorinsky 2014; Smagorinsky 2013a, b; Walker and Smagorinsky 2013), I next describe a corporate initiative in which

Vygotsky's (1993) notion of the secondary disability is potentially diminished as people of difference become incorporated into broader social streams of activity. In the world of commerce, the Walgreens pharmacy chain has pioneered a movement to employ people characterized as having disabilities, a practice taken up by Proctor & Gamble, Home Depot, Wal-Mart, McDonald's, Lowe's, Best Buy, AMC, and other corporations.

The 1990 passage of the Americans with Disabilities Act brought about changes in the USA for wheelchair accessibility, braille options in elevators and other public places, and other efforts to make life more easily navigable for those lacking the full evolutionary set of physical features. The Walgreens Disability Inclusion action was designed to exceed those accommodations by intentionally seeking to provide full employment for those for whom such occupations were rarely available. Although some are concerned that the jobs tend to be low-wage, low-status positions (Otto 2013), the initiative has been widely praised by the government, media, business world, and various groups that view people in terms of abilities rather than disabilities. The general view seems to be that any job is better than none, undermining the critique that the initiative only provides entry-level jobs.

Before reviewing the Walgreen Disability Inclusion model, I will address the concern that low- wage and low-status jobs are demeaning to those who hold them, including those on the autism spectrum. Similar complaints were registered to address Soviet educational psychologist Alexander Meshcheryakov's (1979)methods for engaging deaf and blind people in what some considered menial activities as simple as using the toilet and feeding oneself with a spoon. Bakhurst and Padden (1991), however, see Meshcheryakov working in the sociohistoric tradition of Vygotsky and others in emphasizing *obshcheniya*—interpersonal relationships—as a way of helping to socialize deaf and blind children into their environments through their participation in meaningful forms of activity. Using other terms, they suggest providing a positive social updraft through which new and more complex forms of participation become possible. Bakhurst and Padden argue that "these 'menial' activities are valued as the very basis of future intellectual development for the reason ... that they are activities carried out jointly with others" (p. 208). The key is to engage people in collaborative activities that are worthwhile for the developmental level of the learner such that they both learn how to conduct them independently and develop competencies that enable their graduation to new stages of challenge.

I next focus on the Walgreens Disability Inclusion model given the company's foundational role in providing neurologically and physically diverse people with opportunities to participate in the workforce and become self-supporting and feel affirmed. Walgreens is, of course, a business and not a charitable organization. It was important, therefore, for their hiring initiative to work within the expectations of shareholders to generate profits. Because their pilot programs "didn't move the needle [in the wrong direction] on the business decision," according to company executive David Bernauer, Walgreens expanded the program beyond its test site and made their hiring policy a corporate imperative (Bennett-Alexander and Hartman n.d.).Walgreens has established partnerships with local providers for training, and then considers applications for their retail and distribution centers from this pool, with at least 10 % of their total workforce classified as disabled.

The program is too recent for it to have been a site for disinterested researchers to investigate its process and effects; most reports come from positive media accounts that quote management's optimistic perspective. The program has benefitted from a report authored by the National Governors Association (2012–2013), which concludes that the program achieves what Vygotsky (1993) would consider the laudable aim of having people in the business community view those classified as disabled "not as charity cases but employees with uncommon qualities that can enhance profits" (The Monitor's Editorial Board 2013). This environment, according to Randy Lewis, senior vice president of distribution and logistics for Walgreens, produces benefits not only for individuals considered disabled, but for the workforce in general: "One thing we found is they can all do the job. What surprised us is the environment that it's created. It's a building where everybody helps each other out"(Bennett-Alexander and Hartman n.d.).

The Monitor's Editorial Board of the *Christian Science Monitor* (2013) concluded that studies of the Walgreens initiative have found that those classified as disabled often turn out to be among a corporation's most reliable employees. They are

> more efficient and loyal than nondisabled workers. Absenteeism [at Walgreens sites] has gone down, turnover is less, and safety statistics are up. And the cost of accommodating such workers with new technologies and education is minimal....Many disabled workers are so grateful for a job that they work harder. Some industries, such as software and data testing, prefer workers with certain disabilities, such as autism, because of a person's intense focus on detail. (n. p.)

The Walgreens initiative provides a cultural stream in which those employed may engage in productive labor that has genuine value and in turn allows neurologically and physically atypical people to develop the self-esteem that is so central to living a life of fulfillment. Undoubtedly, the encomium accorded Walgreens would benefit from a critical perspective, few of which are available at this point, in order to verify the impressions of those who have a stake in its success. The program, however, does show potential for providing the sort of useful cultural labor that, to Vygotsky (1993), leads anomalous people to feel included and valued, leading to more fulfilling lives for the individuals employed and to a better environment for those around them. The Walgreens initiative illustrates Vygotsky's (adjusted) tenet that "the task is not so much the education of [the individual] as it is the reeducation of the [social group]. The latter must change their attitude toward [difference] and toward the [different]. The reeducation of the [social group] poses a social pedagogical task of enormous importance" (p. 86).

In programs such as Walgreens', then, the "other" becomes a fellow worker, one who is included and respected for achievements. In the absence of pity and charity, scorn and dismissal, workers are potentially less prone to the secondary disability, achieving instead new social status that enables feelings of success. Undoubtedly, like all panaceas, the program requires continual attention, monitoring, and adjustment. It does, however, provide one channel through which the social goal of inclusion may be realized in the corporate world.

Discussion

In this chapter I have attempted to recast neurodiversity and human difference in general as matters of social inclusion. Most of my research has come in the context of schools, which are relatively circumscribed environments in which policies may control conduct through such initiatives as anti-bullying campaigns. Much of Vygotsky's (1993) writing on defectology similarly is oriented to providing an inclusive education through which atypical children may find acceptance through the opportunities available in productive collective labor. Getting kids in schools to comply with rules, which is hardly easy to do, is much simpler than getting adults in society to voluntarily accept people who exhibit difference. It is especially difficult to change whole social settings that involve people with diverse beliefs so that they are more welcoming and accommodating to those who exhibit difference. Yet given that school ends relatively early in life, the task of reconsidering social practices in the world beyond school so that the whole of the physically, cognitively, and neurologically atypical population feels more included remains a great undertaking.

Vygotsky (1993) argued that society needs to focus less on the pathologized individual and more on the social setting of collective activity. Through the provision of such social spaces, the likelihood of the debilitating secondary disability becomes diminished and the possibilities for leading a life of fulfillment become enhanced. That potential is something that benefits not just the individual but the society as a whole, and is a goal worth striving toward, as indicated by the positive outcomes found by Walgreens executives who see the whole workplace environment changed for the better when a broader range of human types is allowed fruitful participation.

Like the other contributors to this volume, I see the construction of inclusive settings to set the seeds for broader efforts at acceptance. I harbor no illusions that a great societal revolution is underway. Rather, I see the fostering of corporate initiatives, infrastructures such as the Internet that enable spontaneous social channels to emerge (see Part 3 of this volume), and constructed environments such as drama programs (see Part 2 of this volume) serving as exemplars for how others might attend more deliberately to providing social worlds that are less discriminatory and more inviting for a broader range of participants.

Notes

1. The term "defectology" sounds, as readers might have already determined, quite dissonant to modern ears. It perhaps sounded less severe in Russian in the 1920s Soviet Union, yet is discordant in translation, particularly for those of us who are challenging deficit conceptions of difference. Although we strive in this collection to avoid any such terminology, in reviewing Vygotsky I need to employ the terms I am provided in translation. The full title of his volume, for instance, is *The Collected Works of L. S. Vygotsky. Volume 2: The Fundamentals of Defectology (Abnormal Psychology and Learning Disabilities)*, applied to the collection by editors preparing his essays for a modern audience. The three deficit terms in the title suggest an orientation that he systematically dismantles in the essays themselves, yet that at times appear in his own writing, suggesting that

either the terms have become distorted in translation or that, even with his dedication to challenging deficit notions of difference, he could not escape the discursive constructions that his society employed to characterize those damaged physically by warfare. As I note in Chap. 1 of this volume, I fight the same battle to escape the concepts available from the discursive environment that structured my own orientation to neurodivergence for much of my life.
2. The term "dualism" is amenable to other interpretations, such as the Cartesian mind/body dualism in philosophy. Here, I restrict myself to the definition offered by Bozalek by way of Tronto.
3. I would distinguish Vygotsky's conception of self-esteem from the modern US version, in which a child's feelings of importance should not be undermined under any circumstances (see Branden 1969).
4. Vygotsky is often quoted to say that cultural and biological lines of development intersect at age 2, but elsewhere in his writing he sees the two lines as intertwined much earlier. Cole (1996) provides compelling evidence that the cultural line of development begins with a neonate's first human contact, as babies are socialized into gender roles (Rubin et al. 1974).

References

Arendt, H. (1963). *Eichmann in Jerusalem: A report on the banality of evil.* New York: Viking Press.

Bakhurst, D., & Padden, C. (1991). The Meshcheryakov experiment: Soviet work on the education of blind-deaf children. *Learning and Instruction, 1*(1), 201–215.

Bennett-Alexander, D. D., & Hartman, L. P. (n.d.). *Disability discrimination.* Retrieved May 6, 2014, from http://answers.mheducation.com/business/management/employment-law/disability-discrimination

Bozalek, V. (2014). Privileged irresponsibility. In G. Olthuis, H. Kohlen, & J. Heier (Eds.), *Moral boundaries redrawn: The significance of Joan Tronto's argument for political theory, professional ethics, and care as practice* (pp. 51–72). Walpole: Peeters.

Branden, N. (1969). *The psychology of self-esteem: A new concept of man's psychological nature.* Plainview: Nash Publishing Corporation. Retrieved July 24, 2015, from http://ir.nmu.org.ua/bitstream/handle/123456789/113278/82752c2d6efced7dd2ee6a8d6f3200bf.pdf?sequence=1

Cole, M. (1996). *Cultural psychology: A once and future discipline.* Cambridge, MA: Harvard University Press.

Cook, L. S., & Smagorinsky, P. (2014). Constructing positive social updrafts for extranormative personalities. *Learning, Culture and Social Interaction*, *3*(4), 296–308. Available at http://www.petersmagorinsky.net/About/PDF/LCSI/LCSI_2014.pdf

Kotik-Friedgut, B., & Friedgut, T. H. (2008). A man of his country and his time: Jewish influences on Lev Semionovich Vygotsky's world view. *History of Psychology*, *11*(1), 15–39.

Meshcheryakov, A. I. (1979). *Awakening to life* (trans: Judelson,K.). Moscow: Progress.

Moynihan, D. P. (1970, March 2). Memorandum to President Nixon on the status of Negroes. *The Evening Star*, p. A–5. Washington, DC. Available at http://www.aol.bartleby.com/73/1579.html

National Governors Association. (2012–2013). *A better bottom line: Employing people with disabilities. Blueprint for governors*. Washington, DC: Author. Retrieved May 6, 2014, from http://www.nga.org/files/live/sites/NGA/files/pdf/2013/NGA_2013BetterBottomLineWeb.pdf

Otto, B. (2013). Walgreens is not always the answer. *Huffington Post*. Retrieved May 6, 2014, from http://www.huffingtonpost.com/barbara-otto/hiring-disabled-workers_b_2448183.html

Rubin, J. Z., Provenzano, F. J., & Luria, Z. (1974). The eye of the beholder: Parents' views on sex of newborns. *American Journal of Orthopsychiatry*, *44*, 512–519.

Smagorinsky, P. (2011a). Confessions of a mad professor: An autoethnographic consideration of neuroatypicality, extranormativity, and education. *Teachers College Record*, *113*, 1701–1732. Retrieved May 6, 2014, from http://www.petersmagorinsky.net/About/PDF/TCR/TCR2011.pdf

Smagorinsky, P. (2011b). Vygotsky's stage theory: The psychology of art and the actor under the direction of *perezhivanie*. *Mind, Culture, and Activity*, *18*, 319–341.

Smagorinsky, P. (2012a). Vygotsky, "defectology," and the inclusion of people of difference in the broader cultural stream. *Journal of Language and Literacy Education*, *8*(1), 1–25. Retrieved May 6, 2014, from http://jolle.coe.uga.edu/wp-content/uploads/2012/05/Vygotsky-and-Defectology.pdf

Smagorinsky, P. (2012b). "Every individual has his own insanity": Applying Vygotsky's work on defectology to the question of mental health as an issue of inclusion. *Learning, Culture and Social Interaction*, *1*(1), 67–77. Retrieved May 6, 2014, from http://www.petersmagorinsky.net/About/PDF/LCSI/LCSI_2012.pdf

Smagorinsky, P. (2013a). My View: Hear the music—STEM studies aren't the only path to a better future. *CNN Schools of Thought*. Available at http://schoolsofthought.blogs.cnn.com/2013/01/22/hfr-my-view-hear-the-music-stem-studies-arent-the-only-path-to-a-better-future/

Smagorinsky, P. (2013b). *Constructing positive social updrafts for extranormative personalities*. Invited address in recognition of winning the 2012 Sylvia Scribner Award, presented at the annual conference of the American Educational Research Association, San Francisco.

Smagorinsky, P. (2014). Who's normal here? An atypical's perspective on mental health and educational inclusion. *English Journal, 103*(5), 15–23. Retrieved May 6, 2014, from http://www.petersmagorinsky.net/About/PDF/EJ/EJ2014.pdf

Smagorinsky, P., & Daigle, E. A. (2012). The role of affect in students' writing for school. In E. Grigorenko, E. Mambrino, & D. Preiss (Eds.), *Handbook of writing: A mosaic of perspectives and views* (pp. 291–305). New York: Psychology Press.

Smagorinsky, P., Daigle, E. A., O'Donnell-Allen, C., & Bynum, S. (2010). Bullshit in academic writing: A protocol analysis of a high school senior's process of interpreting *Much Ado About Nothing*. *Research in the Teaching of English, 44*, 368–405.

The Monitor's Editorial Board. (2013). Americans with disabilities may be the best workers no one's hiring. *Salon.*Retrieved May 6, 2014, from http://www.salon.com/2013/08/07/americans_with_disabilities_may_be_the_best_workers_who_cant_get_jobs_newscred/

Thomas, P. L. (2014). *Two Americas: George W. Bush and Neil deGrasse Tyson.* Retrieved May 6, 2014, from http://radicalscholarship.wordpress.com/2014/04/19/two-americas-george-w-bush-and-neil-degrasse-tyson/

Tough, P. (2013). *How children succeed: Grit, curiosity, and the hidden power of character.* New York: Mariner Books.

Tronto, J. (1993). *Moral boundaries: A political argument for an ethic of care.* New York: Routledge.

Tronto, J. (2013). *Caring democracy: Markets, equality, and justice.* New York: New York University Press.

Vygotsky, L. S. (1987/1934). Thinking and speech. In L. S. Vygotsky, *Collected works* (Vol. 1, pp. 39–285) (R. Rieber & A. Carton, Eds.; trans: Minick, N.). New York: Plenum.

Vygotsky, L. S. (1993). *The collected works of L. S. Vygotsky. Volume 2: The fundamentals of defectology (abnormal psychology and learning disabilities)* (R. W. Rieber & A. S. Carton, Eds.; trans: Knox, J. E. & Stevens, C. B.). New York: Plenum.

Walker, M., & Smagorinsky, P. (2013). The power of school music programs: Students come for the music and stay for the math. *Atlanta Journal-Constitution.* Retrieved September 1, 2016 from http://blogs.ajc.com/get-schooled-blog/2013/01/01/the-power-of-school-music-programs-students-come-for-the-music-and-stay-for-the-math/?cxntfid=blogs_get_schooled_blog

CHAPTER 3

Adaptation as Reciprocal Dynamic

Peter Smagorinsky

My interest in human adaptation follows from my efforts to understand neurodiversity. This topic has occupied my attention informally for nearly 30 years and has become, within the last decade, a focus of inquiry for me across a series of autobiographical, theoretical, and empirical papers. I was forced to take on this topic during the youth of my daughter, who began exhibiting unusual behaviors early in life, ultimately being diagnosed with a number of what are known as mental illnesses and neurodivergent conditions: Asperger's syndrome, Tourette's syndrome, severe chronic anxiety, depression, oppositional defiance disorder, and obsessive-compulsive disorder, as they are known in the diagnostic community. The charming manner in which she would, as a child, arrange her dolls and other belongings in well-ordered patterns in various rooms of our house eventually manifested itself in other ways that began to get our attention. Ultimately, it led us to consult with medical, psychotherapeutic, and psychological interventionists who provided various combinations of pharmaceuticals and interactive therapies designed to temper her extreme tendencies, which at times could be alarming and destructive.

P. Smagorinsky (✉)
Department of Language and Literacy Education, The University of Georgia, USA

Through our experiences with trying to provide her—and concurrently, to provide her younger brother, my wife[1], and me—with a more satisfying life, I came to understand these conditions from a very personal standpoint. Like other parents of my generation whose children went through a diagnosis, at times I thought that the specialists were talking about me while explaining the results. The more I learned about her makeup, the more I reflected on my own personality, particularly following a major panic attack in 1999 during a conference presentation I was making that resulted in my own diagnosis of severe chronic anxiety, a condition for which I have been taking medication ever since.

That episode and the learning curve that followed my initial resistance to the idea that what was described as "mental illness" could occur in my very own family led me to interpret my own tendencies in light of my daughter's condition. The result was an understanding that much of what characterized her—anxiety, Asperger's, Tourette's, and obsessive-compulsiveness—undoubtedly was part of my own makeup. And I suspect that more than a few people who have attempted to manage, maneuver, manipulate, and supervise me over the years would add an oppositional-defiant temperament to the mix as well.

In conjunction with this recognition, I began writing about neurodiversity—at the time using the term "mental health"—from a very personal standpoint. I began with an autoethnographic reflection (Smagorinsky 2011) in which I related my own and my family's experiences. I argued that although people like my daughter and me are undeniably cut from a different and in some ways less socially acceptable cloth than are most people, we are not deficient, disordered, abnormal, or sick or other characterizations commonly applied to those who experience the world in socially atypical ways. Rather, we had a makeup that, in the right contexts, actually made us assets to social groups and communities of practice, not to mention ourselves. To give one example from my own experience, the combination of Asperger's and obsessive-compulsiveness can lead a person to pursue topics of interest in extraordinary and systematic detail and engage with them with an intense focus that is available to few who are not on this spectrum. We see the world in a grain of sand rather than as one big beach.

In my career as a researcher, this frame of mind, in contrast to being the debilitating abnormality that typically is "suffered" by those with Asperger's, is a tremendous asset that enables me to investigate a line of inquiry exhaustively. In the process I might exhaust some of the people around me, but my publication record has made me, in the academic world in which narrowness and intense focus are rewarded, a valued member of the university culture. I've begun referring to this facet of my personality as a quality, my Asperger's Advantage, rather than the disorder it is generally considered to be (Smagorinsky 2014). There might be accompanying traits, such as interactional bluntness, that some people find dissonant in polite company, but that trait can be tolerated, if not universally welcomed or particularly humored, in a productive university faculty member.

This disposition has enabled me to think deeply about neurodiversity, and to do so through the vehicle of writing, a confluence that has served me well in the production-oriented world of the publish-or-perish environment in which I work by choice. My initial autoethnography was well received and opened the door to my scholarly investigations. In my autoethnography, I had made a brief reference to Vygotsky's (1993) studies of *defectology*, which I review in detail in Chap. 2 of this volume.

As someone with Asperger's, I was not content to write my autoethnography with a second-hand account of Vygotsky's (1993) defectological writing provided by Kozulin and Gindis (2007), my introductory source at the time, and be satisfied with my achievement. Rather, I had to read the whole volume in order to grasp the full breadth of his thinking on a topic that had entered my obsessive mind, and begin writing in relation to this reading (Smagorinsky 2012a, b). These papers hardly satiated my interest, but rather they fed my appetite for understanding Vygotsky's ideas in light of neurodiversity, an issue that he had addressed only peripherally in sections scattered across his writing—in his critiques of Freud's focus on the past rather than on the future, and in Freud's and others' attention on the individual rather than on the social group (e.g., Vygotsky 1927).

This writing also brought me in contact with the work of my colleagues Kyunghwa Lee and Joe Tobin, who were studying other social aspects of human difference. Kyunghwa was interested in how youth from non-White racial classifications were overrepresented in learning disabilities assignments (e.g., Lee 2008), and Joe was in the process of conducting a cross-national study of preschools that enrolled deaf children (Tobin, Valente, & Horejes 2010–2014).We scheduled a semester of discussions with graduate students and occasional visitors. It was a seminar series that included deaf participants, the sort of persons with whom I had had infrequent opportunity to interact during my life. My sensitivity to the problem of secondary disability made me extremely attentive to our deaf participants' needs, such as their need for others to make eye contact with them while they spoke in sign language—even though the vocal sound that translated their signing physically emanated from another person, often in a different part of the room where they could see the signing clearly. Although the deaf speakers and listeners had to make adaptations of their own in order to participate in the discussions, it was incumbent on the rest of us to make adaptations as well.

This phenomenon gave me a new imperative, to investigate the problem of adaptation as one shared by whole groups rather than individuals of difference. This chapter serves as my effort to consider adaptation as a social, rather than solely an individual problem. I first review Darwin's evolutionary theory and the role of adaptation for species, social groups, and individuals, all of which influenced Vygotsky's (1931) attention to the problem of adaptation for people of difference. Not surprisingly, Vygotsky viewed this issue as a social problem not confined to the individual of difference but shared by those in the environment of development.

CO-ADAPTATION IN EVOLUTIONARY THEORY

Most conceptions of evolution and adaptation are motivated by Charles Darwin (1859), a naturalist who was not concerned with human adaptation yet whose ideas have been used to conceptualize social theories of competition and survival. Darwin's contemporary Herbert Spencer (1857), a sociologist who asserted a libertarian perspective on human culture that presumed the "survival of the fittest" in human competition, popularized the notion of *social Darwinism* in the wake of the publication of Darwin's *On the Origin of Species*. Ironically, Spencer's attention to individual monetary competition and Vygotsky's Marxist perspective on collective human labor shared this same source. Given my interest in the role of the social group in accommodating people of difference, it should come as no surprise that I am Vygotskian rather than Spencerian in my appropriation of Darwin to consider the problem of human adaptation.

Fundamental to Spencer's (1857) social Darwinism is the assumption that people are inherently in competition with one another for social and material advantage. His ideas were robustly incorporated into the perspective of US industrialists such as Andrew Carnegie (1889), who said that "while the law (of competition) may be sometimes hard for the individual, it is best for the race, because it ensures the survival of the fittest in every department." Darwin's cousin Francis Galton (1883) further founded the notion of eugenics: the idea that superior human races can be genetically and socially engineered through selective breeding and thinning out the weak. The belief that the strongest survive fits the machinery of American capitalism quite well, or at least its most selfishly motivated version of capitalism that allows for the ruthless pursuit of wealth without regard for the health and welfare of others in society. This conception, while often practiced among industrialists and financiers, is not, however, the only way in which either naturalistic or social Darwinism is practiced.

Stetsenko (2011) argues that Darwin, instead of emphasizing individual competition for survival, was concerned with a species' collective history in that "The relational and historical character of nature, interlinking all living forms through their history clearly comes through in that Darwin employs the notion of *co-adaptations* of organic beings to each other and to their physical conditions of life" (p. 29; emphasis in original). She proceeds to quote Darwin's lament that "our ignorance on the *mutual relations* of all organic beings" overlooks interdependence, the conjoint and reciprocal reliance on others that contributes to the present and future welfare of creatures living in ecological balance. Animals, including humans, do not live in harmonious bliss, given their need to eat and survive, which pits them in competition in what Darwin (1859) called "the Struggle for Existence." He uses this term "in a large and metaphorical sense, including dependence of one being on another, and including (which is more important) not only the life of the individual, but success in leaving progeny" (pp. 63–64).

Darwin (1859), then, was less individualistic about survival than those who claimed to adapt his principles from nature to society. Nature, he argued, provides many examples of mutual interdependence from humans who domesticate dogs to the symbiotic relations between many animals, such as suckerfish who attach to sharks and both groom them and live off the effluvium of their kills. Darwin was among the first to note the complex webs of dependency in nature, exclaiming, "the presence of a feline animal in large numbers in a district might determine, through the intervention first of mice and then of bees, the frequency of certain flowers in that district!" (p. 74).

People's domestication of animals is not always as reciprocal as are their customary relationships with their pets, as is evident in People for the Ethical Treatment of Animals' (http://www.peta.org/) ongoing crusade to persuade people to treat animals used for food, research, and other purposes more humanely. Surviving in light of the human need for food and medical advances complicates the ethics of occupying a crowded planet, including its many and varied human occupants. This ethical component, however, at least in human societies, provides the imperative for accommodating, rather than competing against, other inhabitants of a social and natural space.

Stetsenko (2011) notes that Vygotsky's developmental approach views human growth as a function of engagement with and adaptation to the environment, both in its physical and social senses. This view, she argues, is Marxist in origin, given that it relies on collective labor rather than individual competition. Again, the issues are complicated, in that the USA is a capitalist rather than socialist or communist society, making Marxist arguments problematic in this context, an issue to which I will return.

Vygotsky's conception of collective labor is both historical and immediate. Cultures organize their practices in relation to the environment and through tools designed to enable them to survive its vicissitudes (Tulviste 1991), a process that involves continual transformation and creation to optimize human possibilities. This collective activity is fundamental to social life, resulting in what Stetsenko (2011) refers to as a process in which human development becomes a *"socio-historical project and a collaborative accomplishment…a historical becoming* by people as agents who together change their world and, in and through this process, come to know themselves and their world, while ultimately becoming human" (p. 33; emphasis in original). This point is saturated in the Marxist perspective that capitalism is fundamentally dehumanizing, a problem that Marx believed would lead to its inevitable extinction, superseded by communal social life, an endpoint that has yet to be realized.

From this viewpoint, human society is not necessarily competitive at the individual level, given that intentional, volitional group efforts are available, if not embraced by all. Society need not be ruthlessly oriented to the accumulation of wealth, as those working in Spencer's tradition tend to assume in emphasizing the competitive nature of capitalist societies. A selective reading of Darwin (1859) could easily support Spencer's human version of the struggle for survival. Darwin wrote, for instance, that "the competition [for survival] should be most severe between allied forms, which fill nearly the same place in the economy of nature" (p. 76). Within the same niche, he notes, one species of rat or cockroach might drive out others filling the same ecological niche. What is different about people, however, is their vast within-species differentiation such that they create unlimited societal niches that don't necessarily pit one individual or subgroup against the other for survival.

Rather, humans may work together to benefit not only themselves or their groups but also other people, perhaps even from different groups. Darwin (1859) found it incontrovertible and ultimately axiomatic that "the infinite complexity of the relations of all organic beings to each other and to their conditions of existence, causing an infinite diversity in structure, constitution, and habits, [is] advantageous to them" (p. 119). Vygotsky and others for whom Marx is a starting point thus consider the role of the social group in ensuring survival, even as many societies founded in Marxism have rapidly shifted to totalitarianism (Snyder 2010), suggesting that Marx's critiques of capitalism did not necessarily produce a viable alternative in the actual conduct of human affairs. My own perspective is somewhere in between the extremes provided by Marx and Carnegie, informed by the understanding that cooperative societies, or at least subgroups within societies, are possible if not inevitable, and only when ethical imperatives for mutual care become governing philosophies (see Chap. 2's attention to privileged irresponsibility, the banality of evil, and benign neglect).

Several factors distinguish human evolutionary adaptations from those in nonhuman populations, in particular the availability of cultural-historical adaptations by human social groups, such as the ability to pass down socially constructed knowledge to new generations. I make this observation with the understanding that advances in learning about the complexity of nonhuman life continue to reveal greater intelligence, intentionality, tool use, and social organization than has previously been believed. Vygotsky, for instance, spent a great deal of time distinguishing between people and primates (e.g., Vygotsky and Luria 1993), relying on a knowledge base that now is greatly outdated. He underestimated and mischaracterized the tool use of primates, a phenomenon that researchers have demonstrated in the years following his death (e.g., Ottoni and Izar 2008; cf. Shumaker et al. 2011 for tool use across the animal kingdom; and Wikipedia, n.d.a, for a compendium).

As I have reviewed, people have interpreted Darwin in very different ways. On one hand, his observations about the competitive side of the natural world have been applied directly to human life, with people of superior advantage dominating and at times even eliminating those of lesser or unwanted capabilities, a major project of Stalin in his effort to accelerate the evolution of the "New Soviet Man" in the Soviet Union (Bardziński 2013). This perspective views biological makeup, particularly intelligence, as innate and lacking any sort of malleability. From this standpoint, one is born with physical and cognitive abilities that remain constant across the lifespan. Advantages such as those provided by circumstance—particularly wealth—are viewed in this conception as incidental to one's life potential and trajectory.

On the other hand, Darwin has been interpreted in terms of social group behavior, exhibited in both the natural and human worlds. People need not elevate themselves at the expense of others, but may work cooperatively to produce group potential for survival and welfare. From this perspective, innate biological makeup is elastic, capable of reshaping and growth through social mediation. Those who embrace this view consider members of social groups to be responsible for one another, with those who may lack some evolutionary advantage such as sight or hearing being included in cultural activities through alternative means, rather than being rejected as nuisances in the drive to generate wealth. The unsighted may never see, but they can be provided with tools such as canes and braille texts that enable them to navigate the material world sufficiently to live rewarding lives, particularly when their lives are validated by those around them. They may further benefit others through the contributions they may make when appreciated for the assets that are too often overlooked when they are viewed and essentialized in terms of what they lack.

Adaptation and Social Environments of Development

Early in his career, Vygotsky (1925/1997a) wrote that "Adaptation is the fundamental and universal law of development and life of organisms" (p. 57), available in two types. First, changes are available in the animal's biological structure. These changes are produced over time in Darwin's sense of the evolution of species. The second type of change occurs in behavior, but not in structure. This sort of adaptation is more rapid and flexible, available to individuals but not to species over generations, and it is more a property of mind than body. That is, my thinking is much more amenable to adaptation and change than are my arms or legs, even as both are related to one another.

Vygotsky (1925/1997a) was primarily interested in how mind develops in relation to the environment, calling mind "the most valuable biological adaptation" (p. 57) because it enables a human to gain control over nature. As I have reviewed, it also may produce gains in control over other people, although Vygotsky's nascent Marxist perspective viewed people as more cooperative than competitive, a principle betrayed by Stalin during Vygotsky's lifetime and beyond.

At this early point in his career, Vygotsky (1925/1997a) was strongly influenced by Pavlov, the reigning titan of Russian psychology. Within five years, Vygotsky (1930/1997) had distanced himself from Pavlov's insistence that psychology should investigate the physiology of the brain via the study of nervous associations and related reflexes, unaccompanied by attention to mental phenomena. Pavlov is known today for his "conditioned response" experiments in which dogs were trained to salivate when a light or sound signaled the availability of food. Van der Veer, the translator of the volume in the *Collected Works* in which this essay appears, is among the current scholars who assert that "conditional response" is the more proper translation, a term that suggests the role of the environment—the conditions under which a response occurs—with far greater agency and flexibility than is suggested by "conditioned" in the traditional translation. The notion of the conditional response, argued Vygotsky, bridges biological adaptation as outlined by Darwin and sociological perspectives available through Marx. In this conception, hereditary biological behavior produces social behavior through engagement with the environment.

Vygotsky (1925/1997b) elaborated on this process, arguing that human behavior is predicated on the *historical* ways in which a society has conducted itself and is further shaped by *social experience* of others, such that a person may read or hear accounts of other people's experiences in the world and learn them second hand. People can then adapt the environment to themselves in what Vygotsky, relying on Marx, calls the "doubling of experience that is unavoidable in human labor" (p. 68): the use of the imagination to anticipate material consequences for new actions. He thus situates adaptation in not only personal responses to the environment, but the process of imagining future scenarios, understanding their effects conceptually, and taking the most suitable choice based on this experiential knowledge and capacity for anticipating future outcomes (see Smagorinsky 2013).

In this early work, Vygotsky was operating at the level of Pavlov's theory of reflexes, without positioning the human environment itself as something that may be volitionally changed to adapt such that people with few resources may experience life in fulfilling ways. He took up that project with his work in *defectology*, the study and education of people of physical (e.g., blind), cognitive (e.g., mentally underdeveloped), and what

I would add as neurological (e.g., clinical depression) conditions that produce a poor fit for the construction of mainstream society (see Chap. 1). That aspect of adaptation is central to the issues I address in this chapter.

The Interdependence of Biological, Historical, Cultural, and Social Lines of Development

Lee (2010) argues that biology and culture should be viewed as interdependent in human life, especially given the tendency to argue in Spencerian manner that biology explains cultural difference in deficit terms, an approach that leads to such claims as a bell curve of racial intelligence (e.g., Hernstein and Murray 1994). Just as many dismiss culture in favor of biology to explain human difference and gradations of social value, argues Lee, cultural psychologists are insufficiently attentive to biological factors, perhaps because of the use of biological difference to construct racially hierarchical, deficit-oriented characterizations of society. Drawing on recent work in neurosciences, Lee argues for an integrated conception of human development that accounts for both nature and nurture. She asks, "If adaptation and plasticity are characteristic of human brain functioning, then why are we not doing more to understand the conditions of such adaptation and plasticity, particularly with regard to those who face the greatest exposure to threats or obstacles in our society?" (p. 647). Lee, as an African American woman, is primarily concerned with how youth of color are constructed and treated in educational settings, but her argument applies just as well to any point of physical, cognitive, or neurological difference.

Lee (2010), like Stetsenko (2011), notes that the drive to survive exists at both the level of the individual and the level of the species, both in the immediate communal sense and across generations. Survival, she argues, depends on the adaptive qualities of each organism and the availability of multiple pathways through which survival may be achieved. Pathways may be limited both materially and symbolically. In the corporeal world, one might be limited by geography and weather, as when Laplanders—the indigenous Scandinavian people who live under Arctic conditions—live semi-nomadically in relation to the availability of food sources. Symbolically, speech conventions may discursively limit pathways for those from outside the dominant culture whose members produce its people's definitive texts, such as when Native American people are used as sports team mascots under such appellations as Savages (Wikipedia, n.d.b), suggesting their location on the lower order of the human species.

To Lee, the idea of *adaptation through multiple pathways* has a basis that is simultaneously biological, environmental, and cultural. Germane to my own argument, Lee finds that human stress—of the sort that contributes to Vygotsky's secondary disability (see Chap. 2)—is typically brought on by environmental factors and manifested physiologically.

Lee (2010) goes on to state that one's stress may be manifested at the cellular level to the point that the Lamarckian phenomenon of *soft* or *epigenetic inheritance* may occur, in that this stress can be passed down across generations. Although almost everything about the phenomenon of soft or epigenetic inheritance has been debated since it originated with Erasmus Darwin's 1796 publication of *Zoonomia* and Jean-Baptiste Lamarck's 1809 treatise *Philosophie Zoologique*, and although the jury for the most part is still out on whether or not physiological changes in individuals can be passed down genetically, there is some evidence that at least a partial intergenerational effect of relatively short duration may be available from individual neurological change (Springer and Holley 2012). Lindley (2010) finds that intentional behaviors such as smoking tobacco may have intergenerational cellular effects. Charles Darwin himself appeared to accept some Lamarckian principles, if tentatively:

> We have also what are called monstrosities; but they graduate into varieties. By a monstrosity I presume is meant some considerable deviation of structure in one part, either injurious to or not useful to the species, and not generally propagated. Some authors use the term "variation" in a technical sense, as implying a modification
> directly due to the physical conditions of life; and 'variations' in this sense are supposed not to be inherited: but who can say that the dwarfed condition of shells in the brackish waters of the Baltic, or dwarfed plants on Alpine summits, or the thicker fur of an animal from far northwards, would not in some cases be inherited for at least some few generations? and in this case I presume that the form would be called a variety. (p. 48)

Nonetheless, not all neuroscientists are convinced that Lamarckian effects are real (e.g., Futuyma 2009).I must leave the Lamarckian aspects of these various assertions to those who know better, given my limitations in understanding the science behind the dispute.

Lee (2010) accepts what neurologists such as Immordino-Yang and Damasio (2007) have found regarding the plasticity of human makeup and the availability of somatic (i.e., emotional) influence on neurological makeup. In this conception, one's engagement with the environment is not a function of two static and impermeable entities colliding, but instead produces an interaction through which both environment and the person are amenable to fundamental change. People act on their environments through the use of cultural tools, which may be material (e.g., digging in the ground with a shovel) or psychological (e.g., believing, as do many Native American people that the world is animistic and thus people and the biota emerged from the same source and thus nature should not be exploited). Environments may act on people, with stress following from encounters with nature (e.g., hurricanes) and other people (e.g., through discrimination) or a combination (e.g., when following Hurricane Katrina, Black residents of New Orleans were treated with indifference by government officials charged with addressing their dilemmas). To account for the ways in which people enter into complex relationships with their social and physical environments through an integration of physical, cognitive, and emotional capabilities, Lee employs the metaphor of *braiding* to represent human adaptation.

To Cole (2002), this braiding process is a central aspect of human development. Cole distinguishes natural phylogeny—the evolutionary development of whole species—from evolution, which is infused with cultural mediation:

> In so far as it is dominated by phylogenetic influences, development is a Darwinian process of natural selection operating on the random variation of genetic combinations created at conception. But cultural change operates according to a different set of principles: cultural variations are not randomly generated, they are, rather, descended from the successful adaptations of prior generations passed down exosomatically [i.e., through symbolic means]. While natural selection has the final say, in so far as human behavior is mediated through culture it is "distorted" by a Lamarckian principle of evolution. [Acquired] culture becomes a "second nature" which makes development a goal-directed process in a way in which phylogenetic change is not.... Human beings are hybrids. (pp. 316–317)

Cole's (2002) Lamarckian reference is quite different from Lee's (2010) in that he is making a *cultural-historical* Lamarckian claim rather than a biological one (Cole, personal communication, July 1, 2014). Lee argues that one's cells are altered by a set of emotional of experiences and passed down through genetic heredity. Cole asserts the need for a Lamarckian notion of culture, as opposed to cellular hereditary transmission. What is passed down, while biological at its core, is mediated culturally through the symbol systems that sustain human ways of life, providing cultural groups with a historical purpose in which not only life-forms survive, but ways of living are perpetuated across generations. If survival is available to the strongest, then this principle applies to social groups who assist those who lack what contributes to biological survival in competitive societies, thus gaining strength by cultivating the assets of those who superficially appear characterized by weakness or deficit. Indeed, many scientists assert that the principal reason that a slow, weak, species like humans did not survive their natural environments because of superior intelligence, but they succeeded over generations because they formed societies that pooled their strengths as part of a collective effort to construct lasting communities.

Lee (2010) is interested in adaptation as a whole system rather than a series of separate components that each may be analyzed apart from the others, particularly in terms of how environments may allow for multiple pathways of personal and cultural development for those who are acculturated to see and act on their environments with resilience, knowledge, and agency, and, in many cases, with a collective orientation to problem-solving. This approach requires a conception of human adaptation as malleable, provided that alternative pathways are available. As Daiute (2010) has demonstrated, even those who are considered to be limited in their outlooks by traumatic experiences can become involved in discursive means of envisioning positive social futures through writing and discussing narratives. Cultural practices thus may contribute to the construction of enabling settings that serve those for whom conventional pathways are not apparent or readily available. Such an approach relies on Lee's (2010) argument in favor of multiple pathways for development and practice such that those with advantage, rather than exploiting those for individual advancement, assist others both to help them realize their personal potential and add to their social group's prospects for prosperity by cultivating the possibilities of a wider range of its members.

Qualifying Marxism

My reliance on Vygotsky, a committed Marxist if not a dedicated Stalinist, is problematic in key areas. Vygotsky (1993) considered society from a collectivist standpoint. His understanding of Marxist principles is perhaps most evident in his defectological writing, in which he explicitly embraces nascent Soviet communism as the ideal means through which an equitable society is available. His vision of an uplifting Soviet nation, however, was betrayed by Stalin's repression of dissent in any form (Smagorinsky 2012a), including what was officially interpreted to be Vygotsky's own departure from orthodoxy. The failure of the Soviet Union to realize its claimed potential of an equitable society free of capitalism's harsh inequities surely raises questions about the degree to which Vygotsky's optimistic vision of a society unencumbered by selfishness and personal gain is possible.

In my view, Marxism has made great contributions to critiques of capitalism. However, the social engineering required to produce the Soviet vision of a new human race (Trotsky 1923) appears unlikely to succeed and is ethically questionable from the standpoint of centralizing decisions about what sort of person is optimal and how that sort of person will be created socially, especially given Stalin's approach of violently winnowing people exhibiting the wrong characteristics (Snyder 2010).

Applying Vygotsky's optimistic solution to human difference thus requires a skeptical look at the Marxist principles that he endorsed, while also retaining the communal qualities that he embraced and that are available to people, if not practiced or endorsed by all people. Current US society is deeply polarized, with conservative perspectives continuing to assert the ideals of unfettered capitalism and the individual right to liberty and prosperity (e.g., Friedman 1993), no matter how cruelly the pursuit of that right produces struggles for others. Persuading the most emphatic advocates of this perspective seems unlikely, as does convincing them to contribute to the welfare of people whom they consider to be defective and inferior (Trump 2015).

What I do believe is possible is greater attention to Vygotsky's (1993) perspective on the responsibility of all people for the welfare of their fellow citizens, rather than a remaking of a national people in a mold that fits some but not all. That is, what I offer is not a final solution to the enduring challenges faced by neuro-atypical people, but it is a way to think about considering their potential more than their differences and to think, in conjunction with this view, how channels of activity may become available to them through which to engage in productive, self-affirming, socially valued activity and labor that, in turn, makes the whole society stronger and more likely to benefit from the contributions of the whole of its citizenry.

Adaptation for Neurodivergent People

I next consider the problem of adaptation for cultures that include neurologically diverse people—that is, all cultures, even Stalin's Soviet Union in which he attempted to expel or eliminate people who did not fit his specific mold for the New Soviet Man (see Cheng 2009). In his volume on defectology, Vygotsky (1993) identified two forms of adaptation (see Chap. 2). Consistent with the general outline of the Darwinian and Spencerian conceptions of adaptation, Vygotsky found the need for individuals to adapt to their environments, and environments to adapt to, and in turn construct more accommodating settings for, children damaged by war. Vygotsky's population of concern included people of physical difference, primarily young people injured during war, and people whose cognitive development did not match the pace of the typical person. I adapt his perspective to the population of people labeled as mentally ill and thus considered in deficit to those of modal makeup through the discursive and diagnostic labeling of them as abnormal, disordered, deficient, and other terms of diminishment. Although I reviewed these two forms of adaptation in Chap. 2, I return to them here with specific grounding in the issues I have raised in this chapter.

Individual Adaptation

Adaptation may be undertaken by *individuals* who feel inadequate and become motivated to change such that they feel more fulfilled. Vygotsky (1993) asserted that feelings of inadequacy may serve to motivate a person of difference to appropriate positive new ways of engaging with society. Feelings of inadequacy may thus produce a generative action to alleviate the source of these feelings. Vygotsky (1993) argued, "*Via subjective feelings of inadequacy, a physical handicap dialectically transforms itself into psychological drives toward compensation and overcompensation*" through adaptation (p. 33; emphasis in original). A person may be incapable of walking yet be surrounded by mobile people and become motivated to find possible means of engaging more actively with the world, so as to experience the potentials afforded by kinesis. As Lee (2010) might argue, finding new means of locomotion requires multiple pathways rather than those restricted by the material and corporal world and the symbolic world that pathologizes immobility as deficiency.

Making this transformation requires a concerted cognitive, physical, and emotional shift from believing in a restricted life to envisioning a greater range of developmental pathways. One might, for instance, begin competing in the growing area of wheelchair sports from individual competitions such as tennis and track to team sports such as basketball and football. Or one might undertake water sports that rely on arms and floats, ramps, and other accessories rather than legs. This approach relies on the principle of compensation, which involves a circumvention of obstacles by means of adaptation that allows for full participation in activities central to a culture's social life. To Vygotsky (1993), such adaptations enable one to overcome feelings of weakness and deficiency, instead serving as a unique strength with positive implications for social participation.

Such adaptations are not entirely individual, but they rely on positive social assistance and reinforcement from those who construct both the material and psychological environments of participation. In other words, people's adaptations require a cooperative, supportive perspective on the part of those whose circumstances require them to make few personal adaptations. To Vygotsky (1993), taking advantage of these affordances in order to take part in such compensatory development constitutes a generative response to difference, one that "represents a continually evolving adaptive process. If a blind or deaf child achieves the same level of development as a normal child, then the child with a defect achieves this *in another way, by another course, by other means*" (p. 34; emphasis in original). If one is to overcome obstacles so that compensatory processes serve this generative function, Vygotsky argued that the discursive construction of difference as "defect" needs to be jettisoned and replaced by both psychological and discursive reconstructions of difference that enable generative action and adaptation. What matters most is that human development not be sidetracked by a physical, neurological, or cognitive point of difference. Rather, one should have opportunities for cultural participation such that "the path of cultural development is unlimited" (p. 169).

Feelings of inadequacy can therefore have beneficial effects when people of difference are treated as productive people adapting to their environments. Those who do not have a typical evolutionary human feature, such as sight, must rely on alternative tools and pathways, a condition that requires two dialectical processes. The person of difference must adapt to the world through alternative cultural tools; and the people in the environment must accept these roundabout mediational means nonjudgmentally and respectfully, and in many cases contribute to their construction and development with a communal frame of mind. To reinforce a previous point, individual adaptation requires social support, both in terms of providing alternative means (e.g., braille, wheelchair ramps) and treating atypical people with dignity and support. Failing to do so contributes to the other possible outcome of engaging without the customary assets that evolution has provided human beings, the secondary disability that consists of appropriated feelings of inadequacy.

ADAPTATION AS SOCIAL RESPONSIBILITY

Individual adaptation requires some accommodations by those who surround the person of difference. To Vygotsky (1993), however, simply assisting with the construction of material work-arounds for people of atypical makeup is insufficient. Of even greater significance is the construction of a psychological and emotional environment surrounding the person of difference. Many people in US society view adaptation primarily as the responsibility of the individual with the fewest affordances for adapting, so perhaps it is unsurprising that people whose makeup and development do not follow the evolutionary norm are expected to lift themselves by their own bootstraps and survive, or else sink in a pit of indifference.

The notion of individualism is built into US culture and fits comfortably with its capitalistic economic system. Presidential candidate Herbert Hoover (1928) expressed this value just before his election, saying that after the Great War,

> We were challenged with the choice between the American system of "rugged individualism" or the choice of a European system of diametrically opposed doctrines—doctrines of paternalism and state socialism. The acceptance of these ideas meant the destruction of self-government through centralization of government; it meant the undermining of initiative and enterprise upon which our people have grown to unparalleled greatness.... [Individualistic values] go to the very roots of American life in every act of our Government. I should like to state to you the effect of the extension of government into business upon our system of self government and our economic system. But even more important is the effect upon the average man. That is the effect on the very basis of liberty and freedom not only to those left outside the fold of expanded bureaucracy but to those embraced within it.

Hoover's (1928) concern was primarily oriented to business interests and governmental intervention, but his attention to "the average man" suggests that all Americans, or at least the men who comprised the dominant sex of the era, are individuals first and foremost, free to pursue happiness independent of governmental paternalism. Like most people of his time, Hoover had little understanding of neurodiversity, so my references to his speech are not designed to impugn his sensitivity on this matter. His emphasis on individualism, however, corresponds well with the Spencerian doctrine of survival of the fittest embraced by the most famous capitalists of his day (see, e.g., Miller's 1922 biography of Henry Ford), and of those contemporaneous with the writing of this chapter (see Paul 2011).

This individualistic orientation, while undoubtedly serving the machinery of the economy, has made life difficult for those who by circumstance are not among society's fittest for survival. Not everyone is born equal, at least in terms of their biological and neurological assembly (my concern) or their socioeconomic situations (Lee's [2010] concern with racial and cultural minoritized group members whose lives have been affected by discrimination). The assertion that rugged and fit individuals are society's best hope creates demands for adaptation that in effect produce an underclass of people who are left to flounder in the midst of people more capable of adapting their conduct, yet who feel little social obligation to do so. Of course, not all are so heartless, even as many do consider themselves to have little responsibility for the welfare of others, seeing no personal advantage in assisting others materially or affectively in navigating a world built for the typical majority, producing the sense of *privileged irresponsibility* alluded to in Chap. 2. Those whose makeup departs from the evolutionary norm are viewed as inferior and are vulnerable to appropriating this assumption, and this *secondary disability* of feeling of lesser human value becomes far more debilitating than the original source of difference.

In contrast to this notion of rugged individuals surpassing their circumstances to advance their interests in life, Vygotsky (1993) asserted that the challenge is social and distributed. This insight relies on the Marxist principles of the value of productive labor and the role of mediating settings in human development to provide channels for participation in cultural practice that legitimize one as a valued member of society. In taking Vygotsky's perspective, I of course run the risk of coming across to some as anti-American, or at least anti-capitalistic. I am neither, though aspects of Americanism and capitalism undoubtedly produce the inequities that Marx found so problematic that he believed that at least one of them, capitalism, could not be sustained over time.

Vygotsky (1993) continually asserted the potential of people lacking conventional biological functioning. The blind, he said, only understand that they lack something when the people around them treat them as different and thus deficient. Rather than viewing the blind as being faulty, however, he considered them as competent, capable people who needed alternative, multiple mediational pathways (cf. Lee 2010). Through the creation of future-oriented mediational settings, alternative pathways of development may be opened and cultivated by means of a *positive social updraft* in which to immerse themselves. This postulation transforms the notion of a "defect" into a condition that could conceivably lead to enhanced engagement with the world. Examples include both designed (see Part 2) and informal (see Part 3) activities through which participants take on important roles that allow their personal and social assets to be cultivated, in spite of differences that might limit their possibilities for inclusion in other settings and activities.

This attention to settings and legitimate cultural practice was a critical dimension of Vygotsky's concern for children lacking normative means of engaging with the world. Rather than segregating children to protect them and others from their points of difference, however, he urged their integration into collective life. Focusing solely on what they lack, he believed, would lead to little progress toward this end. Rather, he thought settings must be constructed in such a manner that each person's strengths are cultivated and honored. To Vygotsky, this approach required the majority to consider social consequences primarily in their integration of all people into the social whole.

Vygotsky (1993), like Lee (2010), found that cognition and affect are fundamentally related to one another, to the whole of one's body, and, by extension, to the whole of the mediational context. One's biological makeup is thus inseparable regarding how one feels in relation to how one is treated by others. This attention to the role of affect in overall human development is manifested in his attention to what my colleagues and I (Smagorinsky and Daigle 2012) have called *meta-experience*: the manner in which experience is experienced so as to frame new experiences (see Chap. 2). Those who are treated as defective carry this experience to new experiences in ways characterized by feelings of inferiority and low social status. These feelings frame new experiences such that the belief in one's inadequacy becomes reinforced continually over time.

Yet Vygotsky believed that by treating the evolutionarily different as part of the whole of society's collective work, people may develop the higher mental functions characteristic of general cultural ways of engaging with the world. When difference is institutionalized as defect, society constructs a Matthew Effect in which those with the greatest resources proceed, unencumbered by consideration of the needs of the neediest. As a result, those with the fewest resources are left to adapt to a world that demonstrates little interest in their welfare. They thus are brimming with potential that is suppressed by surrounding beliefs that focus only on their differences as deficits, to both their own detriment and the disadvantage of people who might benefit from their less-obvious abilities.

Discussion

Up to this point I have primarily provided a general overview of the problem of adaptation for the whole atypical population, without a specific focus on the population that has been of greatest theoretical and empirical interest to me, those whose neurodivergence makes them stand out from the perceived norm. This range is quite broad, and the degree of conditions varies, making it difficult to identify a small set of practices that could accommodate all. I will therefore identify what I hope are representative practices that social groups could incorporate into their offerings and operations to provide inclusive environments through which positive social updraft is available for those whose neurological makeups produce a variety of ways of processing their surroundings and acting on them.

My focus on the problem of adaptation includes those undertaken by both individuals and social groups. Individual variation makes simple suggestions difficult to formulate. I will therefore direct my attention to how groups can adapt to reduce stigmas associated with difference, in the process minimizing the secondary disability of feelings of shame, inferiority, and other affective responses that, as Vygotsky (1993) argues, become increasingly enervating over time, providing negative meta-experiences that reinforce one's sense of low social stature and deficiency. Among the broader adaptations required by society is the willingness by the public to invest in such programs, often through taxation, an adaptation toward which many communities and individuals within them are virulently hostile (see Norquist 2015). This problem is exacerbated by the current climate of antagonism toward public institutions in general, from schools to the government itself (e.g., Beck 2009). Once again, the tensions that capitalistic nations such as the USA experience between individual liberty and shared responsibility complicate any efforts to institute programs that benefit people of difference.

My broad approach would be to provide channels of activity that enable participation and validation for people of difference. Often, these opportunities are available in extracurricular activities, particularly at the club level. The young woman with multiple diagnoses of mental illness studied by Cook and Smagorinsky (Chap. 9; cf. 2014), for instance, similar to the youth studied by Black (2008), became involved in the online anime community, although on her own time rather than through school-sponsored activities. Given her family's level of support, she was able to use her own computer and related tools to produce digital art, compose fan fiction, and participate in many other validating activities with online friends. But many young people struggling with neurodiverse atypicality lack the levels of affluence and support available in her home. Schools and community centers could sponsor clubs that allow students to pursue such activities in the company of like-minded peers such that their confluence of interests, rather than their points of difference, becomes the means through which they engage in producing ideas and texts that are highly valued in such settings.

Roles for neuro-atypical children and youth might also be available in more mainstream extracurricular activities. The story of passionate autistic basketball fan Jason Mcelwain (see https://www.youtube.com/watch?v=l2IU1h9sG7U) became an Internet sensation when he, in his role of high school team manager, was put into the final home game of his senior year and, in a four-minute rampage, scored 20 points. Obviously, this event would be difficult to replicate, but I am more interested in the ways in which his coach and team made him feel a part of the team throughout the season, leading up to this inspirational moment. Positions such as team manager, participant in drama productions in appropriate assignments, and other possibilities are available for neurodivergent youth.

Perhaps more complex possibilities would involve sponsored activities that directly concern youth of difference, modeled on the Dynamic Story-Telling by Youth (DSTY) organized and managed by Daiute (2010) for young people who had experienced trauma during the breakup of the former Yugoslavia. Rather than further pathologizing their trauma, Daiute's workshop focused on the construction of positive social futures through narrative writing and the social support available in the group settings. Instead, then, of including her participants in activities such that they fit in with either broadly or locally normative activities, Daiute directly addressed their trauma through a culturally valued medium. Providing such a setting in a community would require the participation of counselors trained in managing therapeutic environments rather than being conducted by well-intentioned but untrained personnel or community members, and it would undoubtedly require some sort of legal counsel given that students' narratives could implicate others in painful experiences. The potential of such an activity, however, might be worth whatever investment in resources is required to maintain it.

The cultivation of seemingly obsessive interests is often discouraged by adults, who seek to broaden young people's horizons; yet for obsessive-compulsives, deep immersion in a topic or activity not only suits their personalities but may produce intensive understandings. Adults, for instance often discourage young people from having narrow reading and writing interests, believing instead that broadening horizons is preferable. Yet those with Asperger's or obsessive-compulsive personalities (or both) often become very frustrated when not allowed to pursue their narrow interests, such as reading all of the books by a single author, or reading entirely within one genre, or reading solely about one topic. Allowing people's makeups to violate social norms in such a fashion might suit their development much better than requiring them to adapt to perceived normative ways of being, as exhibited in Chap. 11, which provides a look at Suskind's (2014) memoir of his autistic son's obsession with Disney characters. It seemed unsettling at first but eventually served a powerful developmental role in his socialization.

Organizing such programs and possibilities often follows from the initiative of dedicated individuals who are sensitive to the needs and interactional styles of neuro-atypicals. What communities need is a broad, systemic commitment to inclusion that provides incentives and support and structural means of achieving it. This project may well face conflict from (1) those who believe that public institutions such as schools have a socializing purpose designed to normalize conventional ways of being rather than to cultivate seemingly obscure interests and pursuits, (2) those who oppose taxing the public to support extracurricular activities, (3) those who advocate individualism to the extent that all adaptation becomes the responsibility of atypical people rather than social groups, and (4) those who simply believe that people who appear weird should be shunned and avoided rather than accommodated. One of our primary goals in this volume is to argue against such conceptions and provide alternative ways of conceiving social life in the hope that we can contribute to some degree of change in perception and process, transforming society into a place of greater acceptance and accommodation for the full range of citizens they serve, without pathologizing them or reinforcing the deficit-oriented ways in which society tends to construct difference.

Note

1. Now, my ex-wife.

References

Bardziński, F. (2013). The concept of the 'New Soviet Man' as a eugenic project: Eugenics in Soviet Russia after World War II. *Ethics in Progress, 4*(1), 57–81.

Beck, G. (2009). *Glenn Beck's common sense: The case against an out-of-control government, inspired by Thomas Paine.* New York: Threshold Editions.

Black, R. W. (2008). *Adolescents and online fan fiction.* New York: Peter Lang.

Carnegie, A. (1889, June). Wealth. *North American Review,148,* 653–665. Available at http://digital.library.cornell.edu/cgi/t/text/pageviewer-idx?c=nora;cc=nora;rgn=full%20text;idno=nora0148-6;didno=nora0148-6;view=image;seq=0661;node=nora0148-6%3A1

Cheng, Y. (2009). *Creating the new man: From Enlightenment ideals to socialist realities.* Honolulu: University of Hawai'i Press.

Cole, M. (2002). Culture and development. In H. Keller, Y. H. Poortinga, & A. Schoemerich (Eds.), *Between culture and biology: Perspectives on ontogenetic development* (pp. 303–319). New York: Cambridge University Press.

Cook, L. S., & Smagorinsky, P. (2014). Constructing positive social updrafts for extranormative personalities. *Learning, Culture and Social Interaction, 3*(4), 296–308. Available at http://www.petersmagorinsky.net/About/PDF/LCSI/LCSI_2014.pdf

Daiute, C. (2010). *Human development and political violence.* New York: Cambridge University Press.

Darwin, E. (1796). *Zoonomia or, the laws of organic life.* Dublin: P. Byrne.

Darwin, C. (1859). *On the origin of species by means of natural selection, or the preservation of favoured races in the struggle for life.* London: John Murray. Available at http://www.literature.org/authors/darwin-charles/the-origin-of-species/

Francis Galton, F. (1883). *Inquiries into human faculty and its development.* London: Macmillan and Co.

Friedman, M. (1993). *Why government is the problem.* Stanford: Hoover Institution Press.

Futuyma, D. (2009). *Evolution.* Sunderland: Sinauer Associates.

Hernstein, R. J., & Murray, C. (1994). *The bell curve: Intelligence and class structure in American life.* New York: The Free Press.

Hoover, H. (1928, October 22). Rugged individualism. Available at http://teachingamericanhistory.org/library/document/rugged-individualism/

Immordino-Yang, M. H., & Damasio, A. R. (2007). We feel, therefore we learn: The relevance of affective and social neuroscience to education. *Mind, Brain, and Education, 1*(1), 3–10.

Kozulin, A., & Gindis, B. (2007). Sociocultural theory and education of children with special needs: From defectology to remedial pedagogy. In H. Daniels, M. Cole, & J. V. Wertsch (Eds.), *The Cambridge companion to Vygotsky* (pp. 332–362). New York: Cambridge University Press.

Lamarck, J-B. (1809). *Philosophie zoologique*. Paris: Librairie F. Savy. Available at http://www.ucl.ac.uk/taxome/jim/Mim/lamarck_contents.html

Lee, C. D. (2010). Soaring above the clouds, delving the ocean's depths: Understanding the ecologies of human learning and the challenge for education science. *Educational Researcher, 39*(9), 643–655.

Lee, K. (2008). ADHD in American early schooling: From a cultural psychological perspective. *Early Child Development and Care, 178*, 415–439.

Lindley, R. A. (2010). *The soma*. Scotts Valley: CreateSpace Independent Publishing Platform.

Miller, J. M. (1922). *The amazing story of Henry Ford: The ideal American and the world's most famous private citizen—A complete and authentic account of his life and surpassing achievements*. Chicago: M. A. Donohue.

Norquist, G. (2015). *End the IRS before it ends us: How to restore a low tax, high growth, wealthy America*. New York: Center Street Books.

Ottoni, E. B., & Izar, P. (2008). Capuchin monkey tool use: Overview and implications. *Evolutionary Anthropology, 17*, 171–178.

Paul, R. (2011). *Liberty defined:50 essential issues that affect our freedom*. New York: Grand Central Publishing.

Shumaker, R. W., Walkup, K. R., & Beck, B. B. (2011). *Animal tool behavior: The use and manufacture of tools by animals*. Baltimore: Johns Hopkins University Press.

Smagorinsky, P. (2011). Confessions of a mad professor: An autoethnographic consideration of neuroatypicality, extranormativity, and education. *Teachers College Record, 113*, 1701–1732. Available at http://www.petersmagorinsky.net/About/PDF/TCR/TCR2011.pdf

Smagorinsky, P. (2012a). Vygotsky, "defectology," and the inclusion of people of difference in the broader cultural stream. *Journal of Language and Literacy Education* [Online], *8*(1), 1–25. Available at http://jolle.coe.uga.edu/wp-content/uploads/2012/05/Vygotsky-and-Defectology.pdf

Smagorinsky, P. (2012b). Every individual has his own insanity: Applying Vygotsky's work on defectology to the question of mental health as an issue of inclusion. *Learning, Culture and Social Interaction, 1*(1), 67–77. Available at http://www.petersmagorinsky.net/About/PDF/LCSI/LCSI_2012.pdf

Smagorinsky, P. (2013). The development of social and practical concepts in learning to teach: A synthesis and extension of Vygotsky's conception. *Learning, Culture, and Social Interaction, 2*(4), 238–248. Available athttp://www.petersmagorinsky.net/About/PDF/LCSI/LCSI_2013.pdf

Smagorinsky, P. (2014, November 26). Taking the diss out of disability. *Teachers College Record*. Available at http://www.petersmagorinsky.net/About/PDF/TCR/TCR2014.html

Smagorinsky, P., & Daigle, E. A. (2012). The role of affect in students' writing for school. In E. Grigorenko, E. Mambrino, & D. Preiss (Eds.), *Handbook of writing: A mosaic of perspectives and views* (pp. 293–307). New York: Psychology Press.

Snyder, T. (2010). *Bloodlands: Europe between Hitler and Stalin*. New York: Basic Books.

Spencer, H. (1857). Progress: Its law and causes. *The Westminster Review*, 67, 445–447, 451, 454–456, 464–65. Available at http://www.fordham.edu/halsall/mod/spencer-darwin.asp

Springer, J., & Holley, D. (2012). *An introduction to zoology: Investigating the animal world*. Burlington: Jones & Bartlett Learning.

Stetsenko, A. (2011). Darwin and Vygotsky on development: An exegesis on human nature. In M. Kontopodis, C. Wulf, & B. Fichtner (Eds.), *Children, culture and education: Cultural, historical, anthropological perspectives* (pp. 25–41). New York: Springer.

Suskind, R. (2014). *Life animated: A story of sidekicks, heroes, and autism*. New York: Kingswell.

Tobin, J., Valente, J., & Horejes, T. (2010-2014). *Deaf kindergartens in three cultures: France, Japan, and the United States*. The Spencer Foundation Major Grant.

Trotsky, L. (1923). From the old family to the new. *Pravda*. Retrieved September 1, 2016 from http://www.marxists.org/archive/trotsky/women/life/23_07_13.htm

Trump, D. (2015). Speech at Bluffton, South Carolina presidential campaign rally. Retrieved July 24, 2015, from https://www.youtube.com/watch?v=kj9xsrhJKOQ

Tulviste, P. (1991). *The cultural-historical development of verbal thinking*. Commack, NY: Nova Science.

Vygotsky, L. S. (1925/1997a). Predislovie. In A. F. Lazurskij, *Psikhologija obshaja I eksperimental'naja* (3rd ed., pp. 5–23). Leningrad/St. Petersburg: Gosudarstvennoe Izdatel'stve/M. K. Kostin. [Preface to Lazursky. In R. W. Rieber & J. Wollock (Eds.), *The collected works of L. S. Vygotsky, Volume 3: Problems of the theory and history of psychology* (trans: van der Veer, R.) (pp. 51–61). New York: Plenum.]

Vygotsky, L. S. (1925/1997b). Soznanie kak problema psikhologija povedenija. In K. N. Kornilov (Ed.), *Psikhologija I marksizm* (pp. 175–198). Leningrad: Gosudarstvennoe Izdatel'stvo. [Consciousness as a problem for the psychology of behavior. In R. W. Rieber & J. Wollock (Eds.), *The collected works of L. S. Vygotsky, Volume 3: Problems of the theory and history of psychology* (trans:van der Veer, R.) (pp. 63–79). New York: Plenum.]

Vygotsky, L. S. (1927). *The historical meaning of the crisis in psychology: A methodological investigation* (trans: Van der Veer, R.). Retrieved from http://lchc.ucsd.edu/mca/Paper/crisis/psycri01.htm#p100

Vygotsky, L. S. (1930/1997). Разум, сознание, бессознательное. In L. S. Vygotsky, *Elementy obshchej psikhologii* (pp. 48–61). Moscow: Izdatelstvo BZO pri Pedfake 2-go MGU. [Mind, consciousness, the unconscious. In R. W. Rieber & J. Wollock (Eds.), *The collected works of L. S. Vygotsky, Volume 3: Problems of the theory and history of psychology* (trans: van der Veer, R.) (pp. 109–121). New York: Plenum.]

Vygotsky, L. S. (1931). *Genesis of higher mental functions*. Retrieved September 1, 2016 from http://www.marxists.org/archive/vygotsky/works/1931/higher-mental-functions.htm

Vygotsky, L. S. (1993). *The collected works of L. S. Vygotsky. Volume 2: The fundamentals of defectology (abnormal psychology and learning disabilities)* (R. W. Rieber & A. S. Carton, Eds.; trans: Knox, J.E. & Stevens, C. B.). New York: Plenum.

Vygotsky, L. S., & Luria, A. R. (1993). *Studies on the history of behavior: Ape, primitive, and child* (V. I. Golod & J. E. Knox, Eds. & Trans.). Hillsdale: Erlbaum.

Walker, M., & Smagorinsky, P. (2013). The power of school music programs: Students come for the music and stay for the math. *Atlanta Journal-Constitution*. Retrieved September 1, 2016 http://blogs.ajc.com/get-schooled-blog/2013/01/01/the-power-of-school-music-programs-students-come-for-the-music-and-stay-for-the-math/?cxntfid=blogs_get_schooled_blog

Wikipedia. (n.d.a). *Tool use by animals*. Available at http://en.wikipedia.org/wiki/Tool_use_by_animals

Wikipedia. (n.d.b). *List of sports team names and mascots derived from indigenous peoples*. Available at http://en.wikipedia.org/wiki/List_of_sports_team_names_and_mascots_derived_from_indigenous_peoples#Savages

PART II

Deliberately Crafted Activity Settings

CHAPTER 4

Social Therapy and Family Play

Christine LaCerva

I have been a practicing social therapist for 35 years and director of the Social Therapy Group, a community-based psychotherapy center in Manhattan and Brooklyn. I am also the lead clinical trainer at the East Side Institute in New York City, which offers postgraduate training in social therapy. My group practice (a rather large one) includes clients from ages 4 to 84. They come from a broad cross section of diverse communities across New York and from all walks of life. Before becoming a therapist, I was a dancer, performer, teacher of the deaf, and, for several years, the director of an experimental Vygotskian school in Harlem.

For 25 years, I have worked with young people diagnosed along the autism spectrum and/or determined to have "disorders": oppositional defiant disorder (ODD), pervasive development disorder (PDD),[1] attention-deficit/hyperactivity disorder (ADHD), and other pathologizing labels. Some have not been diagnosed but are struggling at home and school. In many instances, their families are in turmoil.

To help me support the ongoing emotional and social development of young people and their families, I experimented with new modalities, and over a number of years, I created a multi-family group. Comprising four or five families, the family groups have supported adults and children alike

C. LaCerva (✉)
The Social Therapy Group, Brooklyn, NY, USA

to get better at creating "family plays" where everyone has the opportunity to stretch and grow. In the recounting of this history, I recall some of my conversations over three decades with the founder of social therapy, Fred Newman. The case studies you are about to read are also a major part of my narrative over a 15-year period.

A word about social therapy: It's a philosophical/performatory, group-based approach created by Newman, a philosopher and political activist, along with Lois Holzman, a developmental psychologist. Over the last 40 years, the practice (known across disciplines as "social therapeutics") has expanded into many other areas, including youth, organizational, and community development; early-childhood and adult education; special education; and health care.

There are dozens of articles, presentations, academic books, and popular texts on the approach, which I hope this chapter will inspire you to explore (e.g., Holzman and Mendez 2003; Holzman and Newman 2012; Newman and Goldberg, 1996; Newman and Holzman 2006/1996, 1997). But for the purpose of appreciating the story I recount here, know that social therapy is focused on emotional development. It is a non-interpretative and non-diagnostic approach. It is practical, philosophical, play-oriented, and performatory, and sometimes we refer to it as "radically humanistic," which is a nod to its roots in the radical therapies of the 1960s. As such, it values the revolutionary human capacity to perform, play, create new possibilities, and thereby, transform our world. It's group-based and profoundly relational, and because of that, it has proven to be a powerful antidote to the alienation and narcissism of our culture.

Whether it's a boy labeled autistic or an elderly person struggling with dementia, social therapy relates to all as being "a head taller"—that is, as performers and creators of our lives—able to stretch our performance repertoire with the support of the ensemble. As performers, as environment builders, as creators of the stages upon which we live our lives, we can build new ensembles to engage how we want to be doing whatever it is we're doing. "How are we doing?" asks the group. "Does what we're doing support the group's growth?" It is a process through which we collectively examine the roles, rules, and assumptions we have about our relational lives.

In the narrative that follows you will see that I explicitly use the language of theater and performance to give direction to the group. I talk in terms of "stage," "cast," "play," "scene," "director," and "offer" (a term that is borrowed from improv and refers to whatever it is that another person in the ensemble gives you to work and build with).

The group builds its stage—inventing and trying out performances (some old and stale, some new). Helped by the social therapist, the group is a space for challenging presumptions, assumptions, and the iron-clad identities we have for ourselves and others. In such environments (on our good days), we loosen the grip that the "Truth" and "What's Right" have on us by being more playful and philosophical in how we talk, how we see, and how we feel. Social therapy helps groups of people rediscover their capacity to invent new ways of seeing and new ways of feeling and being. When we undertake this inquiry, we experience our power and emotional growth.

As you will see in some of the texts on social therapy, Newman and Holzman (2006/1996, 1997) were inspired and influenced by the contributions of Karl Marx, Lev Vygotsky, and Ludwig Wittgenstein. Among the many contributions from Marx, they built upon his understanding of the fundamental sociality of our species and of revolutionary activity—that is, the human capacity to change totalities—to "change everything." Marx's identification of the coincidence of the changing of circumstances and of human activity or self-change (Marx 1974) is a key organizing principle of social therapy.

Newman and Holzman (1997) built upon developmental psychologist Lev Vygotsky's (1978) understanding of the dialectical relationship between thinking and speech and the profound sociality of our thinking and speaking. Vygotsky understood human development, including language development, as a lifetime process that we humans create together in "spaces" he called "zones of proximal development," where people of different ages and/or developmental levels relate to one another a "head taller" than they are. Vygotsky appreciated children's play as the engine of development. Newman and Holzman see play as deeply relevant to the growth of people of all ages.

They were inspired by philosopher Ludwig Wittgenstein's (1953) challenges to the concepts of essence and causality, his philosophical inquisitiveness, and his commitment to questioning assumptions about how we understand, see, and talk. These "philosophical investigations" are part of creating environments where we can see and go somewhere new. When we're stuck, we can create "new forms of life" with others, play "new language games," and learn to move around and about to try out something new.

I began to build a family practice with children, many of whom came to social therapy with a variety of issues and labels, including Asperger's syndrome, autism, learning disabilities, attention-deficit disorder (ADD), oppositional defiant disorder (ODD), and other terms laden with deficit and disorder. I disagreed with the psychiatric diagnoses that many of the children came into my office with. And yet I considered that I might have ODD myself, I was so furious at their diagnoses! Fred Newman once said that if you give someone a label and you have the institutions of psychology and psychiatry behind you, that label, and the identity that might follow from it, would follow them forever (Newman and Goldberg 1996). The label becomes who they are, their *essence*. It can limit their creative capacities to perform beyond themselves, and thus produce the "secondary disability" that Vygotsky (1993) found far more debilitating than the source of difference itself (see Chaps. 1 and 2). And yet at the same time, people often need a diagnosis to get services for themselves and their children. This was a complex issue for sure.

My very first patient was five years old. He had been diagnosed as being on the autism spectrum. His family was concerned that he wasn't developing socially; he had no friends. The first few sessions he would not look at me or speak to me. He would come in and yell at me. I said nothing. He then turned to curse profusely at the wastepaper basket for a full 60 minutes. I had no idea what to do. I began to think about the assumptions that might be getting in my way of my helping him. I was holding onto the notion that there was a right way to do this. I decided to join him and stood by his side. Soon, we were both yelling at the wastepaper basket.

In this setting, I had to be fully responsive. This engagement required that I begin seeing the need to view us as "we" rather than as a healthy therapist working with a disordered child. Over a number of weeks, our yelling turned into laughing. We began to create a series of performance games, singing and dancing with stuffed animals. One day, I lined up all the animals in a semicircle, put on some music, and invited him to create a play with me. We had a delightful and hilarious time together. He became more and more relational as we continued our work. His parents reported he was doing better at home and at school.

His family began to refer other families who had children on the spectrum, including those diagnosed with Asperger's syndrome. Families considering therapy, of course, wanted to know if I could be of help. They asked if I could help their child relate to others. Could I help a boy who did not speak catch up to his twin sister, who was already able to have conversations? The sister felt guilty that she could speak and her brother could not. Both had been diagnosed with pervasive developmental disorder (PDD). Could I help them? I had no answer in the absence of creating the conditions to give us all a chance to build something. I don't know if it was hope, desperation, or the relief of experiencing this as a new kind of conversation—but they entered my practice.

Practicing a therapeutic process that focuses on social and emotional development was key in working with these young people. I felt the magic of children and their families performing in new ways that challenged cultural norms of who they were supposed to be and what they thought was possible. Below are several detailed therapy stories from my practice that illustrate the creative evolution of the social therapeutic approach to family therapy and what emerged as the multi-family group.

Performing Jonathon

Jonathon,[2] a 12-year-old boy, was brought by his mother to the Social Therapy Group's center in Brooklyn, NY, on the recommendation of family friends. Mom was friendly and talkative as we walked into my office. She was curious about our work with young people diagnosed on the autism spectrum. "What do you do here?" she asked. Jonathon sat down next to mom and was silent. He looked at the floor. I spoke to him. He did not respond. His mother said he didn't want to be here, but she felt she had dedicated her life to his welfare, and he needed to deal with the intense temper tantrums that were going on at home and at school. He was currently in a special education setting that was not challenging him. His withdrawal from people was deepening. Given that he was getting older, she felt desperate for some techniques to make him stop. Did I have any? I assured her I did not. But I was going to work to build with everything he had to give, including his temper tantrums. "How would you do that?" she asked. "I don't know yet," I replied. "That will be created by me and Jonathon."

She adored him. She prided herself on how very bright he was. He could spout off in several languages. Some of them he made up himself, syntax and all. "He has written a book," she exclaimed. "I think he has Asperger's Syndrome. It is what a psychiatrist said about him, which allowed him to get services in school." She began to cry. "His temper tantrums are ruining our lives. They are him at his worst. What do you have to offer?" Jonathon stiffened, sitting upright in his chair. He was now staring at the door.

I asked him, "What do you think about what your mom is saying?" He responded, "She's talking to *you*, isn't she?" Yes, indeed, he was right. She was talking to me. So I responded to her. I told her that I appreciated her question as to whether I had something to offer. It was an important question. A lot was riding on it. It was terribly important that she and Jonathon knew where they were and with whom they were speaking. This understanding would allow them to decide together to take responsibility for what kind of help they wanted.

I gave them a brief introduction of social therapy, speaking way beyond what I thought Jonathon could understand. "I practice a therapeutic approach called social therapy. It is an alternative to psychology where people can learn to create the conditions and environments they need to embrace our sociality." Jonathon rolled his eyes. I continued.

> What we focus on in social therapy is our relationality to others and the world—not what's inside your head. We help people break out of individualistic ways of thinking and doing that we have all learned. This includes the sometimes frightening, sometimes joyful, sometimes difficult experience of *discovering the other*. In our lives we are always in relationship to others, not just ourselves.
>
> "We play with therapy. How will we do that? Our answer is performance— the human capacity to perform. We perform who we are and who we are not. As children, we performed all the time—as speakers when we weren't, as members of the family before we knew what a family was. Performance is a key activity in growth and development. In social therapy we can grow emotionally when we perform being giving, even if we don't feel like it.

Jonathon shot me a glance. I seemed to be annoying him. "I'm not going to do role play," he said. "So forget it."

"What I have to offer is working with you to perform your life," I responded. "It doesn't have much to do with role play. It has to do with the quality of *how* we do everything. You can learn how to go beyond yourself, learn, play, and grow your capacity to be who you are becoming."

Jonathon was irritated. "Becoming? What the hell does that mean?" he yelled. "Become what?"

I answered, "Becoming is the activity of performing ahead of yourself. It's how human beings develop. It might help you have more control over how you do your anger and frustration. It might even help your tantrums. You did it as a child. You learned to babble with your mom and dad. We learn to babble as part of the activity of learning to speak. We learn, we become, through social/cultural engagement. We go beyond ourselves. Isn't that why you are here today? What you know how to do isn't working anymore."

Jonathon looked at me and said, "I am writing a book."

"Do tell," I said, "I'm interested."

His mother described the novel. He had created a fantasy planet in outer space and a language that was only spoken there. It became clear that Jonathon was well read in many genres. It also became clear that mom had learned not only to speak on his behalf but to speak for him. In the midst of the conversation Jonathon got up and took a seat by the window. His mom made it clear he needed some space right now and that it would not be wise to make any demands on him. "If you do, the tantrums might start," she whispered. "They can last for days." I felt sympathetic to what it must be like to ward off chaos on a day-to-day basis. I thanked her for sharing this information about her son. I could see how important he was to her.

"What kind of help do you want?" I asked. Jonathon would not respond.

She quietly said, "Help him not have tantrums. Don't be too hard on him, though, he can't handle much. He's a genius."

I wondered if being related to as a genius had the same kind of impact as a diagnostic label. What about all the ways Jonathon *wasn't* a genius? Wouldn't being called a genius make it almost impossible for him to ask for help at all the myriad and confusing things he did not know how to do or was simply bad at?

I decided that it would be best for him (and me) to relate to him as an ordinary boy with an ordinary therapist. There were things we were both very good at and things we weren't good at. I mentioned that to his mom. She told me that his identity as a genius was what kept him going. It was all he had. I didn't think so. I told her I was going to relate to him as being able to do things he was not yet able to do. I would look at him through a developmental lens in terms of who he was becoming—that is, more socially and relationally responsive and skillful. What's more, I was also going to relate to myself that way as well. That seemed like a good performatory start for the two of us.

"OK, but what about the tantrums? Can you make him stop?" she asked.

"I can't guarantee he'll stop, but I can help him have many more choices beyond the tantrums," I said. She was OK with that.

I asked her to leave the room for a while. I spoke directly to Jonathon. "Your mom will be back in an hour. I want you to stay with me. Is that OK?" He said nothing.

He decided to stay put. Mom left the room. We heard the front door close. Jonathon fell off his chair and began to scream. I mean, he screamed bloody murder! His mother rushed back. I asked her to go have a cup of coffee. We would be here when she got back. Jonathon was listening to this exchange. He continued screaming, but this time he did not run out of the room. I was very aware that he decided to stay. I decided to relate to what he was doing—staying with me—as the performance of accepting my offer. I said, "OK, let's get back to work."

Jonathon lay on the floor in the center of my office. I said very loudly, "Act 1: The Scream." He looked up and began to howl louder than before. As I was beginning to get a headache, I sat in my chair and was prepared to accept what he had to give at the moment. I thought about Edvard Munch's famous painting *The Scream*. I said to him rather loudly that I thought in fact there was a lot to scream about in the world. I sometimes liked screaming myself.

Jonathon needed this space to scream. It was what he was giving me, like it or not. In social therapy we build with a client's strengths, their weaknesses, their inability to function, and our reactions to all of it. I did not want to begin by telling him what to do. I wanted to help create an environment where we might discover something together. I was wondering what else I might do. Maybe nothing. It seemed just perfect for right now. It might create an opening. Jonathon desperately needed an opening.

As a therapist I often have to resist the impulse to *do something*. There's always the impulse to make something happen. Doing nothing is a lost art in therapy. What about letting something emerge? Yes, create the conditions where something can emerge. Focus on the environment and what it enables.

Jonathon's screaming continued. My assistant in the office next to the therapy room ran in and asked if everything was OK. I assured him that everything was just fine. Jonathon stopped for a moment and looked at me quizzically.

All I knew in that moment was that I wanted to build my relationship with him. He was well read, well spoken, and in pain. He couldn't handle very much. He was unable to be in the world. This sense of isolation mattered the most to me.

What was my job here? Was it to build a safe haven for him? Would that, in fact, help him grow socially and emotionally? I didn't think so. He needed to learn how to be in the world, how to socially and culturally create his life with others. At the moment I was "the other." I would start with me.

What conditions did I think were needed for us learn how to play and perform together? In social therapy we always build the relationship as it lives in the therapy room. We look at how we are affecting each other. Jonathon needed to decide if he wanted to do that with me.

His mother returned and asked me if I thought I could help him. I replied that I did not know if I could. I asked Jonathon, who had stopped screaming, "Are you willing to do this with me, given that I think you might not want to and that I don't know if I can help you?" This challenge caught his attention. He asked, "Why would I do that?" I assured him that he would have to answer that question himself. I wanted Jonathon to take responsibility for what we were doing. He agreed to come back and ran out of the room.

For the next three months, Jonathon lay down in the center of the room and screamed for an hour. In support of his doing whatever he needed to do, I sat in a chair off to the side. I purposely did not sit in the "therapy chair." I had no interest in exerting authority over him. The sessions were difficult for me. How could I help him? I needed to keep going with a methodology that rejected predicting, analyzing, or explaining. We would build with what he was giving as we co-created the conditions where we both could grow. I had no answers. But perhaps that was because there weren't any, other than what would emerge.

What could happen here? For the next few weeks, I began each session by saying "Act 1, The Scream." I thought it was potentially the first performance of a developmental therapy play we were creating together. After a several-week "run" of the 45-minute screaming play we were both starring in, he asked, "Why aren't you telling me to stop screaming?"

"I am not interested in telling people to *stop* anything," I said. "I am interested in helping people become more powerful in their lives. Are you interested? We could do that together."

"What would we be doing?" he asked.

"Creating the therapy together—developing your capacities to be powerful in your life and to go after what it is you want for yourself and others," I said.

"What others?" he asked. I assured him I did not know the answer to that question at this time. The relationships he developed would be his decision. I was working to promote his performatory capacities. I asked if he would sit in a chair, and he agreed to do so.

Over the next six months our relationship grew as we began to create a performed conversation on the latest discoveries in the fields of science, mathematics, and the novel he was writing in a made-up language. I was truly interested and intrigued. As part of these conversations, I introduced him to philosophizing—an activity I had learned from Newman that involves asking "big" questions about little things. He was begrudgingly interested. I would ask him, "What is your language? How does it function here in our conversations?" Jonathon began to play with how to answer. It was a different kind of activity for him—a new language game—and very difficult. It had nothing to do with producing the "right answer"—something that he prided himself on doing well. But at this new game, he was a novice. Knowing was everything to him; he comforted himself with it. It seemed to be all he had. But by making the offer to philosophize, I was relating to him as ahead of himself. I was creating a situation where he would have to perform "a head taller" than where he currently was.

One day, I received a frantic message from Jonathon's mother. The school had contacted her. He had been creating a scene at school—having a tantrum on the staircase to the lunchroom. The principal was considering transferring him to a more restrictive educational setting. He came to our next session and began screaming. I told him he needed to talk in a way that I could hear him, or I wouldn't be able to help. He quieted himself. He told me about a situation where other boys were making fun of him. He started screaming again when he reported that the principal might kick him out because of the tantrums. If that happened, he would not be considered for the prestigious public high school he wanted to go to the next year. He would be moved to a more restrictive special-education-level placement.

Jonathon begged me to call the principal. I told him I did not want to do that. I wanted him to tell the principal in a voice that would allow her to listen to him. Jonathon began to scream at me about the principal: "NO, YOU HAVE TO EXPLAIN TO HER! YOU HAVE TO EXPLAIN IT!" I told him that the explanation didn't matter. What mattered would be building his relationship with her. He had to make a choice, and it was a hard one. He wasn't listening.

Now it was my turn to do a screaming performance. I asked him to sit in the audience in his chair and watch. He complied. I called it "Act 2, The Therapist Screams." I yelled, "PERFORM JONATHON, PERFORM!

PERFORM THE PERSON WHO HAS A SHOT AT GOING TO THAT FANCY ACADEMIC HIGH SCHOOL! START CREATING THE LIFE YOU WANT! *YOU* HAVE TO DO IT!"

He stormed out of the session.

The next day the principal called me. Jonathon had asked for another chance. He assured her that the tantrums would end or be small ones in the bathroom where no one could hear him. She told me that she could see that he had been developing. He actually had some friends now. But she was convinced that he would be incapable of keeping his promise. I thought she was probably right, but I urged her to give him a chance anyway.

Jonathon never had another tantrum at school again. Things weren't perfect, but he had learned that he could create the conditions he needed to perform who he wanted be in the world. We had successfully created a wanting and desire to grow. One year later, he was sitting at his desk at the high school of his choice.

In thinking about the work with Jonathon, I deeply appreciate the importance of the human capacity to perform—to go beyond ourselves and keep building without knowing where or if we were going anywhere. In our therapy plays, both Jonathon and I grew our capacity to be intimate and to respect, honor, and build with the other. We performed.

Building a Multi-family Social Therapy Group

After working successfully with several families individually, I was exploring creating a social therapy group that included children of different ages and with different kinds of therapeutic issues. What might it look like to bring some of the families I was counseling individually into a multi-family group? I spoke to Newman about it. I told him I did not know how to do it. I had worked with children and with families, but only individually. He was pleased to hear about my new adventure. "How could you possibly know how to do it?" he assured me. It was an entirely new undertaking and a daunting task.

As I was embarking on my idea of bringing families together, I wanted to learn the ways that other family therapists had challenged the nuclear family unit and were creating new therapeutic environments. There is the wonderful history of Eia Asen and Michael Scholz's work with multi-family groups (Asen and Scholz 2010). They helped their clients create non-problem-oriented conversations. They made use of a multitude of games and therapeutic exercises that helped individual families get help in a group setting. Anthony Rao (Rao and Seaton 2009) is another psychologist who challenges the plethora of diagnoses given to children, which he views as an alarming social trend. In his family therapy, he helps boys and their parents deconstruct notions of what it means to be a boy in today's world. His approach to "de-pathologizing" behavior is critical to creating environments where parents and children can grow together.

I was also drawn to some of the key developers of play therapy. I found Virginia Axline's seminal work—*Dibs in Search of Self* (1967), which chronicled the beginnings of play therapy—to be important. I was touched by the relationship she built with the young Dibs, who was given the opportunity in therapy to play, unencumbered by adult directives and priorities. His initiative was valued; he was not being driven toward the chute of normality. Central to helping reinitiate Dibs' development was the carefully built relationship between therapist and patient.

Axline (1967) broke the rules to create the first child-centered, nondirective play therapy. Her work was a significant attempt to advance a non-judgmental, humanistic approach that helped children grow. While I did question how she mostly worked with the child alone—separated out from his or her family—her unconditional acceptance of the child and the relationships she built gave young children a shot at growing emotionally.

What would it mean, I wondered, to bring together entire families—children and adults—all of whom identified both as an individual and as a member of their family? Could I support people to create a new social unit—a new group—that recognized, but was not overly determined by, how people relate to one another as family?

I talked with Newman about my observations and new questions. He listened. I shared with him the history of family therapy approaches, including narrative approaches, and we discussed ways to advance the work. We talked about the social therapist's role as the group's organizer—helping the group to exercise its power to keep creating itself.

In order to help the group, I would have to abandon the activity of knowing. I would lead a process that allowed these parents and these children to take a look at their assumptions and biases about themselves and their families, many of which were holding them back. The work wouldn't always feel good, just as working with, rather than against, Jonathan's screaming sessions was often painful. And since people want their family to feel good, the group might have some difficulty going with me.

Could I as the group's organizer engage the group in overthrowing societal roles and rules of what it meant to be a family and create new ways of being together, new ways of talking, and new ways of doing family? Could we evolve as a developmental ensemble where people come together to create its development? I would help them creatively perform living their lives without many of the labels, identities, assumptions, and truth-telling stories that had kept them stuck and in pain. Together we would work to create a new form of life: a multi-family group community. We would play with our strengths, our weaknesses, our joys, and sometimes the exasperation of creating family life together.

In creating this new family play, I wondered if and how we could learn from the children. Could children help the adults grow? Children are, after all, very good at performance and play. They have the luxury of not being fully inculcated into the culture and haven't fully appropriated and learned to abide by the rules of how they are supposed to be. This lack of fixed understandings deepens their capacity to be improvisational and is essential to their growth and development. And to ours!

I began by meeting individually with the five families from my practice, whom I invited to form the group with me. Let me introduce them:

Lila, age 9, was very quiet. Her parents were going through a divorce. She did not have a diagnosis, but she had learned to be ashamed that her parents were splitting up. She hid her face when her mom began to tell me about their family.

Mary, age 10, had made it clear she wished her parents *would* divorce. Too much fighting was going on in the home. At the end of the session, she asked me to go into the office bathroom with her. Her parents were perplexed by this request, as was I. Once we were inside the bathroom, she told me she had something she wanted me to know. I said OK. Mary whispered to me that she thought she was very, very crazy. She said she would never speak about this belief in the group, and I told her that I so appreciated her telling me.

Michael, age 11, had been diagnosed with ADHD. It was hard to be in the room with him. He would move and squirm while his mother would try to get him to sit down. I told them that it was OK if he didn't want to sit. We talked about how this was a brand new situation for everyone, and that I could be pretty "hyper" myself. It drove some of my friends crazy.

Paula, age 12, was diagnosed with learning disabilities. She was outspoken and said whatever she wanted. She interrupted most conversations with off-topic comments. Not sure what to do, her parents often reprimanded her. Every time she would speak, they were ready to ask her to stop talking. In school and often at home, she never quite got it right. I was curious about how we might support her to learn how to talk to the group. I would keep this challenge in mind for sure.

And then there was Benjamin, age 12, who had been diagnosed with Asperger's syndrome. He had difficulty making eye contact and would not speak in the intake session. He was clearly very close to his mom. She was there because she wanted him to gain some social skills. She asked if I could do something about the hours he spent glued to the computer. I asked Benjamin what he thought. He stared at the floor and said he wanted to leave. His mom and I finished the conversation.

During the intake process the parents spoke about how uncomfortable it was for them to talk about the painful aspects of their lives with other families. What if people judged them? What if they were doing it all wrong? They might feel embarrassed. We spoke together at length about the institution of the family and how the family has an enormous impact on everyone in it. I urged them to remember that it would be terribly important that they get the support they needed to use the therapy to create performances that could contribute to the emotional development of them and their children, individually and collectively.

The group, I said by way of introduction, will not be about what was wrong with their family, avoiding the pathologizing that typically accompanies therapies for those with diagnoses of disability. We would work together to create an environment that would allow them to talk about their difficulties, their love and pain, and the exasperation of being a parent or a child who is not related to as "normal." Everything, I told them, that the adults and children give will be available to use as building material for new family plays, new group performances. Group work expands the resources available to families. They would get to know their own child and the other children in new ways. They would no longer have to do it all by themselves.

Some parents were concerned that they would lose their parental authority. "What if I don't like what the group is doing?" asked one mom.

I responded, "Then you will say that, and we will collectively figure out what to do with it." She breathed a sigh of relief. She didn't have to figure out everything by herself.

Now it was time to bring the five families together. Our first group was on a Monday evening. Initially, children and parents sat in a circle. The kids were quite excited. Most of them were socially isolated and had few friends. Here they were sitting with four other children! Michael kept popping out of his seat. His mother was getting upset and trying to get him to sit down. I asked her if she wanted some help. With reticence and awkwardness, she nodded. Other children began crawling around the room or under their seats or going to look out the window. Then came the yelling and admonitions from the parents. One boy went to sit in the opening of a nonfunctioning fireplace. He refused to come out. "Do something!" a parent yelled at me. Feeling a bit insecure, I wondered to myself whether or not family therapy was such a good idea.

A reflective interlude: I was reminded of a quote from the Austrian philosopher Ludwig Wittgenstein (1980), a major influence on social therapy: "When you are philosophizing you have to descend into primeval chaos and feel at home there" (Wittgenstein 1980, p. 65).

I also appreciated how the chaos of this first session might be an important element in freeing us all up to allow something new to be created, something outside the box of traditional therapy and family life. Perhaps out of the chaos, families could see one another from a new vantage point—enabling them to throw "normality" into relief, and allowing them to begin to move around and about the implicit roles and rules. For this reason, I liked the chaos as it jumbles things up and makes it more difficult to slip back into traditional therapeutic responses. For me, the chaos was a reminder of what was needed to "overthrow" ourselves. If you make the decision to go with it, it allows for other possibilities to emerge through play and performance.

I wanted to respond to the mom who was upset by the disorder in the room. I wanted to be careful that I was not performing any attitude of authority or knowing. So often in family therapy, the therapist can fall into the trap of becoming the better, kinder parent. In this group I wanted to organize the adults to follow and create with me. I was not interested in supplanting them, so I had to find out if they were interested in going somewhere new with me.

I said to the parents, "I don't have all the answers. I want to do this with all of you. I will challenge you to go to some new places in how you see your children and yourself. Are you with me on that?" They acknowledged that they were. Their agreement to move with me was terribly important. In the absence of that allowance, the therapy would be coercive. I continued, "Let's philosophize here: What does 'do something' mean?"

Silence.

"Does it mean we want to control what's happening by using our authority as adults? Should we raise our voices and relate to what's happening as a problem that the children have? Or can we create a different response that would help the group develop?" Some of the parents were understandably annoyed. Others were interested.

Now I turned my attention to the entire group, including the children, and asked, "What does the group want to do?" A number of the children spoke up and repeated my question. They were following me! I had their support. I yelled above the commotion, "How should we do this?"

The parents began reprimanding their children. I gently asked them to stop, as I didn't think that at this moment it had anything to do with helping the group develop. This was a very important moment for us. We were shifting the group's gaze away from what the individual parent might need in terms of managing their children toward what the group needed.

I told the children to freeze, as if we were in a playground. They did. I told them I needed them to participate in shaping what we were going to do together. They needed to lead the group. Michael, whose mom was very upset with him, said he didn't want to sit next to his mother. I said to him, "You gave us an opening!"

"I did?" he asked.

"Yes, you are being a leader by saying what is not working for you in the group." I thanked him and said, "OK everybody, sit in the circle next to someone you're *not* related to." All the children jumped up laughing and sat next to a stranger. The parents were having a much harder time with all this. One parent asked me if I knew what I was doing. I assured her I did not. At the same time, I actively focused on what the parents and the children were giving the group to create with. What could we use to create an environment where development toward their goals was possible? I told them that we needed to follow the children's lead and work improvisationally.

The group continued. Mary began to cry. She said she knew her parents wished she was more "together," but she wanted them to promise they would never send her away. They promised. Her mom kept asking if it was OK to be having this conversation. The children began grabbing the opportunity to say things they hadn't been able to say in the privacy of their individual families.

Lila blurted out that she wanted her mother to know that she couldn't handle her parents getting a divorce. Paula added that she had nothing to say about any of this and that she needed the group to know that.

Benjamin's mom said that the chaos in the group was really hard for her. She told us that raising Benjamin was not a picnic. Suddenly Benjamin yelled, "I know it must be a drag to be my mom all the time. I know you hate it. You threaten to send me to boarding school. But it's OK. I still think you are a good mom."

I thought the children's questions and frank and open statements were helping the group expand how we were together. The parents were surprised by the children's thoughtfulness. They commented that they were having a new experience of their own children. The richness and honesty of the group conversation made it clear to all of us that we were breaking new ground. The question for me was how best to keep it going.

Paula, prone to blurting things out, said it would be great if the parents did not yell at their children in the group. This request really annoyed her mother. I wanted Paula to have the opportunity to be acknowledged for saying something of value to the group. My hunch was that this offer, and other offers from the children, would help the group engage how we were sitting, talking, playing, or perhaps even yelling at each other—how we were going to organize family life in the context of the life of our group. I wanted the adults and children to continually be looking at and implementing ideas of how we needed to organize ourselves so our group could grow.

The group decided that any child or adult could ask another group member to stop what they are doing if it was getting in the group's way, as long as they are not related to each other. And any adult could raise a disciplinary issue with a child, as long as it was not their own child. Lila's mom then said to Benjamin, whom she had just met, "We need you to sit down right now." Benjamin obediently sat down.

> I suggested we take the group from the top one more time.
> "How can we begin the group again?" asked some of the children.
> "We can decide ourselves how we want to do things together," I said.

We all sat in a circle, and I reminded them to make sure that they were sitting next to someone to whom they were not related. We played a game with beanbags. I asked that people throw the beanbag in such a way as to make sure the person who would catch the beanbag would look good. This requirement meant that each participant really had to *look at* whom they were throwing the bag to and figure out what they thought the recipient could handle. One parent complained that I was asking too much of the children. I did not understand how impaired they were. She said that her daughter Lila was especially sensitive and could not handle much. I asked the children what they thought about this. Lila was the one who supported the idea of not allowing the parents to yell.

Paula chimed in that we shouldn't make Lila a "special case," since Lila was *already* contributing. Everyone was surprised by Paula's support of Lila. I asked Lila if she was OK with that. I was very moved when Lila responded that she didn't really know how to participate in this way. I assured her she was in good company. And our week-one session came to an end.

Several weeks later, we began to create some new performance activities. Each child would be a director and/or star in a play. Again, Lila's mom told us that Lila would not be able to participate in this activity. I asked why she thought that. She explained that Lila was not social and could not do much with other people.

At this point Benjamin spoke up and said that he had seen Lila reading a book in the waiting room and at other times. "Wasn't that doing something with other people?" Other children and adults agreed that they had also noticed Lila reading in the waiting room. Lila was attentive to the conversation about her, but looked quite frightened. Several parents suggested that if that was a way Lila could be in the group, we should support it. Maybe what Lila could do right now was read a book with us. Lila began crying. Her mom felt she should take Lila out of the room. I asked what the group thought. The group asked Lila's mom to let her stay and do the scene. Benjamin assured Lila's mom that she was doing the right thing by letting the group help her daughter.

I asked Lila where the scene would take place. Lila said the scene would be in the park. She said she was feeling very insecure. Benjamin put a chair in our open performance space where she could sit. The group let her know that reading the book would be a fine performance. Lila sat in the chair. She was asked to give the scene a title. Lila announced in a quivering voice, "The title is *Reading a Book in the Park*." The audience of children and families applauded when the scene was over.

Benjamin yelled out that he wanted to be next. He invited all the children into his scene. They all ran into the open performance space. He announced that he would direct and star in it. "Here's the scene," he said. "We are playing ourselves 20 years from now. We are all camping in the mountains overnight. Everyone is sitting around a campfire toasting marshmallows." As the scene continued, the children pretended that it began to rain and they walked up a hill to a luxury hotel. They paid for a room, drank lots of champagne, and were laughing and fooling around. They were clearly having a good time, relaxing and chatting about their grown-up lives.

The scene shocked Benjamin's mom and several other parents. They had never seen him or the other children like this. "Was this OK?" one mom asked. "Aren't we encouraging drinking?" I reminded everyone that this was a performance. Nor did I think we needed to interpret what it "really meant." I thought we needed to support Benjamin and his friends to perform their play and for the parents to let them be. "We are working to create the conditions where something can emerge," I reminded them.

Benjamin asked that I join the scene and perform as his 20-something friend. What would I do? It was a difficult decision for me. I felt nervous that the parents would not be able to go with it if I joined in. I thought Benjamin was possibly testing me to see if I would stand by my statement that this was all a performance. Conflicted, I decided I needed to have some integrity and be giving to Benjamin. I could not back down. We did the scene again. He gave me an imaginary glass of champagne. I joined in.

When the scene ended, I asked Benjamin, why this scene? What was it about this scenario that mattered to him? He passionately explained that this was the life he would never have. He would never be independent. He would never have friends. So could we just let him be? He was very upset.

The group asked how he knew all this. He told us that he had Asperger's syndrome. He was smart and at the same time, he could barely function socially. He had no friends. His mother began to cry. Another child went over to her to comfort her.

One of the children yelled out, "You have the group Benjamin. You have all of us!" Benjamin nodded. The group ended for the day. Benjamin did the scene over and over again for weeks. The other children loved Benjamin's play. I was now in the audience. I had passed the test. Not surprisingly, the parents were conflicted. I urged them to let it be what it is, a scene in a therapy play. With all of our conflicts, we marveled over the power of performance.

The group continued for another year at the parents' request.

During this time, I was asked to train mental health professionals in how to work with children therapeutically. I asked Benjamin to assist me. He was incredulous, as was his family. His parents felt it was way too much pressure, but Benjamin was adamant that he be allowed to participate. His parents finally gave him permission. I began the training by talking about social therapy. After an hour or so, Benjamin got up from his seat and announced that he was going to do a series of performances. He would play a therapist and instructed people attending the workshop to be the patients. He asked that I perform as his first patient. This direction was not where we had planned to go. I was unsure of this detour, but I decided to go with it.

We arranged the chairs for the scene. Benjamin sat in the big therapy chair. I entered his therapy office and sat down. My "therapist" was playing with finger puppets. He did not make eye contact. I was getting nervous about how this performance would go. I wondered whether I was making a mistake here.

I finally asked if he was the therapist. He said he was. He kept playing with the puppets and not looking at me. He asked quite competently what I wanted help with. I told him that I had no friends. He looked up from his puppets. He asked me what I wanted him to do about it. I was taken aback. He asked me about my life. I told him I was isolated. I didn't go out much. I was on the computer most of the time.

He said quite clearly, "You do not have the conditions to grow. Create those conditions. Make a friend and come back. I will help you keep your friend. You need to take responsibility for your life."

For the rest of the training Benjamin continued performing as the therapist and had a great deal to say to everyone. It was an emotional experience for everyone there. His mother had stopped by and could not believe what she saw. She was discovering that there were ways she had not been able to see her son's growth toward becoming more socially engaged and engaging.

In the weeks following the workshop, however, Benjamin became withdrawn. His teachers reported that he was regressing. I thought he had had a big reaction to the performances he had become capable of. Often mumbling to himself, Benjamin would say, "I trained those therapists. I have something to say." He became less participatory in the family group. His silence was noted. The family group ended months later.

Throughout those weeks and months, I was concerned that perhaps I had taken too big of a leap with Ben. I spoke to Newman about it. Had I missed something here?

He agreed that I had. I had missed that one cannot predict the twists and turns of how development emerges. I had missed that development cannot be explained by some linear accounting of how this young boy was responding. I should stop trying to make sense of what had gone wrong.

Perhaps nothing had gone wrong, and this episode was part of a fascinating performance of Benjamin coming to terms with the complexity and conflictedness of who he was and who he was becoming. Development can be hard, as it brings new demands to all of us.

Trying to make sense of it all, I was distancing myself from this young boy who had discovered that he could go way beyond what traditional paradigms of growth and development could explain.

What was so perplexing for him and his family was that this non-rule-governed activity of play and performance had allowed him to leap ahead of himself, to perform as if he were a head taller. And now he was withdrawing. With the support of the group, he had become a leader. He clearly experienced himself as the creator of his life with others. He had improvisationally participated in the group's social growth and they in his. He had worked with others to shape the group as a laboratory for new life performances. He was learning how to work with others to shape the group and, in turn, allow himself to be shaped by it. This social-cultural experience had allowed him to go somewhere he had not been before. He was right. He *had* trained those therapists, and he did indeed have something say.

Many months after his family therapy group ended, Benjamin wanted to talk about the training. Did I really think he had taught them something? I passionately answered that yes, he had. The trainees had learned and grown from the conversations he had performed with them. The workshop he had helped me lead challenged their assumptions about what therapy is. They had learned more about how to philosophize, and they were better clinicians for it. Benjamin had a hard time processing his new, more adult role. He had gone way beyond what he thought was possible for himself. Soon after these conversations, he formally ended his therapy with me.

His social withdrawal lasted over a year. His parents lovingly stood by him. Benjamin told them he needed time. In various phone conversations, I urged them to give it to him. It was very painful for everyone. They were worried about the many hours he was glued to the computer. They had always known what was best for him. They didn't now.

Almost a year later, Benjamin called a family meeting at the kitchen table. He said he felt he could not develop any further living at home. They had helped him with everything. They shielded him from harm. They gave him whatever he wanted. They understood him. But he wasn't growing. He needed a situation where he had to stand on his own two feet the way he was able to when he performed in the group. Would they consider sending him away to school?

It was painful yet moving to them that he was working to take responsibility for what he needed to go further. Still, they were conflicted about responding to his request. What if it didn't work? On the other hand, perhaps he needed to live at a boarding school with other young people. He might have the conditions there to do more growing. His mother was very emotional as she told me the story in one of our conversations. She had grown tremendously too. She felt he should be given the chance to make a go of it.

The next fall they placed Benjamin in a residential school. He did remarkably well. He made friends. He built relationships with his teachers. Sometimes he came home on weekends. Often he did not. He was living his life.

Discussion

This chapter has centered on social therapy with families and how the developmental paths of children and parents were reignited through their engagement in a form of therapeutic performance and family play. This experience required them to reenvision and reinvent new roles at home and in other social settings and work through how these ways of relating might unfold in the many scenes of their lives. The narratives illustrate how the philosophical/performatory activity of questioning familiar roles and relationships in the course of performing new ones can open up new possibilities and contribute to environments where all can grow emotionally.

Playing, imagining, and performing on a therapeutic performance stage of the participants' own making allowed families to grow. And while the growth process was often chaotic, challenging, and even threatening, the social therapist as the group's organizer helped the group power onward to create itself.

Upsetting social roles and rules in the process of devising new "language games" can indeed be chaotic and emotionally tumultuous. The unfamiliar and chaotic process, however, forged a new intimacy both within and among families. New relationships and new social channels helped adults and young people alike access resources and create new possibilities for being together. They were less alone. They had more social resources. The social therapeutic process allowed for more satisfying family and interfamily dynamics and personal developmental pathways, even (and especially) when in one instance they required a departure from the family's immediate oversight and regulation to be realized.

The cases reported here illustrate how, under the direction of the social therapist, the group was related to and emerged as the unit of growth. And while the child provided the impetus for the family seeking therapy initially, it was ultimately the family group that developed.

As the therapist, I always had my eye on the group—the relationship. When that "group" was a group of two, I worked to be completely responsive to the young person sitting (or screaming) across from me. My focus was our relationship. I had to go with him or her, even when that involved enduring very disturbing behavior. This decision to let the children lead the activities was a key part of building the "we" that would be indispensable to that child's emotional growth.

Although parents bring children into social therapy to "fix" something about their child, social therapy focuses on development, on spontaneously constructing the settings that provide the positive social updraft through which such development becomes possible. We build with the totality of what the child gives us—their strengths as well as their weaknesses. Children on the autism spectrum are typically highly intelligent and can learn through appropriate sorts of engagement and challenge. In social therapy, the opportunity to play and perform allowed these assets to become foregrounded, with the children being given the responsibility to lead the adults in the activities, thus shifting attention to what they do know and can do rather than what they lack.

The process of development had many twists and turns. As I have reviewed, the tensions that arose during the therapy sessions were often significant, leading parents to question my competence. But those tensions ultimately indicated where the greatest performative needs lay, and provided the impetus for helping the young people with their difficulties in relating to others and with developing their capacity to lead a relational life.

Through the exploration of these tensions in a playful, imaginative environment—one in which the play could be chaotic and threatening—new rules of engagement (new performances) emerged that families came to rely upon. In the end, families constructed a new form of life in their therapy group that unexpectedly reinitiated everyone's emotional development. Often disruptive (there was no way around that), this shift allowed for a process where all—children and adults alike—could contribute to creating a therapeutic play and performance space to premier a new family play.

Each family's hopes for socializing their child were realized, although not necessarily in the direction they had ever imagined when they decided to enter therapy with me. That uncertainty is central to the drama of human development—as disconcerting and disorderly as it might seem at the outset of a therapeutic journey undertaken for the purpose of creating a more satisfying life.

NOTES

1. "The diagnostic category of pervasive developmental disorders (PDD) refers to a group of disorders characterized by delays in the development of socialization and communication skills. Parents may note symptoms as early as infancy, although the typical age of onset is before three years of age. Symptoms may include problems with using and understanding language; difficulty relating to people, objects, and events; unusual play with toys and other objects; difficulty with changes in routine or familiar surroundings; and repetitive body movements or behavior patterns. Autism (a developmental brain disorder characterized by impaired social interaction and communication skills, and a limited range of activities and interests) is the most characteristic and best studied PDD. Other types of PDD include Asperger's syndrome, childhood disintegrative disorder, and Rett's syndrome. Children with PDD vary widely in abilities, intelligence, and behaviors. Some children do not speak at all, others speak in limited phrases or conversations, and some have relatively normal language development. Repetitive play skills and limited social skills are generally evident. Unusual responses to sensory information, such as loud noises and lights, are also common." National Institute of Neurological Disorders and Stroke (2015), n. p.
2. All names are pseudonyms.

REFERENCES

Axline, V. (1967). *Dibs in search of self*. New York: Ballantine Books.
Asen, E., & Scholz, M. (2010). *Multi-family therapy concepts and techniques*. New York: Routledge.
Holzman, L., & Mendez, R. (2003). *Psychological investigations: A clinician's guide to social therapy*. New York: Routledge.
Holzman, L., & Newman, F. (2012). Activity and performance (and their discourse) in social therapeutic practice. In A. Lock & T. Strong (Eds.), *Discursive perspectives in therapeutic practice* (pp. 184–195). New York: Oxford University Press.

Marx, K. (1974). Theses on Feuerbach. In K. Marx & F. Engels (Eds.), *The German ideology*. London: Lawrence & Fishart.
National Institute of Neurological Disorders and Stroke. (2015). *NINDS Pervasive Developmental Disorders information page*. Bethesda: Office of Communications and Public Liaison, National Institute of Neurological Disorders and Stroke, & National Institutes of Health. Retrieved August 23, 2015, from http://www.ninds.nih.gov/disorders/pdd/pdd.htm
Newman, F., & Goldberg, P. (1996). *Performance of a lifetime: A practical-philosophical guide to the joyous life*. New York: Castillo International.
Newman, F., & Holzman, L. (1997). *The end of knowing: A new developmental way of learning*. New York: Routledge.
Newman, F., & Holzman, L. (2006/1996). *Unscientific psychology: A cultural-performatory approach to understanding human life*. iUniverse. Originally published by Westport: Praeger.
Rao, A., & Seaton, M. (2009). *The way of boys: Raising healthy boys in a challenging world*. New York: HarperCollins.
Wittgenstein, L. (1953). *Philosophical investigations* (trans: Anscombe, G. E. M.). Oxford: Blackwell. Retrieved October 21, 2015, fromhttp://gormendizer.co.za/wp-content/uploads/2010/06/Ludwig.Wittgenstein.-.Philosophical.Investigations.pdf
Wittgenstein, L. (1980). *Culture and value* (trans: Winch, P.). Oxford: Blackwell.
Vygotsky, L. S. (1978). *Mind in society: The development of higher psychological processes* (M. Cole, V. John-Steiner, S. Scribner, & E. Souberman, Eds.). Cambridge, MA: Harvard University Press.
Vygotsky, L. S. (1993). *The collected works of L. S. Vygotsky. Volume 2: The fundamentals of defectology (abnormal psychology and learning disabilities)* (R. W. Rieber & A. S. Carton, Eds.; J. E. Knox & C. B. Stevens, Trans.). New York: Plenum.

CHAPTER 5

Shakespeare and Autism: Reenvisioning Expression, Communication, and Inclusive Communities

Robin Post

The Hunter Heartbeat Method (HHM), created Kelly Hunter, is a theatrical performance-based program designed for children on the autism spectrum. This chapter will describe the practice and processes involved in the implementation of the method and also discuss the recommended programmatic elements that comprise this innovative technique. The HHM features a series of games that bring the unique characteristics of and interactions between Shakespeare's characters into focus as children on the spectrum portray the characters and tell the story of the selected play. The method transforms the complexities of Shakespeare's plots into a sequence of games that are specifically tailored to address the communicative challenges that accompany autism.

The HHM provides children on the spectrum with a "positive social updraft"(see Chap. 1) through which they are able to develop and strengthen their communicative and interactive skills and places children on the spectrum within a supportive context for developing greater possibilities for engagement and interaction. The method is flexible and adaptive and makes it possible for those on the spectrum to explore various modes of

R. Post (✉)
The Department of Theatre, The University of North Carolina-Wilmington, Wilmington, NC, USA

© The Author(s) 2016
P. Smagorinsky (ed.), *Creativity and Community among Autism-Spectrum Youth*, DOI 10.1057/978-1-137-54797-2_5

communicative expression that facilitate social interaction. As a result, they gain access, familiarity, and ease with a wider variety of cultural activities.

A critical component of the activities is their provision of opportunities for playful, performative engagement. The children get the opportunity to perform scenes between characters who, at times, express heightened dramatic emotional states or unwittingly negotiate communicative strategies as a means to understand and belong. The children begin to understand the limits and boundaries for social engagement through this dramatic reenactment. Significantly, rather than curbing their autistic traits through imposed limits, the games open up channels of activity through which social skills are acquired and adopted of their own accord as they come to experience and embody the successes and failures and the emotional highs and lows of the characters. The approach is thus asset-oriented rather than deficit-centered.

The Hunter Heartbeat Method, Shakespeare, and Autism

I served as director of a three-year longitudinal research study, *Shakespeare and Autism*[1], from 2012 to 2015. During this time, I had the opportunity to observe, implement, and assist in creating some of the games that comprise this innovative technique. In this chapter, I will speak from my perspective as director of the applied research component of the study. In an effort to support the ongoing inquiry into the efficacy of the work through its replication and study, I will also be sharing the novel and original methodology that introduces new ways of working and playing with children and adults on the spectrum and that supports the notion of creating more inclusive communities. I will share some of the theoretical underpinnings of the HHM and describe some of the dynamic features of the method that occur in a live setting. The structure and pedagogy of the HHM require and result in the creation of a safe social space, wherein Shakespeare's text, rhythm, and storytelling are used to playfully explore a wide range of vocal, emotional, and physical expression, with the children's attention to their own heartbeats helping to ground their use of Shakespeare's verse in their own organic rhythms.

The objectives of the research were to provide weekly 60-minute sessions of the HHM to the same group of children, in grades four through seven, over an extended period of 42 weeks. The overarching goal of the project was to determine, through protocols and parental questionnaires, whether change had occurred in the children's presentation of the core features of autism. Specifically, the research inquired into change in social and adaptive functioning, emotional facial recognition and expression, and verbal skills. Preliminary findings of the pilot were very promising, specifically indicating notable growth in social and adaptive functioning.

During the course of the research, Kelly Hunter wrote and published *Shakespeare's Heartbeat: Drama Games for Children with Autism*, an instructional guide for implementation of her work using Shakespeare's *The Tempest* and *A Midsummer Night's Dream*. The games used for the research project I describe relied exclusively on *The Tempest*. A majority of the games that comprise the techniques of the HHM can be demonstrated by two actors in just a few minutes, and the games enable the children to enjoy both playing them and watching others play them.

The HHM is an experiential exploration that specifically addresses some of the communicative barriers experienced by those on the autism spectrum such as challenges with eye contact; spatial awareness; social skills (e.g., taking turns, leading and following, receiving and giving, etc.); emotional facial recognition and expression; verbal skills; and integrating vocal, physical, and emotional expression. For example, one of the initial games involves greetings between children and all participants sitting within the activity's circle (see Fig. 5.1 for an example of the circle). Each child takes his or her turn to sit on an "x" in the center of a circle and says "hello" to each of the participants who are sitting in the outer circle, while simultaneously tapping out the rhythm of the heartbeat on his or her chest. The participants sitting in the outer circle reply with their own "hello" after being greeted.

This game addresses challenges with a variety of challenges facing young people on the spectrum:

- *spatial relationships* (remaining in the center),
- *mobility* (moving one's body around the circle to face each participant in the outer circle while tapping the heart),
- *eye contact* (with each person receiving the "hello"),
- *turn-taking* (children on the outer circle must wait for the child in the center to get around to them, and each child takes his or her respective turn in the middle),
- *receiving and giving* (sending "hellos" and waiting to receive a "hello" before moving on),
- *emotional facial expression* (the "hellos" are often accompanied with an emotion such as happy, sad, and angry), and
- *verbal expression* (saying the word "hello").

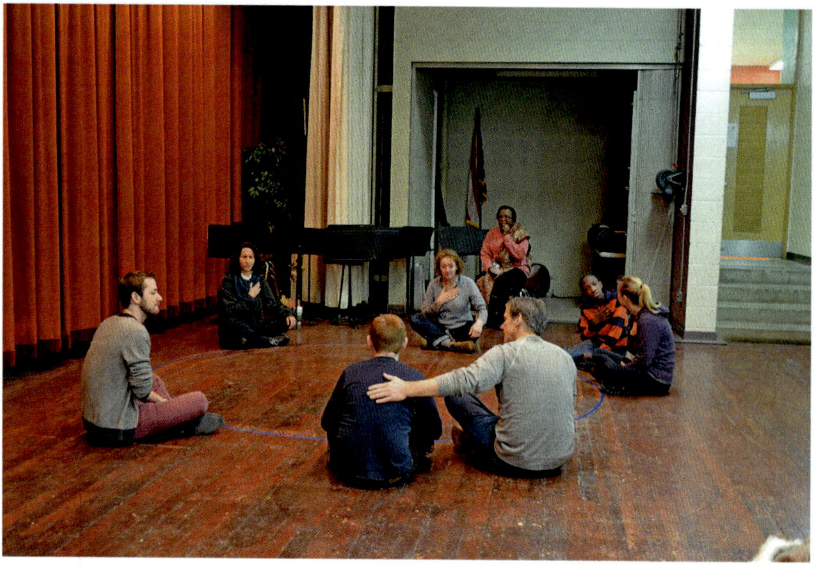

Fig. 5.1 The HHM circle. (Photo by Ji Rye Lee)

This introductory game establishes the structure for the methodology and is typically repeated at the beginning of each session, which allows the children to build their skills.

Bidirectional Focus of Teacher/Learner

The HMM emphasizes the recognition of unique individual differences for those on the spectrum, with a focus on inclusion and accepting the meaning-making perspective of each participant. The method encourages those who lead the work to broaden their concept of communication and connection to include nonverbal, physical, rhythmic or music-based, and kinesthetic communication grounded in role-play and character exploration. Inclusive communities are constructed through acceptance, compassion, communication, and human connection. Introducing new ways to communicate and connect with different types of people will broaden the range of people included in social activity and build inclusivity among the neurotypical[2] population.

The connections being made when engaging in the games that comprise the HHM benefit not only those on the spectrum, but also the teachers, actors, social workers, parents, and others who must expand their own modes of communication by learning and expressing themselves in ways that may initially feel foreign to them. In this way, negotiation of social constructs and adaptation are shared by the children and their guides alike rather than being the sole responsibility of the children (see Chap. 3). The method requires adults in the setting to construct a fluid environment within the HHM structure such that a positive social updraft is available, one whose flexibility is responsive to the needs of the children. An honest and truthful attempt to connect and communicate is a two-way street, and both parties must strive to meet in the middle. This mutual adaptation creates inclusive communities where everyone involved, including those on the spectrum, determine the ways in which communication and connection will occur.

"Teachers" of the HHM must become students as much as, if not more than, the children on the spectrum. They must observe and listen with heightened awareness and focused attention on learning from those with whom they are playing. They must also be willing to share their playfulness during the process of listening. The HHM's reliance upon this bidirectional focus of teacher as learner and learner as teacher contributes to the manner in which the structure of the work and the games create safe social situations in which to explore expression and communication for both parties. Of critical importance is the need for mutual adaptations to be undertaken by both the adults and children so that the parameters of activity remain flexible (see Chap. 3).

The work requires teachers to rethink their instruction and accept the risk of being vulnerable, a dynamic that places a primary means of adaptation on those who construct the social setting of the activities. The performative experience is *not* one where the teacher knows the rules of the game and diligently presses the child to adapt and adhere to them. More accurately, the actor, teacher, parent, aid, and others in teaching roles serve as guides who facilitate and introduce new ways of exploring expression, while simultaneously waking themselves up to that expression with each participant. I will refer to teaching artists as "guides" for the remainder of the chapter.

One example of the shared experience between the guide and the child is evidenced through the HHM game "Lovestruck" (Hunter, 2015, p. 33), which is based on the moment in *The Tempest* when Ferdinand and Miranda *see* one another for the first time. When the two characters—one played by a guide, one by a child—find one another's eyes, they share a choral, "Doyoyoying!" This sound is accompanied by a gesture of their hands in front of their eyes as if their eyes were popping out of their heads (as seen in many cartoons). The game (see Fig. 5.2) is repeated a few more times until the final time when they say, "I love you."

This expression of love can be very genuine between the guide and the child, and the vulnerability that characterizes this event is experienced for both guide and child alike. Without the guide's willingness to be vulnerable, a rehearsed and almost blocked expression of care is more likely. I have seen this reluctance to engage with openness in teaching artists who keep their emotional walls up and "pretend" at the expression, thus doing what many acting teachers affectionately refer to as "acting badly." Pretending to express the emotions involved in the games limits the possibilities for connections. Investing in truly experiencing the expression has much greater rewards for all involved. The HHM is, like other approaches described in this volume, *relational* at heart.

To illustrate how vulnerability plays a role in the process, I would like to share a workshop fragment from the primary research that I observed over a period of several weeks with one with one of our teaching artists, Genevieve Simon[3] and Jake,[4] a 12-year-old boy on the spectrum:

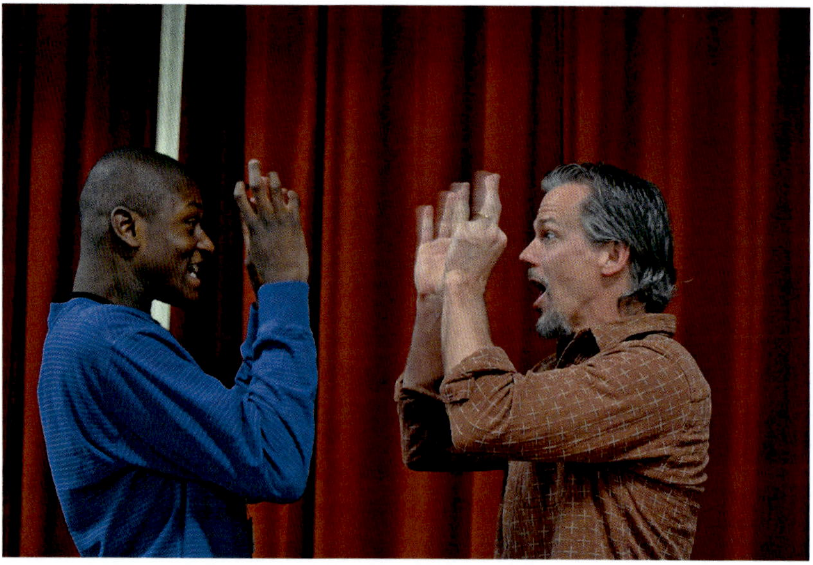

Fig. 5.2 The Doyoyoying game. (Photo by Ji Rye Lee)

On more than one occasion, I was brought to tears by the connection between [guide] Simon, who played the monster, Caliban, who is learning to speak, and [child] Jake, who worked patiently and lovingly to teach the muttering Caliban the syllables of his name. Simon's vulnerability encouraged Jake to comfort her and make her feel safe and he began to say things like, "It's OK, you almost have it," or "Very close, try again." Simon's willingness to be genuinely vulnerable in these moments increased the possibility for Jake to experience a sense of connection, care, and empowerment when teaching his partner. Prior to our work with Jake, he made little to no connection with those around him, often muttered things under his breath, making no eye contact and remaining in a world to himself. After working with Simon for a several weeks, this child who had very minimal verbal skills was able to focus his attention on Caliban and made a concerted effort to teach him his name. He also grew ever-more vigilant in his effort to get Caliban's attention by making eye contact with him. Genevieve wrote about her work with Jake in her field notes: "[Jake] is making such huge strides each week, it's blowing my mind. Today I suddenly remembered how long it took for him to look directly at me last year and I almost can't believe it now, since he looks right at me every single session. He does such a great job teaching Caliban how to speak as Miranda!"(see Fig. 5.3)

There is no way to prove that Simon's vulnerability led to this outcome, and arguably the game itself, regardless of the guide's vulnerability, would have had the same results. However, playing Caliban requires the guide to listen and learn from the child teacher, Miranda, which inherently places the guide in a vulnerable position. The level of vulnerability experienced by the guide may be determined only by the guide herself. However, I would argue that both guide and child benefit more from a willingness to let down their walls and really invest in the evolving relationship between the characters.

The HHM encourages guides to practice living in the unknown with children on the spectrum and allow the process of the work to lead them through the uncharted world of emotional, physical, and vocal expression. Rather than trying to force conformity to an arbitrary norm, the HHM acknowledges the wide range of characteristics for those on the spectrum and incorporates and works with those characteristics as a means to connect, rather than working rigidly in opposition to them. In terms of the process of constructing a positive social updraft, the manner in which the autistic child experiences social norms and expressive interactions is constructed, in part, by the guide's ability to perform and playfully engage with the child in a way that is flexible yet enacted such that socially viable means of interaction are cultivated.

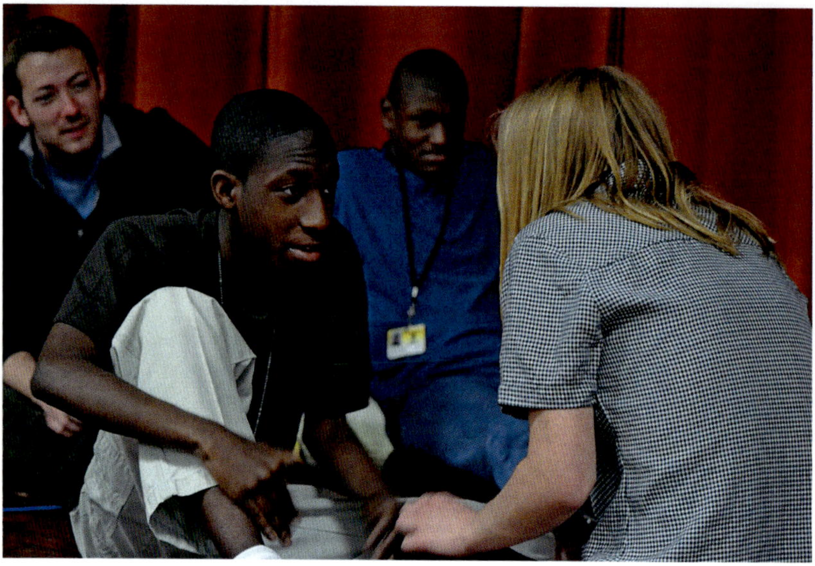

Fig. 5.3 Teaching Caliban his name. (Photo by Ji Rye Lee)

Structure, Empowerment, Praise, and Play

Structure, empowerment, praise, and play are central concepts or principles embedded within the HHM, and the content and performance exist synergistically. These principles create an inclusive environment that can be applied easily to teaching in general. Those who are implementing the HHM can and should refer back to these principles as pedagogical benchmarks for self-assessment. In other words, one should ask, "Have I provided the necessary structures? Have I truly played with the children and with my fellow guides? Have I offered consistent praise to the children for their efforts? Have I been consciously empowering the children through the work?" Although there is considerable flexibility with this structure, some aspects of the program's features are not open to reconstruction. For example, the work must open and close with the heartbeat hello and goodbye so that the opening and closure of the sessions are explicit.

Structure

Structure provides the boundaries within which it becomes safe for participants to explore. Providing a clear structure or parameters within which creation is possible is a common pedagogical principle for most techniques serving the performing arts. Graham and Hoggett (2014) emphasize the importance of structure when creating new works, asserting, "We are firm believers that limitations create freedoms and breed creativity. Asking performers to improvise in a void can be really counterproductive" (p. 16). Structure brings order to social engagement and is a staple of programs designed to support the development of autism-spectrum children (Howlin 2000). In the HHM the structure of the setting provides safety, reliability, and a protective environment that frees the participants to explore play. Without structure or order, chaos can result, and although this principle applies to anyone engaged in play, it may be of heightened sensitivity for many children on the spectrum who are often more comfortable and feel safer if they know the specific rules of the environment in which they are to function.

For example, Clare Sainsbury[5] realized she was on the Asperger's spectrum when she was 20 years old while studying at Oxford. She (2004) emphasizes her need for structure and the predictability of the day's events while in elementary school:

> [I]t is important to ensure that the day and the week have a predictable shape and order, and that any alteration or interruption of the schedule (for example, different events to mark the last day of term) are talked about and explained well in advance. If promises of any sort are made, then they must be honored and when statements which cannot be guaranteed in this way, then this should be made clear by adding "probably" or "maybe." Not knowing what's happening or not being able to predict what's going to happen next, even when it comes to apparently "trivial" details, can generate anxiety. (p. 57)

Another example of this need for structure occurred during our pilot project. The start of every session began, like clockwork (an appropriate phrase for those aware of the significance of time for many on the spectrum), with the "heartbeat hello." Field notes report the following:

> A 10-year old boy named Nicholas had taken to sitting next to me during the sessions and could be counted on to remind me when the hour was almost up by showing me the minutes left on his watch. While waiting for children to arrive on one particular day, I decided to try something new. Typically, the guides and I had short conversations with the children next to us about anything and everything while waiting for the work to begin. However, after one of the children mentioned the previous week's work and meeting Titania, the queen of the fairies [in Shakespeare's *A Midsummer*

Night's Dream], I tried to have a conversation with everyone about who she was and what she was doing. This was met with a stern "no" from Nicholas accompanied by a firm gesture with his arm as if to say "this is out of bounds." It was clear to me that he was not at all comfortable changing the structure of things. I quickly moved directly into the heartbeats and he calmly settled in and gained the reassurance that the structure he had come to rely upon would be maintained.

Nicholas was, however, able to demonstrate variations when portraying characters in the games. His ability to be pliable and flexible within the structured framework supports the concept that the freedom to explore new expression is much more likely when the frame that holds that structure is solid and steadfast.

HHM Workshop Space

The ideal space for a HHM workshop is one with limited sensory input or distraction from lights, sound, and extraneous objects. This type of space—whether it's a theater stage, a classroom cleared of its contents, or an empty studio space—reduces distractions and brings everyone together in a "neutral" and equalizing space where neither the guide nor the child has more ownership or belonging in the space than does the other. Guides and children alike come to know and take ownership of the new space that they will share and create for the duration of the workshop(s). Providing familiarity limits transition distress. A foreign space is just that, and this factor must be acknowledged and taken into consideration when negotiating its impact on the children and the work being done.

The Circle as Activity Boundary

A circle demarcated on the floor with masking tape delineates the space where the HHM activities occur (see Fig. 5.1). This circle circumscribes a literal boundary outside of which the participants sit, within which the participants perform, and on the edge of which the participants place the tips of their toes when standing and playing full-group circle games. This taped circle on the floor alleviates any confusion about where the play space exists and where the observation takes place. Some activities require each participant to take his or her turn around the circle.

This simple yet essential boundary provides clarity to the children, enabling them to understand whose turn it is. It further provides a literal line for the facilitator or guide to refer to as needed. Children will occasionally drift into or away from the circle taped on the floor; the tape clearly defines parameters for playing space, whereas a circle without this explicitly designated border is much harder to maintain. An unmarked circle, where many theater artists practice their art, results in fuzziness or formlessness and is more likely to cause an ambiguous experience that can then lead to anxiety and discomfort for all involved. Adaptations to the circle can be made for specific populations; for example, a teacher in the UK who works with children who are blind has modified the arrangement by replacing the tape with a rope to outline the circle.

Roles and Processes

An optimal HHM workshop includes a facilitator who offers *brief* and succinct plot points from the play and then introduces and facilitates each game. Additional members of the workshop may include a group of guides who may be actors, teachers, aides, parents, or those involved in other roles, all of whom help to illustrate the story and engage in play with the children. Hunter (2015) says, "Ideally the children play one to one or two to one with actors, whilst a leader facilitates the workshop—but it is also possible to lead and play with the children alone" (p. 9).

Although Nicholas—the boy on the spectrum who insisted that a game's structure not be violated—needed for the configuration of the activity to remain predictable, he observed actors and children perform the Shadow Game with a large disparity and range of expression, which enabled him to do the same. In this game the invisible Ariel follows Caliban around the island and shadows his every move. Some performers may enact pushing through a bramble of trees or jumping over an imaginary river, while others eat an imagined fish from the river or scratch an itch on the backside (a favorite for many children). The range of expression modeled by the guides allows children like Nicholas to play with a variety of materials and ideas and explore the imagined journey without strict adherence to the "right" way to act out their journey. Barring any harm or disruption to self or others, performance allows for and encourages any and all expression. As such, the anxiety about acting correctly is significantly diminished, whereas the opportunities to celebrate success are abundant. Similarly, "errorless learning" is a recent neuroscience and educational practice based on the principle that eliminating the possibility for error among those on the autism spectrum will increase their success (Fillingham et al. 2003).

The order in which the activities occur must be equally dependable. In each workshop, the children watch pairs or groups of three guides play/model a new activity inside the circle (see Fig. 5.4); afterward the children work one-on-one with the guide, outside the circle, in order to learn and practice the game. Each pairing of child and guide returns to the circle and has a turn to show the whole group what they've been working on. This process repeats itself with each new game until the close of the workshop. Additionally, games are revisited and repeated if and when workshops take place over a period of weeks, months, or years. The level of skill involved in the games increases over time and acts as a series of building blocks wherein the original games are continually reviewed. Although only a few of the HHM games are described in this chapter, Hunter (2015) provides the "how to" for upward of 50 games in *Shakespeare's Heartbeat*.

Just as each workshop session begins with the "heartbeat hello," where the participants place their hands on their hearts and literally tap out the rhythm of their heartbeat, each session ends with the "heartbeat goodbye." There is a comfort created by the dependability, familiarity, and repetition of a workshop that opens and closes with an almost identical activity. As simple as it may seem, the children know that they can and do depend (as evidenced by Nicholas) on this consistency for every session.

There is also one facilitator who leads the games while the guides partner with the children. Again, this arrangement lets the children know that they can rely on the leadership of the facilitator to adhere to the structure of the games and to hold and direct the shape of their journey each time they engage in the activity. They also know that they can depend on the guides to join them in a role that fluidly moves to and from mentorship to partnership.

Empowerment

Many games involve a trade-off in who "holds" the power, meaning that when the children pair up with their guides, the games create an opportunity for the children to both lead their guides and to follow them. The children always have a guide as a partner as they explore the opportunity to "control" an adult within the boundaries of the game. This reversal in roles not only strengthens the dynamic of teacher as learner and learner as teacher, but empowers the children by giving them responsibility for guiding

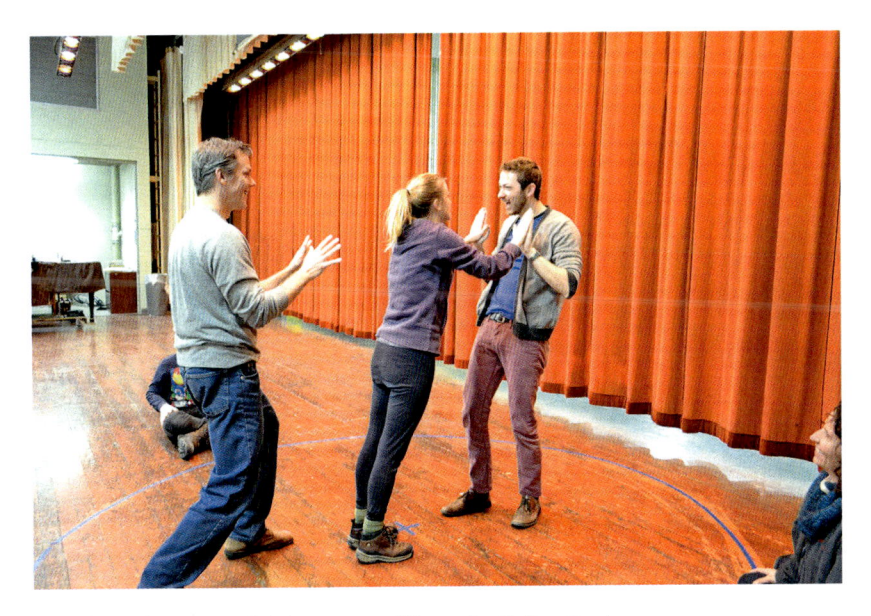

Fig. 5.4 Actors model the games. (Photo by Ji Rye Lee)

their adult partners and reinforces a mutual relationship built on trust and a negotiation of leadership (see also LaCerva and Feinstein, this volume).

For example, during one of the games from *The Tempest*, Ariel leads Ferdinand around the island in a musically induced trance. The person playing Ariel holds the power in this game, leading Ferdinand around the island with the palm of his/her hand while making musical sounds. Ferdinand must follow Ariel's hand with his eyes and body. Each person has a turn in the role of the leader for this game, a feature that empowers and builds the children's confidence in their leadership. As children grow and develop in their lives, they often struggle for a sense of control. Children on the autism spectrum, in particular, may have a difficult time with what they experience as a lack of control or power. In particular, says Sainsbury (2004), for children whose behavior can be challenging for others,

> It is important to differentiate between "structured" and "directive" environments, as the two are often confused. … [R]eferences to "structured" environment often indicate one which is tightly controlled, with strictly enforced rules. The "structure" needed by children with Asperger's syndrome, in contrast refers to order, not control; in fact, it is important to share control and involve children in planning. (p. 57)

The flexibility of a guiding structure, as opposed to a structure that limits the possibilities for the child on the spectrum, leads to empowerment within social boundaries. The following narrative depicts a scenario from our middle-school intervention where the control during the games was negotiated between the guide and the child:

> Bradley was a 12-year-old boy who consistently tried to assert his control and change the way a game was played by inserting new and different pieces of text or by pushing his face aggressively against his partners. His guide and partner, Assistant Professor Kevin McClatchy, recognized that Bradley's provoking behavior seemed to emerge from the need to be heard, understood, and given a chance to control some part of his day. McClatchy's insight and empathy allowed him to work patiently with Bradley and to effectively negotiate with him for control. Specifically, he allowed Bradley to change slight details or to put his "trademark" on a game as long as the game's targets remained intact. Bradley and McClatchy's give-and-take developed into a friendly, strong relationship between the two that made it possible for Bradley to trust and take more risks in the work. Furthermore, the willingness of McClatchy to adapt Bradley's additions into the games highlighted the flexibility within the games and demonstrated the concept of partnership to other children.
>
> Bradley was accompanied by teaching assistants who had the primary responsibility of "watching" him during our sessions. Bradley initially found entering the circle for the "hellos" particularly challenging and typically opted out of this part of the session. On several occasions his assistants would convey a look of disapproval for his behavior or perceived opposition and demand that he comply. Although participation is encouraged in the games, no child is ever required to participate, and the stern reactions from Bradley's assistants heightened his discomfort and stress. Alternatively, when McClatchy offered to join Bradley in the circle, he was able to participate in this game, albeit with some initial reluctance to do so. Bradley consistently requested McClatchy's presence in the circle for this game, which demonstrated his need for physical and emotional support as well as McClatchy's ability to provide this support simply sitting by his side while simultaneously encouraging his participation. This small adjustment gave Bradley some personal control over the experience while accomplishing the targets of the games, not the least of which included engagement in the activity.

Each game is flexible enough to allow small changes to be made to accommodate these unique individualized differences in readiness without sacrificing the overall foundation and intentions of the games or methodology.

The Heartbeat Hello

There is a sort of magic in the practice of the "heartbeat hellos" as they open each session and serve to empower the collective. The rhythm of iambic pentameter, the metrical line Shakespeare used to write his plays, is very similar to modern-day speech patterns. Master of Voice and Shakespeare scholar, Patsy Rodenburg (2002), discusses the relationship between the emotional life of Shakespeare's characters and the rhythm of their speech: "[The iambic] releases the physical pace and momentum of the verse, and illuminates the meaning through the stress. It also charts the heartbeat—including the stoppages or skips—of the character" (p. 84). In other words, variations of the iamb coincide with changes to the emotional quality of what is being expressed. Similarly, the heartbeat, which marks the rhythm of life, ebbs and flows according to one's emotions and in turn affects the rhythm of language. This initial heartbeat game, rooted in in the use of the iamb, introduces the connection among heartbeat, emotion, and language (see Chap. 10). As the group taps out their heartbeats, they simultaneously say hello with the accompaniment of a suggested emotion such as happy, sad, angry, surprised, fearful, or other feeling. Depending on the emotion, the rhythm of the heartbeat will be either the regular da-DUM emphasis of the iamb or it will change, which often happens with anger or surprise where the heartbeat may skip a bit, speed up, or be irregular.

All participants engage in tapping out their heartbeats, an action that sends the message, "We are all beginning together, we are beginning our day by acknowledging our own internal rhythms and then attempting to sync up our internal rhythms. Therefore, we are joining our life forces together and tuning into our internal rhythms, which change and grow in response to our emotional states."

It is worth mentioning that actors spend long hours working to make the connections between the shifts in Shakespeare's meter and the corresponding emotional life of the character. The technique and practice of the "Heartbeat Hellos" introduces the universality of experience for all involved in making the connection between shifts in rhythm of speech and the corresponding emotional life. *All* participants share in an awakening of the internal, emotional, physical, and vocal life and what may appear as a seemingly simple activity can actually be quite profound, equalizing, and empowering for all involved.

The Introduction

Another deceptively simple activity is the introduction. Establishing a foundation of trust at the very outset is critical to the success of the HHM. In every culture there is a custom for greeting or meeting a new person that is inherently vulnerable and significant for both parties. Although it may seem to be an obvious or simple piece of advice, making an effort to learn and remember an individual's name must be emphasized. One should always strive to learn the names of the children upon meeting them and then remember them or have some readily available system for name recognition and recall of the children. As discussed before, the parallel roles of teacher as learner and learner as teacher are present throughout the entire process. Not only does learning and remembering the names of the students support all subsequent work, it also immediately introduces the children to the significance of names.

This initial conversation can provide helpful information about the children such as whether or not they want to talk and engage; whether they appear shy, quiet, or introverted; whether they require some physical and emotional space; whether they seem frightened or anxious or apprehensive; and in general, how they are experiencing the moment emotionally. Gathering whatever pertinent information might be available will facilitate a better connection with the children, but the primary objective of the initial meeting is learning the names of the children and then using them when communicating with each other. The tending to names and rhythms of their lives in the "Heartbeat Hellos" sets the foundation for inclusion and empowerment and helps them enter the "updraft" of the activities.

Praise

Praise is embedded in and repeated throughout the process. Guides are encouraged to praise their child partners consistently throughout their work together and very specifically when a child masters a specific task. Praise and reinforcement may be provided with physical signs. For instance, a simple "thumbs up" indicates success when a child has completed a task such as making brief eye contact or reciting a sequence of text. Additionally, verbal praise, such as "You've done a wonderful job of waiting your turn before speaking" or "You are doing a great job of sitting and staying behind the line," is helpful clarification if either has been difficult for a particular child to master. After each pair shares their work in the circle, everyone sitting in the circle applauds and the facilitator often prompts, "Let's give ourselves a round of applause" following a group activity.

There is a general feeling of having done good work together in the space. There should never be any sense that someone has not done well even if he or she wasn't ready to participate; the emphasis is always on the positive and on the feeling of achievement. The HHM provides the sort of meta-experience that enables social comfort and confident performance in the future. Meta-experience is not to be confused with meta-theater, which refers to occasions when a theatrical play comments on itself. Rather, it refers to how an experience is experienced such that it frames new experiences (Smagorinsky & Daigle 2012). Success, in this conception, produces confidence that provides a frame of mind in which new successes seem possible.

Placement in the space, even if only to watch, equates with participation. Watching may be all a child is ready for, and even that level of participation deserves applause and appreciation. Individual readiness is recognized, and all participation regardless of degree and scope of activity is praised.

A sensitive and skilled guide will include children's contributions without enabling them to dominate or change the entire experience. A guide should provide the structure and the goals for each game and work flexibly within them, and thus be able to determine how and when to break or modify a rule in response to a child's suggestions. For those who appear to be exhibiting challenging or destructive behaviors, the guide can try a new and different approach. Searching for the appropriate communicative fit for any particular child is inherent in the process. Guides must listen to what their child partners seem to need and to what they may be struggling with, and then trust the method's processes to explore the approach that seems to address these needs and challenge their growth. Again, learning from the children provides insights about how to reenvision communication and build inclusive communities.

The pedagogy of this work requires the power to listen patiently and meet the children where they are without the guide feeling rejected or taking things too personally when things get challenging. A child's challenges rarely equate to something being "wrong" but instead invite an opportunity to gain more information and try something new. Heathcote (1984) asserts that in her approach to drama,

> I must not be afraid to move out of my centre, and meet the children where *they* are. The ability to go forward to meet people gives me the opportunity

to vary my approach and my responses. If I do this, I shall not be afraid to try unfamiliar things, because I'm not afraid of being rejected. Rejection is not a part of trying to meet someone. Even if some rejection must take place, let that be of the idea and not of the person. I think we—the teachers and the pupils—often feel rejected in the school when it's really our ideas that are being rejected.

I must also have the ability to see the world through my students, and not my students through it. (p. 18; emphasis in original)

A child may resist or reject an activity due to anxiety, vulnerability, or confusion about what is asked of them. The guide may need to adjust the activity or the delivery of the activity. The guide is thus always a learner, exploring and trying something new with the children, and adapting to the unfolding events. This stance requires deep and intentional listening. This level of listening and being present conveys a message to the children that they are valued and deserve the time it takes to find a fit that works for them. It further encourages that fit through adaptations to the games, while staying within certain parameters (e.g., the circle, the hello, and the goodbye) of the method.

Play

Additionally, when guiding a child in a game, deep listening must be coupled with deep character immersion. Immersing oneself into a character is about play, a dimension that is at the core of the pedagogy. A guide must truly partake in the joy of the games as much for themselves as for the children. Merely "demonstrating" playfulness, without the congruence of experiencing the giddiness and excitement of portraying Shakespeare's characters, will likely result in uninventive, flat expression and will diminish the "coming to life" that attentive, engaged, and riveting play can birth Hunter has referred to the work as a medium by which the children "wake themselves up to themselves." Guides will also wake up parts of themselves that may have been dormant for some time if they commit to play.

This sort of play requires adults to abandon their inhibitions. The practice of releasing inhibitions and taking playful risks is at the core of actor training where significant time is spent undoing behavior that is the direct result of socialization. Specialized voice and movement pedagogies such as those of Arthur Lessac or those explored in Movement techniques such as Laban, Feldenkrais or Viewpoints, are similar in that their guiding principles are connected to a search for those instinctive inclinations, intuitions and rhythms that are much more likely to occur in the toddler of youthful behavior of the young child. The idea is that we are socialized in such a way that our bodies, voices and emotions operate under duress and adapt in ways that deter optimal health and operation and that we must reclaim the instincts, impulses and abilities that were accessible prior to these aspects of socialization. Arthur Lessac's (1990) Body Wisdom, describes the physical, emotional and vocal disconnect at great length and the following passage begins to introduce the cause and effect of socialization:

> We are so conditioned by the outside environment that our very bodily processes have been taught to keep pace with chaos. While keeping pace with chaos might seem to be an achievement, it is in fact a programmed escape – from both environments. Even our intellect has become part of the outer environment, divorced from its birthright in Body Wisdom. Unconsciously caught and unaware of a conflict between the body's native, instinctive response mechanism and the environment's chaotic stimuli from the outside, the problem-solving choices at our disposal only contribute to producing fear, anxiety, conflict, and tension, further advancing the deterioration of the body, its balance and its relationship to feelings and thought.
>
> The outer environment's influences and controls, shaped and shaded as they are by ritual, by convention, by economic considerations, by physical standards, and by imitative self-images, are all too casually tolerated as understandable, and therefore, acceptable, in the adult world. (p. 14)

Actors practice techniques that are meant to bring them back to their natural state prior to socialization, allowing them to access their innate abilities to move, vocalize, and emote. Similarly, the HHM requires that guides engage in the kind of serious play that young children unconsciously engage in with regularity.

The children on the spectrum are not told that they will be working on making eye contact, practicing emotional facial recognition, learning turn-taking, and learning other social conventions, but rather they are told that they will be playing games. Just as the children focus on play and storytelling, the guides concentrate on the children, a focus that frees them up to drop their heightened attention to their own risk-taking and character exploration. This stance results in deeper listening; greater moment-to-moment awareness; and authentic, open, and playful engagement.

Many acting techniques attempt to remove actors' focus from themselves to perpetuate a release into "the moment." This phrase was made famous by acting teacher Sanford Meisner, architect of the *Meisner technique*—wherein the attention of the actor is on the other rather than the self and intended to lead to authentic instinctive responses. Several actors guiding this work have found that they are able to explore playfully and achieve "living in the moment" with the HHM because they are so intensely focused on the experience of their child partners. The result is a freedom to play joyfully, an experience often missing in traditional actor training methodologies. The release from the rigors of traditional training allows actors to relax into the work and enjoy the process, which in turn paves the way for new discoveries and strong emotional connections among participants. When children observe teaching artists enjoying their own creative choices (see Fig. 5.5), they witness the range of possibilities open to them, and the joy of discovery becomes contagious. The children begin by imitating what they see until they feel comfortable expanding options on their own, enjoying the freedom to explore their imaginations.

The HHM creates a social space where children on the spectrum can experience a sense of belonging and shared ownership of the space and all that occurs there. Empowerment emerges through a freedom to exist and unabashedly share exploration of vocal, physical, and emotional expression. The HHM games create an environment where the children, facilitators, and guides come together and receive the same set of criteria to practice play and connect with a shared sense of meeting in the middle. The games that comprise the HHM diminish the internalized sense for someone on the spectrum that he or she is "deficient." Concurrently, the work encourages those in positions of leadership to expand out and rethink how to reenvision the community of people in which they live and begin to adjust their communication and interactions accordingly.

The concepts of structure, empowerment, praise, and play provide the foundation and design of the HHM. Although these concepts and principles are integrated into the process and delivery of the HHM, reinforcement and consistent reminders of their significance provide the guides more fluency when bringing them to bear. Investing in these principles makes it possible to communicate with fresh and new perspectives and makes it possible for all to wake themselves up to themselves and to each other.

Immersion into the HHM challenges the notions of what the broad society has defined as "normalcy" and "deficiency." Those who have spent some time in this work will find themselves questioning the presumed need and validity for such labels. As Heathcote (1984) says, "When children come to us with labels—this is a slow learner, this is a non-reader, [this is a child with autism]—we tend to shut our minds to change: but the ability to preserve an interest in children prevents teachers from stereotyping them in all sorts of ways" (p. 18). The transformative work challenges and questions what we have come to accept or been expected to comply with as societal labels for "normalcy." My own learning through this work has changed the way in which I perceive every individual I meet. I no longer make quick assumptions about how anyone will interact with me or what their level or style of engagement means. The HHM has encouraged me to expand my awareness and has provided me with knowledge about the wide spectrum of difference among all of us.

Reenvisioning the Professional Theater Experience: In Here Out There and The Tempest

The HHM led to two innovative, original theater productions that contributed to reshaping the identity of theater nationwide and internationally as well as providing local communities with education about autism and the need for more inclusive thinking. *The Tempest*[6] was the first of its kind production, bringing professional actors from the world-renowned Royal

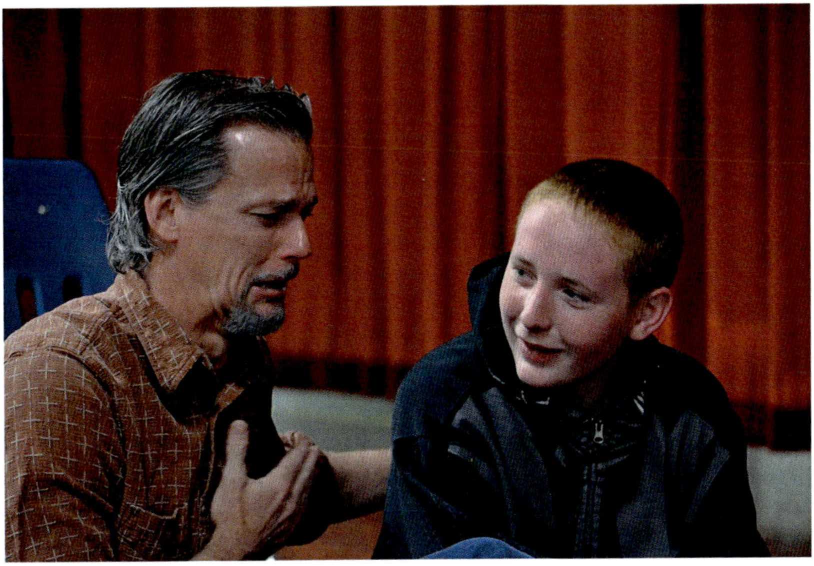

Fig. 5.5 Actor modeling emotional expression. (Photo by Ji Rye Lee)

Shakespeare Company together with professional actors from The Ohio State University. The play was adapted and directed by Kelly Hunter, who incorporated the games into a live professional theatre experience whereby children on the spectrum joined the actors on the edge of a ground cloth, painted in a spectacular montage of color, which represented Caliban's island.

The story of *The Tempest* was told by the actors and the children who attended each performance. This show was not a typical audience participation performance but a true melding of children who were immersed into the magical world with the actors while their caregivers and others observed in a circle of seats outside the world of the play. This groundbreaking performance opened in Stratford Upon-Avon at the Royal Shakespeare Company's and The Other Place Theatre in June 2014, and it had its North American Premiere at The Ohio State University's Wexner Center for the Arts in July 2014. This type of production advances the potential for new and innovative professional theatre traditions and expands social and community opportunities for those on the spectrum.

The second performance, *In Here Out There*[7], was a new work, and the main stage production was created by The Ohio State Theatre's Master of Fine Arts (MFA) class of 2014. The performance was a theatrical response to the MFA's work with the Shakespeare and Autism research project. Their focus, when devising the piece, and the overarching theme of the production revolved around the question, "What is normal?"

The nine MFA actors, and the number of students who have had the opportunity to implement the HHM with children on the spectrum, have a new perspective about "normalcy," community, inclusion, and difference. The HHM has led to this type of creative scholarship, which is changing the way this ever-growing segment of our population is viewed and making it possible to express and connect in new places and in new ways.

The HHM makes vocal, physical, and emotional expression familiar and comfortable; it creates the possibility of ownership and provides the safety to explore and play with new ways of being in the world. The work fosters a more inclusive and diverse understanding of the world where labels that tend to divide us become blurred in our appreciation for the importance of coming to understand each individual. The HHM and the supporting national and international research is far-reaching in its influence on inclusive thinking when engaging those on the spectrum and in making social and creative space for more pliable and interactive strategies for instruction.

Notes

1. The empirical research study began in 2012 at The Ohio State University (OSU) and was supported by a collaborative partnership between Kelly Hunter (creator of the HHM and an actress with the Royal Shakespeare Company), the Department of Theatre at the Ohio State University, the Nisonger Center (Center for Excellence in Developmental Disabilities at Ohio State) and several schools (names withheld to protect anonymity) within the Central Ohio area.
2. *Neurotypical* refers to those whose neurology follows the evolutionary norm; *neuro-atypical* refers to those whose neurology is different from this norm, often as part of the autism spectrum (see Chap. 1).
3. Genevieve Simon, an undergraduate theatre major at OSU, was one of the five core teaching artists who led the work for the research project.
4. All children's names in this chapter are pseudonyms.
5. Clare Sainsbury is the daughter of Lord Sainsbury, science minister and founder of Sainsbury's markets in the UK.
6. The Department of Theatre at The Ohio State University and the Royal Shakespeare Company co-produced *The Tempest*, adapted and directed by Kelly Hunter, at The Other Place in Stratford-upon-Avon from June 24 to July 4 and in Columbus, Ohio, at the Wexner Center for the Arts on July 16 and 17 and WOSU@COSI on July 19 and 20, 2014. The acting ensemble was Greg Hicks (RSC), Chris MacDonald (RSC), Kevin McClatchy (OSU), Mahmoud Osman (OSU), Robin Post (OSU), and Eva Tausig (RSC). Production personnel included Anthony Lamble (designer), Vince Herbert (lighting designer), Paula Salmon (company stage manager), Claire Birch (RSC producer), Lesley Ferris (OSU producer), David Tanqueray (RSC production manager), Eric H. Mayer (OSU production manager), Matt Hazard (OSU technical director), and Ji Rye Lee (creative ensemble/photographer).
7. The Department of Theatre at The Ohio State University produced *In Here Out There*, the MFA Outreach and Engagement Project, in the Roy Bowen Theatre, November 13–23, 2014. The actors were Sarah Ware (Callie), Camille Bullock (Celia/Mac), Jane Elliott (Katherine/Ben), Brent Ries (Edward/Toby), Sifiso Mazibuko

(Anthony), Melonie Mazibuko (Olivia), Meg Chamberlain (Bea), Aaron Lopez (Captain H), and Patrick Wiabel (Red). Production personnel included Maureen Ryan (project director), Robin Post (director of outreach), Sheree Greco (production manager), Zachary Bailey (stage manager), Joshua M. Quinlan (scenic designer), Sarah Fickling (costume designer), Matt Hazard (lighting designer), Eve Nordyke (sound designer), Elizabeth Harelik (dramaturg), Chris Zinkon (technical director), Jim Knapp (technology manager), Ji Rye Lee, and Artem Vorobiev (poster design).

REFERENCES

Fillingham, J. K., Hodgson, C., Sage, K., & Lambdon Ralph, M. A. (2003). The application of errorless learning to aphasic disorders: A review of theory and practice. *Neuropsychological Rehabilitation: An International Journal, 13*(3), 337–363.

Graham, S., & Hoggett, S. (2014). *The frantic assembly: Book of devising theatre* (2nd ed.). New York: Routledge.

Heathcote, D. (1984). *Collected writings on education and drama*. Evanston: Northwestern University Press.

Howlin, P. (2000). Autism and intellectual disability: Diagnostic and treatment issues. *Journal of the Royal Society of Medicine,93*, 351–355. Retrieved July 27, 2015, from http://www.ncbi.nlm.nih.gov/pmc/articles/PMC1298058/pdf/10928021.pdf

Hunter, K. (2015). *Shakespeare's heartbeat: Drama games for children with autism*. New York: Routledge.

Lessac, A. (1990). *Body wisdom: The use of and training of the human body*, 2nd ed. San Bernadino: Lessac Institute Publishing Company.

Rodenburg, P. (2002). *Speaking Shakespeare*. New York: Palgrave Macmillan.

Sainsbury, C. (2004). *Martian in the playground: Understanding the schoolchild with Asperger's syndrome* (10th ed.). Chicago: Lucky Duck Publishing.

Smagorinsky, P., & Daigle, E. A. (2012). The role of affect in students' writing for school. In E. L. Grigorenko, E. Mambrino, & D. Preiss (Eds.), *Writing: A mosaic of new perspectives* (pp. 293–307). New York: Psychology Press. Retrieved September 1, 2016 from http://www.petersmagorinsky.net/About/PDF/BookChapters/AffectInWriting_Grigorenko_Mambrino_Preiss_Writing.pdf

CHAPTER 6

We Don't Want to Fit in: A Reflection on the Revolutionary Inclusive Theater Practices of The Miracle Project and Actionplay for Adolescents on the Autism Spectrum

Aaron Feinstein

The teenage years are miserable. The classic presentation: weird pus-filled bulges announcing themselves from the skin, sexual confusion and desire, and the general awkwardness of learning to fit into an adult body, and adult responsibility. This ungainly confluence is only the beginning for those of us who were outcast, ridiculed, or bullied by our peers because of a physical or developmental difference. A vast majority of the work that I have been involved with in my adult life has involved serving people with a range of psychological and developmental diagnoses, most notably teens on the autism spectrum. My theater work with teens on the autism spectrum has been rooted in the fact that I got through the loneliness of my own teenage years because I made my way to one of the safe places for those who don't fit in within most schools: the Drama Club.

I was a teenager in the mid-90s, the attention deficit hyperactivity disorder (ADHD) era, when the common diagnosis doled out by the psychological

A. Feinstein (✉)
Actionplay, Brooklyn, NY, USA

© The Author(s) 2016
P. Smagorinsky (ed.), *Creativity and Community among Autism-Spectrum Youth*, DOI 10.1057/978-1-137-54797-2_6

establishment for teenagers who did not fit the norm was ADHD. I certainly fit into this category from the psychological diagnostic criteria as presented by the *Diagnostic and Statistical Manual of Mental Disorders IV* (American Psychological Association 1994). I was fidgety and forgetful; I had a difficult time following verbal directions; and in noisy or overwhelming classes that were packed with students, I typically fell apart. Through the years, I have gone back and forth on the necessity of the diagnosis. The diagnosis gave me a feeling of a recognized modality of difference, but as I finished school and learned my own ways of dealing with some of these issues, the importance of this label seemed to slip away. I realized that many of my differences, conceived by others as "disorders," were also my strengths. In my adult life, I was able to acknowledge these differences as strengths. The diagnosis seemed to only pathologize the differences.

The diagnosis was the thing my parents were looking for, and it certainly made my life a bit easier. It was a seal of approval from the psychological establishment that I was different. I was not just "lazy, hyperactive, stupid," or whatever other terms could have been projected onto me. No, I was ADHD, which meant that I was tested, and officially different. Through the diagnosis, I was able to advocate for some of the things I needed to help me in a rigorous academic environment. I was able to sit in a quiet space for testing, and was given first priority for smaller class sizes.

At this point in my life, I feel incredibly privileged that my mother was an educator and that I received some basic accommodations that so many more children with the same diagnosis need. It is deeply disappointing that in the 20-plus years that have passed since I was a teenager, little has changed in the education establishment. Large class sizes and lack of individualized education continue to be the norm in most school districts, and studies show that the growth of class sizes has had a harmful effect on children's learning (Schanzenbach 2014). If kids fall outside the dominant school culture, there is a great possibility that they will slip away into further isolation, and the damaging effects of this isolation are well documented in the increasing teen suicide rate (Cutler et al. 2001), projected feelings of isolation among teenagers, and rising truancy rates in many school districts.

In terms of the bigger issues that I was dealing with on a social and emotional level, the ADHD diagnosis was of little help. I was lonely and bullied, I rarely felt as though I had a person to talk to, and I had a difficult time making friends. I wanted deeply to be accepted, and to find a place in which I could transcend the mundane and cruel horrors of adolescence.

I remember making my way to the Drama Club, which met on Thursdays at my middle school in Los Angeles. I had an interest in acting, but I remember walking in the first day and thinking that this was not where I wanted to be. The kids in the club were the biggest outcasts of the entire school. There was nothing remotely "cool" about this group, and the last thing I needed for my fledgling social life was to hang around with a group of kids who were sometimes even bigger outcasts than I was. I was more concerned with the idea of acting and theater as a platform to stardom, not a place where I was going to be moving myself down the rungs of the "caste system of American adolescence" (Milner 2006).

Our Drama Club attracted a gender-diverse, racially diverse, sexually diverse, physically diverse, and neurodiverse body of students that came together for a variety of reasons. The Drama Club provided a space where, as Vygotsky (1978) characterized the process, "Play creates a zone of proximal development for the child. In play a child always behaves beyond his average age, above his daily behavior; in play it as though he were a head taller than himself" (p. 102). The Drama Club was a playful zone of proximal development. It was an environment in which my identification with the diagnosis of ADHD and my poor academics did not have to define me, because I could perform as someone who was other than myself, or beyond my conception of self through the group-based collaborative process of playful dramatic reinvention.

The playful process of reinvention was encouraged through the rehearsal process, and the Drama Club developed its own unique identity outside the school's mainstream. We didn't need to fit in to the dominant school culture, because we were part of a community that acknowledged the idea that we did not fit in. Even if being a "thespian" wasn't always a primary form of identity that was communicated to the masses, we still shared the unique intimacy of being part of a separatist culture of our school. We fully embraced our own theatrical, silly, and exaggerated way of interacting with one another. We became friends through separating from the normative elements of school culture, and we relished our weirdness.

Performance was incredibly liberating through my teenage years, during which my notion of self seemed to be all-important. The Drama Club gave me the experience of being part of a community in which diversity could thrive. It was a powerful enough experience to keep me going back to the rehearsal room for the rest of my life. I was challenged by the rigor and playfulness of rehearsal. I shared intimate conversations with my peers in the darkness of backstage. I learned the discipline of ensemble performance, where I had to rise above my own individuality and become part of the group. The applause from the audience was confidence building. For me, and for those of us deemed "the other" by the dominant culture, the ability to find a community built on acceptance and diversity was essential to our development and survival.

The Miracle Project

The Miracle Project was an experiment started by my colleague Elaine Hall, an energetic, intensely positive, and respected acting coach for kids, known by her students as Coach E. It started as an inclusion group of 12 autistic teens ages 4–18 who often had additional diagnoses, five of their neurotypical peers and siblings, five adult volunteers, and four adult staff members including me. We were tasked to create an original piece of musical theater based on Jewish culture. I was one of the directors of the program, but I had little experience with the autism spectrum. The class had many features of an elective Drama Club. It was a place where children and adults who were considered by the dominant culture as different could come together with the goal of creating something as a community. It seemed to be an impossible task as well. The idea of creating an original musical from scratch with a group of autism-spectrum children over 22 consecutive Monday evenings seemed to be a daunting challenge.

I was a young theater director, freshly graduated from UCLA's MFA Theater Directing program. I came to this space because I disliked how conventional the professional theater world was. I always regarded the theater, and theater people, as unconventional, and when I entered into my early professional theater experience, much of that unconventionality was missing, replaced with an emphasis on the storytelling aspects of theater for an educated upper-middle-class audience. I was still searching for the revolutionary, unconventional, and community-building aspects of theater, and I was (and still am) up for a challenge. Coach E's idea sparked my love of the possibilities of theater in its assembly of people who were definitely from outside the norm.

Coach E created The Miracle Project out of her experience of parenting her non-verbal autistic son Neal. She was an actress and found that other creative types (musicians, actors, dancers, painters, etc.) had a better ability to reach and connect with Neal than the more traditional approaches of occupational, speech, psychological, and behavioral therapies (Hall 2010). Coach E believed that creative types could connect with autistic-spectrum kids because of their natural flexibility, their acceptance of difference, and their resonance with feeling outside the normative culture in the same ways that many on the autism spectrum do. She also had a belief in the theater as a place where differences could be appreciated, and viewed The Miracle Project stage as a celebration of the unique individuals on the autism spectrum.

The parents who showed up the first day of class with children on the spectrum were incredibly grateful for the opportunity to participate in an activity outside the realm of therapy. The stress of constantly trying "to fix" their "disordered" child overwhelmed and isolated many of the parents. These parents wanted an opportunity for their kids to do something outside the various office visits and doctor's appointments, where they could meet other Jewish families and kids who had the shared experience of autism. At The Miracle Project, we were not attempting to fix anyone. We were there to create a musical.

Working with Sensory Experience

This group's uniqueness can be illustrated through a snapshot of the first day of class. I witnessed a diverse range of children on the autism spectrum. There were kids crawling under the desks, spinning in circles across the floors, and waving their fingers in front of their face as kids on the spectrum sometimes do. I learned that many of these behaviors were rooted in an individual autistic's sensory processing differences, which make the barrage of sensory information available at every moment difficult to process.

Children on the autism spectrum present the same features as do neurotypical children in terms of the functionality of their sensory organs (eyes, ears, nose, tongue, etc.), but in their sensory neuroprocessing there can be more extreme differences in reactivity (Cerliani et al. 2015). People have seven senses (not 5): sight, smell, taste, hearing, and touch; and then the two that are typically left behind but are incredibly important in understanding the autism spectrum: the proprioceptive and vestibular senses.

The proprioceptive sense is a discriminative sense (Ayres 1973). Proprioception is the sense of the relative position of parts of the body and their strength of effort being employed in movement. This sense is important as it lets people know exactly where their body parts are, and how they are positioned in space to plan and coordinate their movements.

The vestibular sense is a totally unconscious sense if it is functioning normally. It develops prenatally and provides information about changes in position and about movement. Receptors for this sense originate in the inner ear, which contains fluid and hair cells (Bear, Connors, & Paradiso, 2007). The vestibular system explains the perception of the body in relation to gravity, movement, and balance.

Many children on the autism spectrum present with differences in proprioception and vestibular sensory processing compared to the general population (Baranek et al. 2006). Studies haves shown that spinning, hand-flapping, rocking, and other autistic motor movements are an attempt to regulate proprioceptive and vestibular sensory systems, and they are part of the process of bringing the autistic person to a feeling of regulation or balance. Regulation techniques such as repetitive motor movements, aimless running, self-stimulatory behaviors, and self-injurious behaviors have also been strongly correlated to sensory processing abnormalities (Case-Smith and Bryan 1999; Watling and Dietz 2007).

Autistics (and neurotypicals) also may exhibit patterns of behavior that are over-reactive, under-reactive, or sensory-seeking to information received by the seven senses and processed by the brain (Liss et al. 2006). Autistics often describe themselves as being oversensitive to certain stimuli to the point of being impelled to withdraw from them (Grandin 1996). Many individuals on the autism spectrum also underreact to stimuli, for instance, ignoring painful bumps or bruises (Ornitz 1988). A typical example in the media of the extremity of autistic sensory processing concerns autistic children who cover their ears because of everyday sounds being too loud. These children may be over-reactive to sound, but the same children could be visually sensory-seeking and crave visual stimuli (bright colors, flashing lights, etc.). This example illustrates only one of the ranges of sensory profiles that exist on the autism spectrum.

Autistics use many techniques to compensate for their sensory processing differences. Many autistics rely on predictable routines, repetitive phrases, and singular interests that help them to create order and familiarity within a sensory overwhelming world (Dunn 2001). Coach E encouraged us to "follow the child's lead," the words of the late and prolific Dr. Stanley Greenspan, a developmental psychologist and the co-founder of the DIRFloortime® therapy model (DIR stands for Developmental, Individual-differences, and Relationship-based approach) for working with children on the autism spectrum and related conditions (Greenspan, Wieder, & Simons, 1998).

Greenspan defined autism as a neurodevelopmental difference of relating and communicating. The DIRFloortime® therapy model involved a relationship-based approach that encouraged parents, therapists, and educators to engage with their children's individual interests and sensory needs by "following the child's lead" or engaging the child's communication by tapping into their unique interests, and supporting each child's individual differences and sensory needs. Greenspan also encouraged parents, educators, and therapists to emphasize high affect (facial and body language expressiveness), creativity, and inventiveness (Greenspan and Wieder 2006). Greenspan encouraged Coach E to bring her passion for acting and the theater arts to the autism community because he thought that actors' natural expressiveness and ability to use high affect would be a tremendous benefit for engaging autistic children (Hall 2010).

A Relational Approach

Coach E encouraged The Miracle Project staff to engage the children, and not to judge the behaviors that we were observing as the children being avoidant of relationships. In Coach E's eyes, the spinning, flapping, and singular interests were opportunities to connect, deepen communication, and form relationships. On the first day of The Miracle Project, the staff and volunteers were joining the children during their spinning across the floor. We were spinning with them and creating dances. Our music therapist sat calmly under a table, and strummed her guitar with an overwhelmed child in an attempt to engage him. I was a bit hesitant at first, but I also was eager to connect and meet the individuals in the group.

There was a particular individual, Ari[1], who was drawn to me, or maybe it was the other way around. Ari was a lanky 13-year-old boy, with a burst of black hair that jetted out from his head in the style of a punk rocker. He kept approaching me to share his exhaustive knowledge of Pokémon (a popular anime show, toy, and brand in the early 2000s; see Cook & Smagorinsky, this volume), by announcing enthusiastically in alphabetical order every possible manifestation and name of the Pokémon characters in perfectly articulated Japanese. This outpouring was confusing to me, but Coach E encouraged me to "follow the child's lead." Rather than run away from the barrage of information being produced by Ari, I chose to engage him.

It was tough going at first. Ari would become frustrated, flap his arms, and start over every time I disrupted his flow of the Pokémon characters in an attempt to engage him in a conversation. I had to figure out another way to engage because I was not allowed to communicate verbally during his listing of the characters. At first, my desire to connect with Ari and my patience with him (a disposition that I quickly realized was quite useful), and his own patience with me, were the personal qualities that were essential for us to learn how to relate to one another. I could have viewed Ari as a human Pokémon Encyclopedia, delivering information only to entertain me and increase my knowledge and understanding of Pokémon. I knew that Ari was sharing his knowledge because he was attempting to connect with me in his own way.

The rules that Ari established were relatively simple. I was not allowed to interrupt the entire alphabetical flow of Pokémon characters to ask questions, or say anything. I did my best to respect this regimen. When I interrupted, Ari became visibly frustrated. He would become red in the face and would walk away flapping his arms and hands, and then he would start over at the first "A" named Pokémon, "Araragi-Hakase, Professor Oak." As an adult, I needed to adapt to his need for uninterrupted time to detail these characters. In the setting of The Miracle Project, adult rules were typically jettisoned so that kids' rules helped them to establish the norms for their conduct.

Opening Moves

We always started each Miracle Project session with an opening circle performed in the same way every week. There was a name-game activity and song, which created familiarity and routine for the group. The music of our song leader filtered into the class, indicating that it was time for class to begin. This explicit signal seemed to quell the anxiety of the group. When Ari heard the guitar, he would typically stop reciting the Pokémon characters, and would sit next to me for the opening activities.

Coach E would have us start the class with our staff and participants introducing themselves with their name and a movement of their choice corresponding to their name. The entire group would then repeat the name and movement of the person. It was a great opening activity because it created ensemble by giving all participants (staff, volunteers, and kids) the chance to perform their own unique name, and then have their name performed by the group. Some of the children would develop skits, routines, and monologues for their name introductions.

There were a couple of participants who had verbal communication challenges, two non-speaking participants who would introduce themselves only through movement, and one child who would use assistive communication technology to introduce himself by tapping a trigger on an electronic communication device. We created an opportunity for all participants to perform some element of their individuality in some way, and then had each person's individuality performed by the group through repeating it, or copying it, in an act of full acceptance of the chosen identity. I remember one of the teens singing her name in the melody of a Shakira pop hit and performing a wild dance, and then the whole group attempting it (even though I think it made all of us pretty uncomfortable). Every kind of individual self-expression was accepted and performed by the ensemble.

Ari usually only said his name under his breath, but sometimes I would suggest a movement to him. He was not particularly eager to try new things. I could always tell that he enjoyed watching the movements of the other kids, and through his enjoyment of their movements, he was beginning to connect with the group. He occasionally would go up to certain children and repeat their name and movement verbatim in the same way they expressed it in the opening circle. Sometimes he would tell one of the children that their movement was different than it had been the week before. Ari always noticed the little differences and nuances.

The routines and rituals were very important to Ari. One day, we started late and we skipped singing our opening song. Ari paced around repeating Pokémon slang in frustration. At one point, he walked up to our musical therapist and grabbed her hand and dragged her to the guitar to play music for our opening circle. For Ari, it was impossible to start the group without the opening music. Routines, in this context, do matter.

Performative Activity

The next part of class took us through a series of exercises that included a movement activity in which we moved across the floor in different ways, and what was loosely defined as a play-building exercise. Ari had a difficult time engaging at first, but during the movement activity, I had an idea to move with Ari in the manner of various Pokémon characters. He wasn't sure at first, but he got a kick out of other kids in the group who were moving across the floor in their own unique ways. I asked Ari whom he wanted to move like. He did not want to do the activity, and was ready to leave the room. I told him that I was going to move like Pikachu, the one character I could remember; I had learned from my young nephew that Pikachu was the gold standard of Pokémon characters. I did what I thought was an excellent Pikachu movement, and Ari shook his head and said, "No no no, that isn't it." Some other participants caught on and encouraged Ari to show his movement of Pikachu. Coach E asked Ari if he was ready to share with the group. "No, no, not today!" I respected the fact that he knew he was not ready to perform for the group.

Over the next couple of weeks, I watched Ari open up to the group on his own terms. I tried various ways of asking Ari questions about the Pokémon characters, and Ari would rightly assume that I was interrupting his list, and he would start over. It was extremely frustrating. I wanted to connect in a more reciprocal way (what the DIR/Floortime® model calls *circles of communication*; see Greenspan et al. 1998), but I could not figure out how to connect with him. At the end of our rehearsals, we typically had a staff and volunteer meeting in which our staff would process the day's class. I frequently would discuss Ari, and how I was frustrated that I still could not connect with him in a way in which I felt the shared excitement of a relational back and forth conversation. It was mostly Ari speaking a monologue, and I was commenting on it. The reciprocity just was not there.

After several weeks of attempting to connect, and giving Ari the respect and space he needed, I figured it out. As long as I did not interrupt his list, Ari would let me perform the movements of the Pokémon characters. The moment I tried this, Ari immediately took notice and would correct my movements. He would say "Araragi-Hakase, Professor Oak" and I would create with my body and face a wooden, stoic, and respectable Professor or how I imagined the great "Professor Oak" to look. I would usually perform the physicality of the character completely wrong, but this mischaracterization also gave Ari the opportunity to correct me and show the way he interpreted the character. I would ask questions, and occasionally he would show me, or he would manipulate my body into the correct position. Sometimes I would even make sounds that were vaguely anime-ish or faux Japanese, and Ari would giggle. Sometimes he took out a pack of the Pokémon cards, and showed me the character and how he thought they would move. We were suddenly relating! It was a breakthrough that happened because I did not force Ari to communicate with me. I finally figured out how to relate with Ari by respecting his rules, by adapting to his ways of engaging with the world.

This movement activity also translated to the group. One of the activities that I introduced to the group was a statue-making theater game (Boal 2002) in which one of the players (the sculptor) creates a physical statue by manipulating the body of another performer (the statue) with movement and gesture without touching the other person. We evolved the activity so that sculptors could talk to their statues (not part of how Boal described the activity), because we found that some of the children had a difficult time with the subtlety of their sculptor's gestures, and we adapted the exercise so that the entire group could feel successful in the activity. This flexibility meant that one could say, "Make an evil menacing grin" as a sculptor and then manipulate the partner with gesture and movement to match the way the grin was designed to look. I went on stage with Ari, and he surprised me by stepping up and sculpting me into the great Professor Oak. During the sculpting, Ari studied his Professor Oak Pokémon card so he could create the image of Professor Oak in great detail. The group and Coach E loved it, and I was hamming it up by making my gestures particularly bold. At the end of the day, we performed for the parents, who were participating in their own Miracle Project support group. Ari's mom was in tears. She had never seen Ari interact with so much joy and intent.

BUILDING RELATIONSHIPS THROUGH COLLABORATIVE PERFORMANCES

The next session, I realized that I could use Ari's knowledge of Pokémon to help him relate to other children in the group. I convinced another kid in the group who had an interest in Pokémon to suggest a Pokémon character, and then Ari would sculpt one of the other children in the group into its form. He loved the game and saw that the other kids in the group accepted his ideas. He could be exactly whom he wanted to be, and because of this acceptance, he started participating in having himself sculpted into other children's non-Pokémon-related ideas. The simple act of accepting Ari as the genius Pokémon cognoscenti that he presented himself as, and of respecting and adapting to the rules that he established, allowed for Ari to begin to trust the group and accept other children's ideas. It was exciting to see him relating, enjoying, and playing with the other children in the group.

The acceptance and expansion of children's unique ideas was only further represented in The Miracle Project's performances. The collaborative process of connecting to the children's ideas and passions and then performing those passions as a group was presented on stage. Ari played a Pokémon-esque character in our musical performance. The Fire (what he titled himself) transformed into the great kings throughout Jewish history as part of our show. It was wonderful to see many of the children's interests incorporated into the show, from show tunes to invisible pets. The staff wrote the show, and we did our best to stitch together the ideas of the children in the group. Ari had the opportunity to perform and show his passion of Pokémon by making all sorts of fighting noises, expressing proclamations of power, and sharing his love of Japanese popular culture. At the same time, he also sang the songs that other kids had inspired, and participated in the ensemble performance on stage.

Ari's Pokémon interest did not take away from the production. The ensemble's acceptance of Ari's Pokémon passion encouraged Ari to perform in the numbers that were inspired by other children. Ari and all of the children had their moment to shine on stage, and to be completely, unabashedly, who they were. During rehearsal, I watched kids who were very isolated from one another join together in the devising of the play. The performance was a celebration of the many different personalities and differences apparent in the rehearsal room.

Actionplay

This inclusion-based work at The Miracle Project inspired me to launch my own company Actionplay, relying on performance and improvisation for teenagers and young adults on the autism spectrum. Actionplay's work is similar in its scope to that of The Miracle Project, but focuses on the idea of being a community with rules and ideas defined by the performers, outside any methodology, and rooted in revolutionary practice.

I moved to New York in 2006, and was excited to bring what I learned from my time with The Miracle Project and the work of the DIR/Floortime® model to a new city and a new time in my life. I was becoming established in the autism community as someone who was known for doing unconventional performance-based work. The Miracle Project was the focus of the two-time Emmy Award winning HBO documentary: "Autism: The Musical" about our Los Angeles-based Miracle Project. The popularity of the HBO film opened up the possibilities of theatrical work with people on the autism spectrum to a much wider audience.

I started Actionplay as an inclusive drama club for teenagers in New York City with the emphasis on play and creative improvisation, rather than creating plays and productions. My goal was to not define the creative projects that we took on and not to directly employ any established methodology. Of course, without a clear goal or direction to head in, we were in for a far messier process. It meant that the group had to actually come up with their own ideas and ways of working together. Over time, we devised a structure that worked for our participants. I saw my own role as a leader and participant, with just enough of an outside eye so that I could monitor the progress and create opportunities for our burgeoning community.

Although I decided not to push the idea of performing, it turned out that almost every group wanted to culminate their Actionplay experience with a performance. I was reluctant at first because I saw through my work at The Miracle Project that the performance could be challenging because it sometimes came with unreasonable expectations from the schools, parents, and community. Although it was an exciting and rewarding experience for parents to see their children on stage, some of the parents and members of the community would criticize the show, feeling that their child seemed to be acting too young, too disabled, or too babyish. Many parents had the expectation of The Miracle Project to challenge and advance their child's interests so that they could see on stage a more advanced and socially acceptable version of their child. The expectations of the parents were quite stressful, and Coach E attempted to keep the shows positive and joyous. The difficult part about this emphasis on positivity was how to honor the improvisational work that was occurring during the rehearsals. Much of the improvisational work expressed pain and sadness, and I wanted to present this reality without sanitizing the performance for our audience.

At Actionplay, I chose to work with teenagers and adults on the spectrum, and I found that most of them had been ridiculed and bullied throughout their lives. I could personally relate to the harshness of bullying from my own grade school experience. Our inclusive group was composed of teenagers and young adults on the autism spectrum, neurotypical performing arts high school students, adult volunteers, and adult staff members. It was a diverse group of individuals with an extraordinary range of passions and preferred interests including pop star Michael Jackson, the 1960s rock band The Monkees, zombies, and existentialism. I learned that many of the teens were bullied because of their unique interests, and many of them acknowledged the feeling of being identified as having a "disorder." Our devising of an original performance was based on improvisations that reflected our performers' passions, interests, and range of talents.

Music's Role with Autism-Spectrum Youth

I was fortunate enough to find a fantastic musical therapist and song leader to help build Actionplay's programs. Gabriel Lit, our musical therapist, was a graduate of NYU's Musical Therapy program and did his internship at the Nordoff-Robbins Center for Music Therapy. The Nordoff-Robbins method favored an improvisational and communicative approach to working with music, in direct contrast to the more passive music-for-music's-sake approach to music therapy (Simpson 2009).

Music therapy group improvisations are a powerful tool for working with groups of adolescence on the autism spectrum who do not communicate successfully using verbal means. Music therapy can also offer safety because of its complementary relationship with words, with the music oftentimes containing the more conflicting emotions that may not be easily expressed through language (McFerran 2010). Gabriel used music as a form of radical communication to connect with the teenagers in our group. The music became the glue that bonded our Actionplay group together, and a way to create safety of self-expression in our group improvisations. Gabriel's unique ability allowed him to improvise musically with our group, and to create original songs with our Actionplay performers based on their individual passions and preferred interests. He also had an ease with connecting musically with our non-verbal communicators, and respecting all forms of expression as a form of communication.

Building Community

Early in our process, I established that the people in the rehearsal room, adults and teens, neurotypical or diagnosed, were a part of the performance. This collaborative emphasis seemed to remove the exclusivity component that I observed in many other programs that did performance-based work with people of difference. Inclusion meant that everyone was responsible for performing on stage and bringing the play into existence. When our performers on stage had a difficult time because of autism or any other reason, the adult volunteers or staff members could help them by continuing to perform. I had witnessed many programs in which the adult support staff was reduced to crisis management, physical assistants, and microphone holders, and they were certainly not an active part of the performance. At Actionplay, every child and adult was a performer, and their support came from singing the songs, showing up to rehearsals, and being part of the production.

Our performance-based approach to building community also translated into our parent and sibling community. I never understood the idea of "support groups" because the support groups I participated in were usually groups in which people would compete with each other in a Darwinian contest of despair and tragedy. I took a different approach to Actionplay's parent community. I encouraged our parents and siblings who were not directly involved in the performing to help build the sets, create the programs, and support the aspects of the performances that needed to be supported. Through this process, the families were supported, and many of them developed personal relationships with one another, extending the notion of community beyond the bounds of the activity.

Resisting the Culture of Normativity and Compliance

A vast majority of the teens in Actionplay were enrolled in school programs that employed applied behavioral analysis or ABA, which is a research-based approach to behavioral modification (Baer, Wolf, & Risley, 1968). Prizant (2015) describes these programs as attempting to "measure progress as the reduction or elimination of behaviors considered to be autistic behaviors. The focus is also often on building positive skills" (Prizant 2015). Without over generalizing ABA, which may be helpful for many families depending on the practice (there are many forms of ABA), ABA is deficit-oriented, serving inherently as a compliance-based therapeutic model that views behaviors as an inherent part of the autism-spectrum *disorder*. These behaviors can be altered through behavioral modification. The Lovaas ABA model, one of the most common forms of ABA used in autism, has a stated goal of making children on the spectrum "indistinguishable from their peers" (Shea 2004). It thus pathologizes difference as a problem to be cured, focusing on difference as deficit at the expense of assets to build upon.

There has been much criticism from groups of autistics regarding ABA's relationship to compliance. Williams (1996), an autistic writer, scholar, and artist, writes about ABA:

> Compliance is not learning, because you do not connect with your own thoughts, feelings or intentions. Compliance is mindless. Compliance may appear to achieve things in the short term but the arrest in the development of connections to thought, feelings and intention may not only create extreme (generally compliantly repressed) chronic stress, but may ultimately result in physical, emotional or mental breakdown if the effects of pervasive compliance are not properly addressed. (p. 52)

Actionplay's solution to address the culture of compliance that many autistics are subjected to came in the form of comedy. Orwell (1945) wrote that "A thing is funny when it upsets the established order. Every joke is a tiny revolution" (n. p.). Humor acts as a form of subversive resistance for many oppressed groups. Bryant (2006) describes how humor was used as a form of resistance by Czech nationals under an oppressive "Germanizing" Nazi regime. If compliance-based cultures in schools and in home life were limiting to our teens' thoughts, feelings, and intentions, Actionplay's productions were a form of active resistance against the dominant autism culture of compliance and conformity.

At Actionplay, our team decided that all ideas, behaviors, and intentions, however autistic, "disordered," wild, bizarre, inappropriate, or silly (as long as they were not meant to be physically injurious of oneself or another), were completely accepted, and in the true improvisational tradition, served as the groundwork for further performances. The creation of a performance was more than just the enactment of our participants' passions and interests in a celebration of autism. Actionplay performances were action-based and encouraged our performers to take their power back from the dominant culture's insistence that they fit in. Our group needed to be allowed the opportunity to express their negativity toward the limitations of the cultural idea of autism as disorder, and comedy served as a powerful form of active resistance. Actionplay's version of theater was completely unsanitized. Our participants' feelings of having a disorder—indicative of the secondary disability described by Vygotsky (1993)—became the basis for subversive comedy, and comedic techniques were used to take the power back from the dominant culture that attempts to make autism-spectrum youth comply with neurotypical standards and become "indistinguishable from their peers."

In learning about the teens in our group, we discovered that many of them were not allowed to discuss their passions and preferred interests in a school setting. They were frequently told that their ideas and ways of communicating were babyish, inappropriate, or not suitable for a school setting. We created a platform in which our performers' ideas could be accepted and then expanded upon, and also challenged by others in a group setting. The individuality of our performers was encouraged, and the Actionplay performances were a culmination of our ensemble-based work.

Action in Actionplay

The framework that defined each of the productions came out of the improvisational activities that occurred during rehearsals. Our staff, led by me and our Educational Director, Sara Hunter Orr, a graduate of the Applied Theatre Graduate Program at the City University of New York (CUNY), devised games and activities that would allow our performers to be experts and leaders of their own unique interests, and then to create scenes out of these interests and incorporate them into the group structure. Sara's devising skills incorporated a clarity and tight framework for the improvisations, and were rooted in improvisational games and a respect of each of our performers' individual means of communicating and self-expression.

In our original musical comedy production, "Revenge of The Godz," the idea of resistance against the culture of compliance was apparent in the story, subject, and songs. When our group of teens began devising "Revenge of The Godz," the group decided that the characters of the play were ancient mythological gods that had been turned into statues by Zeus, the leader of the gods. Zeus cast a spell on this particular group of rogue gods because he was jealous that they were becoming too powerful. The creation of the God characters was an individual process for each performer, and each of our performers had the opportunity to define and name his or her character. The God character identities were rooted in our participants' unique interests. There was a god of Zombies, a god of Rock and Roll, and a god of unbridled strength among our motley crew (among many other interests). Zeus was played by one of our participants who was excited by the idea of playing the villain.

In the play, Zeus's spell wore off, and The Gods woke up from their statue existence and found themselves at The Museum of Deities in

New York City in 2015. They attempted to break out of the museum and realized that they had lost their powers. Once they figured out how to work the weird elevator thing (they are ancient gods!), the Gods visited the floors of the museum that corresponded with each of the characters' individual interests. For example, the God of Zombies found a floor of the museum dedicated to horror movies and memorabilia, and announced with excitement when she found her monster friends, "I'm back!" a line of her own creation. The Gods escaped the museum and were thrust into modern day New York City. As they walked around New York City, they were overwhelmed with the sensory environment and the intensity of the sights and sounds, a plot element rooted in the autistic experience of sensory overload.

As the Gods dealt with this new world, they met the villainous leader of a Mega Corporation, Martin Whitebox, who sang a song about having to "fit in," a difficult concept for the once all-powerful Gods. The performer who played Martin Whitebox wrote the song, and it was full of ABA tinged anti-sentiments like "quiet hands," which is a common ABA phrase used for children who flap their arms and hands, and other statements that are used to normalize the autistic population in compliance-based therapeutic approaches. This addition was based on this particular performer's own experience of compliance-based therapy. The performer had never had the opportunity to play a villain, and enjoyed getting to play a person who makes the others comply. In speaking to him after the performance, he expressed the enjoyment he had over the opportunity to "act evil."

Martin Whitebox brought all of the gods back to his mega-corporation and turned them into minions, forced to construct his sterile technological device, The Whitebox. The Gods complied because they thought Martin Whitebox was a decent person because he helped them to fit into the modern world. The Gods soon learned that the modern world's expectations of them were quite limiting and in full denial of their "God given powers," a sentiment reflecting the feeling of being identified as disordered by the dominant culture.

The experience of working in Martin Whitebox's assembly-line factory was tinged with the overarching theme of compliance. The Gods built The Whitebox product in a robotic assembly line using mechanical movements, which were part of the stage choreography. One of the gods named Fernanda Diaz, a conquistador-inspired god who loved gold and jewels, led a workers' revolt in the fashion of a *Les Miserables* musical number, where the cast hoisted flags and smashed The Whiteboxes that they were forced into making. The musical number "Down with The Whitebox" was a true act of breaking out of the narrowly defined "boxes" or the limitations of the dominant culture. The song was also written solely by the performer playing the goddess Fernanda Diaz and featured lyrics pertaining to her own experience of being stigmatized as having a disorder.

In the end, Martin Whitebox was actually Zeus in disguise (played by the same performer). Zeus's intention was to control the gods because he was afraid of them "becoming too powerful." Toward the end of the play, the gods embraced their own uniqueness and regained their powers to fight and take down Zeus once and for all. The Gods were not going to have their uniqueness challenged ever again!

The final number of the Musical was called "We Don't Want To Fit In," which is an appropriate song about the Actionplay experience with the lyrics: "So we're not the same, it's our uniqueness. Difference isn't weakness! We don't want to fit in!"

Discussion

Actionplay is about embracing one's individuality, and serves as a radical form of acceptance of each of our performers as healthy individuals, rather than the societal view of them of being identified as disordered because of an autism diagnosis. There is an understanding among our staff, parents, and participants that the differences that make our performers unique are not only important, but potentially the passions and interests that will lead them to a more hopeful future of employment possibilities and happiness in life. The idea of disorder is dangerous, and only adds pathology and limitations to the essentially limitless possibilities of all individuals.

A show or stage performance, even one that is based on uniqueness and individuality, is also an attempt to become part of an ensemble and develop something that is greater than the sum of its individual parts. The autistic teens who were onstage and performing in front of an audience chose to control some of their little utterances, flapping, and other autistic behaviors in order to bring "Revenge of the Godz" into existence for an audience. The difference is that our performers chose to exert this level of control and focus on themselves during the stage performance. There is no one on stage forcing anyone to change his or her behavior or to comply with any perceived standard of how a performer should appear on stage.

Actionplay's staff, parents, and volunteers help each individual adapt to the stage environment. Because Actionplay is adaptive, our performers help design their own costumes to take into account individual sensory needs. The cast and crew also maintain an open dialog about performance jitters and nervousness before going on stage. It is nothing short of remarkable to see the transformation from an individual-based process to a collective process during the rehearsals, with the culmination of this process being a stage performance that is inclusive of the larger New York City community. The ensemble-based performance gives each individual the opportunity to be celebrated, but also upholds the idea that the performance is a group effort, in which the "we" is much more powerful than the "I." There is a strong relationship of sharing our cast's collective experience of being othered with a mostly neurotypical audience, and then receiving the approval from our audience in the form of applause. The performance is a form of integration with the community, and an active process of challenging the stigmas surrounding difference.

"We don't want to fit in" is a rebellious and revolutionary statement against the normative culture's insistence on "fitting in" and compliance. Lobman (2012) wrote of a recent production I directed called "A Brief History of All Things":

> I appreciated the ways the kids were able to be who they are—they stared off into space, they spoke under their breath—and at the same time they were able to perform as other than who they are. At times I could literally see them choosing to support the play, rather than to just do what they "normally" do.

As Vygotsky (1978) states, the performers were acting on stage as if they "were a head taller" and at the same time being exactly who they are in all of their vibrant individuality.

Actionplay and The Miracle Project are both inclusive groups that rely on ensemble-based performance to build social communities that rise above the feeling of being excluded and othered. In that sense, they provide their participants with a positive social updraft through which they become valued members of a community of practice. In difference, there is great strength. The meaningful and supportive relationships that are formed in the rehearsal room are essential for those of us who don't quite fit in. Recently, one of our performers came up to me after rehearsal and said, "At Actionplay, I found my people." Such is the power and potential of designed settings that produce a positive social updraft for those generally considered too disabled to grow in the company of others.

Boal (1985) maintains that "the theatre is not revolutionary in itself, but it is surely a rehearsal for the revolution. The liberated spectator, as a whole person, launches into action. No matter that the action is fictional; what matters is that it is action!" (p. 98). The Miracle Project and Actionplay are built on the revolutionary idea that all people should be respected and valued for their differences. Psychological, developmental, and mental health diagnosis can be meaningful for a variety of reasons, but the double-edged sword of diagnosis is that it also comes with the damaging social stigma of disorder and pathology.

Inclusive theater and performance provide those of us deemed "the other" the opportunity to be part of communities built on self-expression and developmental growth, and the opportunity to directly challenge these damaging stigmas and the secondary disability (Vygotsky 1993; see Chap. 2) that they inevitably produce. For neuro-atypical teenagers and young adults, the "revolution" is rehearsed by forming communities that create a microcosm of a more functional society. The practice of the revolution will happen in inclusive rehearsal rooms, inclusive performance venues, and outside the compliance-based systems that make us all feel that we have to fit in. *We don't want to fit in.*

Note

1. The names of all children are pseudonyms.

References

American Psychiatric Association. (1994). *Diagnostic and statistical manual of mental disorders* (4th ed.). Washington, DC: Author.

Ayers, J. (1973). *Sensory integration and learning disorders*. Torrance: Western Psychological Services.

Baer, D. M., Wolf, M. M., & Risley, T. R. (1968). Some current dimensions of applied behavior analysis. *Journal of Applied Behavior Analysis, 1*, 91–97. Retrieved August 10, 2015, from: http://approaches.primarymusic.gr/approaches/journal/Approaches_1(2)_2009/Approaches_1(2)2009_Froudaki_Review_ENG.pdf

Baranek, G. T., David, F. J., Poe, M. D., Stone, W. L., & Watson, L. R. (2006). Sensory experiences questionnaire: Discriminating sensory features in young

children with autism, developmental delays and typical development. *Journal of Child Psychological Psychiatry, 47*, 591–601.
Bear, M. F., Connors, D. W., & Paradiso, M. A. (2007). *Neuroscience: Exploring the brain* (3rd ed.). Baltimore: Lippincott Williams and Wilkins.
Boal, A. (1985). *Theatre of the oppressed.* London: Pluto Classics.
Boal, A. (2002). *Games for actors and non-actors.* New York: Routledge.
Bryant, C. (2006). The language of resistance? Czech jokes and joke-telling under Nazi occupation, 1943–45. *Journal of Contemporary History, 41*(1), 133–151.
Case-Smith, J., & Bryan, T. (1999). The effects of occupational therapy with sensory integration emphasis on preschool-age children with autism. *American Journal of Occupational Therapy, 53*, 489–497.
Cerliani, L., Maarten, M., Thomas, R. M., Martino, A. D., Thioux, M., & Keysers, C. (2015). Increased functional connectivity between subcortical and cortical resting state networks in autism spectrum disorder. *JAMA Psychiatry, 72*(8), 767–77. doi:10.1001/jamapsychiatry.2015.0101.
Cutler, D. M., Glaeser, E. L., & Norberg, K. E. (2001). Explaining the rise in youth suicide. In J. Gruber (Ed.), *Risky behavior among youths: An economic analysis* (pp. 219–270). Chicago: University of Chicago Press.
Dunn, W. (2001). The sensations of everyday life: Theoretical, conceptual and pragmatic considerations. *American Journal of Occupational Therapy, 55*, 608–620. Retrieved August 10, 2015, from: http://www.aota.org//media/Corporate/Files/Publications/AJOT/Slagle/2001.ashx
Grandin, T. (1996). *Thinking in pictures.* New York: Vintage.
Greenspan, S. I., & Wieder, S. (2006). *Engaging autism: Using the floortime approach to help children relate, communicate, and think.* Cambridge, MA: Da Capo Press.
Greenspan, S. I., Wieder, S., & Simons, R. (1998). *The child with special needs: Encouraging intellectual and emotional growth.* Reading: Addison-Wesley.
Hall, E. (2010). *Now I see the moon: A mother, a son, a miracle.* New York: HarperCollins.
Liss, M., Saulnier, C., Fein, D., & Kinsbourne, M. (2006). Sensory and attention abnormalities in autistic spectrum disorders. *Autism, 10*(2), 155–172. Retrieved September 1, 2016 from: http://www.kinsbournelab.org/uploads/1/4/3/1/14315208/liss_saulnier_fein__kinsbourne_2006.__sensory_and_attention_abnormalities_in_autistic_spectrum_disorders.pdf.
Lobman, C. (2012). The Miracle Project: Not acting normal. *East Side Institute Community News.* Retrieved August 10, 2015, from https://esicommunitynews.wordpress.com/2012/05/21/the-miracle-project-not-acting-normal/
McFerran, K. (2010). *Adolescents, music and music therapy: Methods and techniques for clinicians, educators and students.* London: Jessica Kingsley Publishers.
Milner, M. (2006). *Freaks, geeks, and cool kids.* New York: Routledge.

Ornitz, E. (1988). Autism: A disorder of directed attention. *Brain Dysfunction, 1,* 309–322.

Orwell, G. (1945). *Funny, but not vulgar.* Retrieved September 1, 2016 from http://orwell.ru/library/articles/funny/english/e_funny.

Prizant, B. (2015). *Uniquely human: A different way to see autism and create pathways to success.* Webinar available at http://presencelearning.com/blog/dr-barry-prizant-in-conversation-with-clay-whitehead/

Schanzenbach, D.W. (2014). *Does class size matter?* Boulder: National Education Policy Center. Retrieved July 15, 2015, from http://nepc.colorado.edu/publication/doesclasssizematter

Shea, V. (2004). A perspective on the research literature related to early intensive behavioral intervention (Lovaas) for young children with autism. *Autism, 43,* 49–67.

Simpson, F. (2009). *The Nordoff-Robbins adventure: Fifty years of creative music therapy.* London: James and James Publishers Ltd..

Vygotsky, L. S. (1978). In M. Cole, V. John-Steiner, S. Scribner, & E. Souberman (Eds.), *Mind in society: The development of higher psychological processes.* Cambridge, MA: Harvard University Press.

Vygotsky, L. S. (1993). *The collected works of L. S. Vygotsky. Volume 2: The fundamentals of defectology (abnormal psychology and learning disabilities)* (R. W. Rieber & A. S. Carton, Eds.; trans: Knox, J. E. & Stevens, C. B.). New York: Plenum.

Watling, R. L., & Dietz, J. (2007). Immediate effect of Ayres's sensory integration–based occupational therapy intervention on children with autism spectrum disorders. *American Journal of Occupational Therapy, 61,* 574–583.

Williams, D. (1996). *Autism: An inside-out approach.* London: Jessica Kingsley.

CHAPTER 7

The DisAbility Project: A Model for Autism-Specific Creativity and Civic Engagement Within the Broader Context of Difference

Joan Lipkin, Marcy Epstein, Paula Heller, and Peter Smagorinsky

In discussing how theater humanizes societies, Woodruff (2010) notes that theater requires rules for behaviors—when to be quiet, when to applaud, when to arrive, when to leave, and how to listen—that establish societal norms. Woodruff cautions that without these public events, individuals become isolated and societies become non-cohesive. In essence, segregation kills the sense of belonging, and societies can be destroyed once individuals no longer feel they can relate to other members of the society.

J. Lipkin (✉)
That Uppity Theatre Company, St. Louis, MO, USA

M. Epstein
University of Michigan, Ann Arbor, MI, USA

P. Heller
That Uppity Theater Company, St. Louis, MO, USA

P. Smagorinsky
Department of Language and Literacy Education, The University of Georgia, USA

© The Author(s) 2016
P. Smagorinsky (ed.), *Creativity and Community among Autism-Spectrum Youth*, DOI 10.1057/978-1-137-54797-2_7

Whether or not a society integrates individuals with behavioral, developmental, and physical "disabilities" into the larger society shapes societal expectations both for people with and without such points of difference.

This general relationship between societal mores and diverse manifestations of what are considered disabilities in performing arts or applied theater practice is the focus of an emerging research area, one that combines disability[1] and performance studies. Sandahl and Auslander (2005) argue that the representation of disability on stage or as a subject of performance is intrinsically connected to the perceptions of disability in everyday life, and vice versa.

This chapter provides a look inside the DisAbility Project, a touring theatrical ensemble based in St. Louis that has performed for over 100,000 people. Its work has been archived in the permanent collection of the Missouri History Museum. The DisAbility Project has attracted visitors from as far away as Afghanistan, China, and Bangladesh to study techniques for group process, specifically through designing and modeling integration both for rehearsal and performance and generating material. By documenting the theater company's history and creative development, then exploring major themes of disability and theatricality, including its work with autistic children and adults, we hope to demonstrate the wide-ranging potential of integrative theaters like the DisAbility Project in enriching the public understanding and inclusion of autistic people.

The ensemble was founded in 1995 by theater artist and educator Joan Lipkin and the late occupational therapist and Washington University professor Fran Cohen. The DisAbility Project is housed under the umbrella of That Uppity Theater Company, an award-winning company dedicated to cultural diversity and social justice. This program, unlike those featured in other chapters in Part 2 of this volume, is not specifically designed for children and youth on the autism spectrum. Rather, it was founded to provide a larger theatrical window into the lives of people labeled as having mental or physical disabilities, to promote cultural diversity and integrative theatrical practice of the highest quality and civic engagement.[2] However, their techniques and strategies are useful in exploring how others can adapt the social environment to help human development through play and performance. The company describes what they do as "edutainment," valuing art and education in shared measure.

In writing this chapter about autism-specific theater, we continue to be struck by the challenges of language and labeling. Many of us working within the field of disability are faced with an on-going tension of language and label that autism makes even more palpable. It is difficult to create a space for our work with adequate resources without naming things, and yet, this standard practice can be reductive and divisive and cannot easily stay in step with shifting popular cultural attitudes about language. For example, in recent years, there has been a shift in agreement around "people first" language in the field of disability studies. We have noted especially in reference to autism that there is a growing rejection of "people first" language, for example, saying "person with autism," because this linguistic attitudinal nuance suggests that they can be separated from their autism, which is an essential aspect of their identity.

Thus, in some circles, there is a preference for identity-first language, which is seen as a more positive identification as an autistic person. Or, some people may prefer to be described as autistic. This language has evolved from the *moral* and *medical* models, which used terms such as "cripple" or "imbecile"; to the *rehabilitation* model, which looked at disability as a medical problem in need of fixing; to a *social* model of "person-first" language, which worked toward fixing the environment with ramps and other accessibility issues and labeled the people with disabilities; and finally, to an "identity-first" language that is more positive and culturally powerful, in that the identifier language suggests a whole individual whose point of difference is simply part of the whole (Dunn and Andrews 2015, p. 255).

Debates like this are on-going because they establish both who we are and what we are creating with theater in a world of changing understanding and appreciation of our specific differences, in this case, disability-specific and autism-specific difference. Moreover, this tension is crucial to the ways in which people communicate with each other and advocate for social change. We acknowledge that it may be an impossible task to find language to explore these issues that feels acceptable to all. The DisAbility Project deconstructs its own name and its connotations by the way it is spelled, capitalizing the "A" as if to question the concept of ability/disability and even make it ironic. Consider the dynamics, too, of being an "actor with autism" or an "audience member with autism." The considerable range of neurodiversity and subjectivity among autistic people further complicates language. In the arena of civic engagement, the dominant culture has yet to communicate in some cases at all and at most sufficiently with the range of autistic citizens in their community. Thus, the issue of naming is a crucial place to begin a discussion of the DisAbility Project's history, since it explores the more general disability language as it evolved, as the language of autism is developing now.

Origins

When Lipkin and Cohen launched the DisAbility Project in the mid-1990s, the language of physical and mental disability was remarkably absent from public theater, except for the objectifying narration heard at the carnival, surgical theater, or charity tel-a-thon. There were few if any people with disabilities seen on stage, or in the audience. At the start of her career, however, Lipkin became familiar with avant-garde theater director Joe Chaikin, who had a heart condition that required three open-heart surgeries. In 1984, during the third of these surgeries, he had a stroke that left him with partial aphasia, a condition resulting in struggles with speaking, reading, and writing, but no apparent loss in intelligence or creativity. Following the loss of his ability to communicate easily through spoken language, Chaikin continued to act, direct, and produce plays in collaboration with other playwrights, performers, and directors, increasingly featuring disability themes. Learning of his latest focus, Lipkin traveled to the Atlantic Center for the Arts, where Chaikin was an artist in residence, to work with him as an artistic associate.

Chaiken's practice sparked a creativity among his actors and audiences that questioned the fluidity and adaptability of bodies and characters, even the anticipation of the audiences. Unusually, the experience of people in all their diversity could be explored on new, powerful terms. This experience was so profound that Lipkin returned to St. Louis motivated to continue creating work about disability. There she connected with Cohen, who had significant contacts in the local disability community. Together, they determined that they did not want a conventional ensemble. Instead, they saw their work as a respectful and fully invested experiment in which they brought together people with disabilities to create their own world. They wanted to be free of debilitating assumptions from society at large, and to see if they could construct a context for creating something theatrical and compelling. They wanted to create work about the culture of disability and to help people with disabilities represent their own experience for a wider public.

Among their early supporters was Max Starkloff, a St. Louis native and a nationally recognized disability rights activist who had become paralyzed in a car accident in 1959 at age 22. Although not previously involved in theater—his activities centered on promoting independent living, a need for which he founded three major organizations—he shared interests with the founders and wanted to promote cultural representation of people like himself who had physical limitations. Starkloff was happy to have theatrical allies to help develop a program for bringing attention about disability rights to a broader audience. As happens in all emerging marginalized communities, this process faced some opposition, including pushback from those who did not want to emphasize disability. Lipkin realized the seriousness of the historical moment of forging theater with a community who was emerging, like the larger autism community now. At an initial information-gathering meeting with disability leaders in St. Louis, the founders shared their vision for a traveling disability theater ensemble to deliver their message in ways both educational and entertaining.

Mission

In terms of theater arts and education for autistic people and their communities, it is worth exploring life experiences and trajectories, individually and collectively. Programs such as the DisAbility Project bridge the gap between the cognitive and the emotional needs of people, thus promoting a higher quality of life. Greenspan and Greenspan (2010) argue that imagination, self-control, and planning all come from play. Theater uses organization and imagination, requires intellect through analysis, demands emotional empathy and self-control, and cannot take place without the social skill of collaboration with others. Through theater, autistic participants particularly—who may be stressed by the demands of conventional speech, communication, and social expectations—can practice and even redefine social interactions through art in a safe place both as actor and audience member. Rather than escorting individuals experiencing autistic symptoms out of the sacred space of theatrical performance for such behaviors as talking out, the project invites them into a welcoming space where all can equally participate in the theatrical process.

The work of the DisAbility Project exceeds the scope and definition of modern research on the brain, even as it reflects some of its learning. According to Siegel (2011), many parts of the brain can be strengthened by what he calls "Mindsight" tools. He maintains that people need time to look inside their minds and train themselves to be in the moment. Neurons mirror minds; thus, Siegel claims that people can intentionally activate these circuits, and they become the root of empathy. "By viewing mind, brain and relationships as fundamentally three dimensions of one reality—of aspects of energy and information flow—we see our human experience with truly new eyes" (p. 58).

Unlike some art forms, theater takes place in the present tense. The DisAbility Project, through the actor/audience relationship, grew its practice into a refined production of shared experience and dialogue in order to create changes in perspectives and promote empathy. Actors take the audience on a journey so that they can see human experience with new eyes. Actors who have disabilities use their own voices to help the audience see their world through their eyes. And by having the audience actively participate, actors are given the opportunity to share the experiences reciprocally. Lipkin, relying on audience self-report, has been able to document a shift in empathy through a post-show survey that measures changes in attitudes and predictable behavior among children and youth after seeing a DisAbility Project performance.

Thus, the Project's mission fills a major gap in the cultural representation of difference in society reflected in theater. Roughly 20 % of people in the USA—approximately 56.7 million people—have been diagnosed with a legally defined form of what is known as a disability, whether it is sensory, cognitive, or mobility related (United States Census Bureau 2012). Unemployment is high among those in this category; stable data on the presence of disability, including autism, among the US population that does not meet the legal definition are difficult to establish, but it is generally understood that disabled people comprise the largest and most financially challenged demographic group in the country. The DisAbility Project brings awareness and sensitivity to issues in the disability community through a combination of art and advocacy, touring and performing before audiences at diverse venues: educational institutions (primarily schools, the ensemble's most frequent location for performances), conferences, special events, festivals, religious and civic groups, and corporations.

People classified as disabled, like most marginalized, minoritized social groups, have been denied roles in the society in which they live, on and off the stage. While this treatment is changing, with certain disabled people finding increasing representation in mainstream industry, there are important reasons that some people's experiences as disabled have not advanced as quickly as those of some of their allies. Autism can be one of the most difficult conditions to address. General understanding of autism is still inadequate, even stigmatizing. Autistic children and adults often get steered away from the arts and toward other cognitive and social forums, and are subjected to increased medical experimentation. Moreover, the original tension we discuss here—the adaptation of communication and identity needed to transform the social environment represented by the theater—is not usually brought forth for autistic individuals who seek the arts.

In short, autistic people are still overwhelmingly asked to bend toward a society that does not yet understand autism or people on its spectrum. Autism presents our society and our theater with a promising call toward adaptation and cultural richness (see Chap. 3). Adaptation can easily be made for many disabilities, such as wheelchair accessibility, American Sign Language, real time captioning, descriptive services, and so on. With these adaptations, one size does not fit all, and the interface between the person and the accommodation does not always result in the most productive synthesis for inclusion. Autism challenges the existing social environment of theater to an even greater degree, in part because of the ways in which it affects social interactions. Our project is designed to cultivate three relational dimensions of the theatrical experience: the performer, the audience, and education.

Participants

The DisAbility Project ensemble and its other personnel—choreographers, directors, and office staff—are themselves comprised of people with and without disabilities. At most of their performances, these ensemble members perform a collage of 8–12 short pieces that feature issues and scenarios that present challenges about the culture of disability. Some of the themes explored through their performances include transportation, employment, architectural barriers, the history of disability, societal attitudes, and other obstacles to leading a gratifying life. All of these themes invite an audience encounter with the world that they inhabit; the autistic ensemble members stand to gain a collective expression of the world they inhabit as well.

DisAbility Project performers include people with a variety of physical conditions such as spinal cord injuries, degenerative arthritis, Ehlers Danlos Syndrome, myelopathy, epilepsy, blindness, alcoholism, amputation, asthma, autism-spectrum diagnoses, bipolarity, blindness, brain injury, cancer, cerebral palsy, cognitive delay, depression, Down syndrome, epilepsy, HIV/AIDS, multiple sclerosis, polio, spina bifida, stroke, and other diagnoses, depending on the year and particular cast. Unlike more conventional theater, the theatrical experience changes dynamically with this kind of diversity in the cast. Many of those involved with the DisAbility Project, regardless of personal makeup and typicality, have experienced discrimination and oppression for their sexuality, race, physical status, neurological makeup, or other form of difference. Their lives have stood in contrast to those of society's *normates*, a term attributed to Thomson (1997) that represents the notion of the definitive human being as idealized in a fully functioning body, mind, and neurological system. This position requires its antipode, including autistic people, in order to establish its own sense of optimal existence. It is the task of autism-positive creatives to re-present this normativity and its impact on people defined and objectified by it. Nearly by definition, this task is similar to that of autistic people who must re-present their "neurotype" in an environment that has already labeled them as antipodals, when they demonstrate repeatedly that they exist.

By design, in order to diminish the privilege of norms and neurotypes, the DisAbility Project advances a wide range of disability experiences, using its institutional memory to honor the history of all the people who have crossed its path. The performances are designed to help all in attendance consider life from multiple perspectives. Furthermore, they engage audience members in challenging the general notion that those labeled disabled are deficient, incomparable to non-disabled people, and thus not privy to the opportunities that life affords to those of typical physical, neurological, and cognitive makeup. The program draws attention and support to the differences in the whole range of human experience rather than normalizing certain physicalities and mentalities while marginalizing others.

A Disability Aesthetic

The DisAbility Project uses theater to portray circumstances that provoke audiences and performers to consider challenging social issues from new perspectives. Disability and feminist studies inform this aesthetic, as well as the community struggles that might shape life in a Midwestern US city. Fox and Lipkin (2002) discuss how feminist theater and disability studies offer an alternative to theater that uses disability symbolically. As conceived, the DisAbility Project rejects the common practices of theater that so displaces autistic and disabled people. The academic expression of the artificial relationship in which the disabled community is often forced out of the theatrical environs comes from Mitchell and Snyder (2001), who term this phenomenon *dramaturgical prosthesis*: the manner in which dramatic narratives may serve as a means of response to the notion of the normate, the fabulous idealized human form as opposed to an appended, flawed, disabled form. This prosthetic addresses the need to fix anything that departs from this optimal form.

The ubiquitous use of disabled characters in literature and film contributes to the marginalization of disabled people, turning real people "dramaturgically" into metaphors that subject the same individuals and occlude the meanings they would construct for their own lives. Conversely, portraying accurate representations of the disability narrative to examine and reshape the prosthetic relationship can transport the audience to an empathic understanding to integrate the individuals with disabilities into the society that currently marginalizes them.

To reshape the theater's social relationship, Lipkin supervises and edits the development of most of the scripts in order to draw on the perspectives of the ensemble, both disabled and normate. Ultimately, the audience (whose feedback after shows contributes to the evolution of the scripts over time) is led on a journey through disability culture that entertains and educates by supporting the disability experience. This type of *devised theater* originates with some combination of writers, actors, directors, choreographers, and other contributors who identify a starting point such as a title, a theme, an incident, or other germ of a storyline and work out a plot or subject from this point of origin. In recognition of different forms of learning and creating, some work is generated through a sharing circle with the whole group, paired sharing, and individual writing. Lipkin maintains that there are many ways to "write" a story, and these approaches might include writing orally and having the text transcribed. Another of our techniques that might be useful for autistic people is to be interviewed on a topic and then have another ensemble member turn the text and perspective into a piece. Importantly, the production of each storyline is also reviewed for potential distress or alienation, since theater tends to push at limits, and "limits" can be as potent and dynamic as names in an autism-specific and disability world.

The ensemble's revised work also reflects the aesthetics of experimental theater as a form. As such, it is often deliberately malleable in its narrative structure and does not necessarily employ conventions of dramatic storytelling or theatrical rules. Instead, it is a unique form of theater that could never have existed in the form it takes without the specific performers who generate it. This particular strand of experimental form is highly flexible and context-dependent, but it is also designed for re-enactment and familiarization. Lipkin refines the loosely constructed story to produce a script. Devised theater is especially appropriate for community-based work because people are not pigeonholed into a prescribed notion of what they can play. The diverse composition of the ensemble insures that no single life experience epitomizes the others. Further, rather than serving as symbols of disability by using able-bodied actors to portray disabled characters, the performers typically embody their own conditions and thus speak from the experience of disability.

The Theatrical Model and Process

The DisAbility Project is complex and interactive, so to illustrate its theatrical model, it is useful to examine the subset of experiences attached to performances, beginning with setting the stage with educational activities before the show begins. This stage of the overall model includes planned interruptions and interludes, providing audience members the opportunity to be active participants in the theatrical process.

Pre-performance Activities

Although the Project performs for a variety of ages, including adults, we focus here on the young audiences to meet the objectives of this volume. Each performance is tailored for the needs of particular groups of youth. In order to focus these audiences for participation, the project's directors prepare thought-provoking pre-show activities. These pre-show activities serve to calm young audience members from the stimulation of traveling to and entering a possibly unfamiliar auditorium. To observe a show in a place filled with many new people and sounds can be a potentially disorienting, overstimulating experience for autistic children, as well as other youth who usually function best with order, predictability, and familiarity. Simultaneously, those who need stimulation have a place to discharge their energy; so this activity benefits and unites a wide range of theatergoers to atypical environments.

As students gather outside the performance area, they are given a worksheet with several options, including to write an answer to the question "Why am I a piece of art?" and to draw a portrait of themselves as well as a portrait of a family member, classmate, friend, or teacher, the latter helping to ground and connect them to significant others. They are given such sentence-starters as "I am a piece of art because" and "When I think about disability, I think about." This theme will be revisited later in the scripted performance. By giving students a choice of activities to express themselves through drawing or writing, the participants' multiple intelligences (Gardner 1983) are subtly engaged through the young people's composition across sign systems (Smagorinsky 1995). In working with students of mixed abilities, giving them choices is especially productive.

Lipkin often begins a show by asking the audience what their experience is with disability. Do they have any friends, neighbors, or family members with a disability? She opens up a space for sharing, and often children and youth with learning disabilities or who are autistic will self-identify and seem eager to do so. As Lipkin gets a feel for the audience, this episode may be followed by leading the audience in a round of "Hello My Friends," sung to the tune of "Shalom Havarim." If a number of schools are present, she may ask them to give a rousing shout out for their school and to wave at their new friends. Rather than trying to diminish energy, she embraces it and deliberately provides several outlets for harnessing the energy. Thus the students are independently and collectively engaged in the process before the show even begins. The pre-performance activities prepare the audience members similarly to the ways in which English/Language Arts teachers might use introductory activities that promote reflection on background knowledge for literary themes (Smagorinsky et al. 1987). Both contexts draw from the initiation of language—sometimes difficult for autistic children—to create meanings from words but also meaning from being. There is no failure in this practice, so young audiences need only to anticipate the excitement of live performance.

Humor is a central aspect of the ensemble's engagement with their audiences, in part to sustain a variety of connections, which humor allows. Lipkin and ensemble members use humor as they interact with the audience, and it is also an important part of the scripts. Proximity of shared emotions, especially through laughter, allows for the expectation of emotional guarding and emotional release. Self-defined ambassadors of goodwill who educate and entertain their audiences, the ensemble members rely on humor to help people relax and open themselves to the themes of the plays and the project overall. According to Lipkin:

> I try to do things with humor and grace because I know that people are uncomfortable with other people's differences. Unfortunately, the need to reach out and to adapt falls to those who are different, when it should fall to the normates, who have power and represent the dominant culture. [See Chap. 3.] Adaptational responsibility should fall to normates, but they are often afraid of difference, so we are put in the position of comforting our audience so that they can hear us. In one of our opening pieces, several performers who use wheelchairs in their daily life say, "We're here to have a good time, and we can't if you don't. So relax, sit back, enjoy yourself, and feel free to laugh. Deal?"

Autism-Inclusive Performance

The show often officially starts with a piece called "Are You Going to the Show?" (see Appendix 1), in which three people talk about attending a show on disability and what it might involve. Autism adds particular richness to an opening scene such as this, because the tension of involvement itself is central to both the autistic and theatrical experience. The script raises questions that will resonate through the remainder of the repertoire, challenging the audience to foster empathy for how the world is experienced from the perspective of someone with a disability classification. Thus the audience is welcomed into representation of autism, the broader culture of disability, and the themes of the day's performance.

During the scripted version of "I Am a Piece of Art," ensemble members present their own responses to the prompts previously given to the students as pre-show activity. They share what they consider to be their strengths, disrupting the notion that they are disabled and deficient, first and foremost. For example, an actor says, "I am a piece of art because I can move mountains with my wheelchair." The text of the ensemble is then enacted as a kinetic group sculpture. Through *narrative transportation* as defined by Gerrig (1993), the audience identifies with the disability culture by immersion in new stories of the disabled to replace possible pre-conceived ideas and attitudes. According to Bailey (2009), the shared live theater experience connects individuals and constructs community. Adaptations toward training the eye for the "narrative transportation" around the autism spectrum present their own challenge, but now there is a tool, a kinetic process that potentially "transports" the voice of the ensemble member and relocates its story, expanding the focus of how communication is operated on stage.

Building on new concepts at the same time, Lipkin or another ensemble member guides the audience on its journey, closing the gap between audience and performer, and introducing various pieces. Through this brokerage role, she normalizes difference by sharing statistics about disability as well as statistics about the general population, encouraging the audience members to share their personal stories beyond stereotypes. Fixed ideas become more fluid; the audiences begin to feel that difference is desirable and exciting rather than simply acknowledging it. Finally, Lipkin constantly scans the audience to see how the performance is received and checks on the energy and focus of the audience. This monitoring becomes a crucial part of any autism-specific experience, helping to manage a place that feels safe for the child who, psychoneurologically *or for any other reason*, feels unsafe. During this portion of the program, children and youth can safely volunteer their experiences and be recognized, a form of attention they are often denied in public spaces. Children watch each other as they dare to speak or come on stage to problem solve. Many times there are more volunteers to share than can be accommodated.

There are some theater elements easier to execute than others; the key is to manage a threshold for safety while still inviting dialogues, stories, and themes that point to the social injustice that many theatergoers are already experiencing. Throughout the performance with the DisAbility Project, Lipkin leads discussion generated by questions to the audience. For example, preceding the piece "Employment" (see Appendix 2), the audience is given facts, such as how disabled people in the USA comprise the largest unemployed and underemployed demographic, even though they have the largest retention rate. Most adaptations cost $500 or less. After this piece, the audience is acknowledged for their enthusiasm and commitment to the process of problem-solving. This recognition encourages further participation as the performance evolves, while lending the statistics more personal meaning.

This threshold of safety and social justice framework must be maintained, which can be challenging, but the by-product of a safe environment is the extraordinary transfer of disability culture strength, the empathy of difference. Through the witnessing of actors and audience, the DisAbility Project shares personal experiences throughout the show, validated at each interlude. These breaks are more or less scripted and come as often as necessary to include the audience in an exploration of themes for the various short plays to follow. They serve as an artistic channel for empathy to mirror the prominent gift of the audience: the potency of their empathy. Through interruption of the dramatic action, audience members may experience and channel empathy for others. This technique engages the whole body and allows time for the audience to digest one experience before moving on to the next. Finally, a number of audience members, including those on the autism spectrum, are welcomed on stage at intervals built into the production.

Through these exchanges, the DisAbility Project both calls attention to and distances its participants from the notion of disability; the audience and ensemble could be readily directed more specifically to one difference, such as autism, but the DisAbility Project company's discussions situate the specific experience more widely within a civic theater. They lead to a questioning of the cultural framing of disability in terms of the public perceptions and the specific challenges to the disability community. Jettisoning the more typical terminology of disability with which the audience is likely familiar and replacing it with potentially awkward and alienating new language might be of long-term benefit to, but immediate estrangement from, the performances and their intent.

Lipkin thus uses extant, familiar terms while simultaneously questioning their connotations, providing a conundrum common to challenges to the status quo: by calling attention to the oppressive terminology familiar to most people and often in circulation, a vocabulary that we have used throughout this chapter, she calls attention to its oppressive nature and the ways in which it marginalizes people. In educating the audience on the deep-seated connotations of these words, young audience members gain an understanding of the power of language. According to the company's post-show surveys (explained next), audience members leave with an intention to speak differently.

These practices break radically from conventional theater and require careful and purposeful experimentation if the artistry based on disability and difference is to grow in substance. The DisAbility Project integrates actors and audience members of mixed abilities by shared participation in the performance, but the interactivity of ensemble and audience is key to the transference of disability (and specifically autistic) authenticity. Rather than spectatorship, the audience reacts during the performance about what they are seeing as the action unfolds. Project directors adapt the shows and the environment for different audiences at different performances (see Chap. 3), "keeping it real." Simultaneously, access to the content of the plays and interludes needs careful tending, since the accommodation of youth with disabilities often flags, and optimal inclusion is lost. Adaptations could include dimming auditorium lights and lowering the sound level for autistic youth who could become overstimulated. These adjustments alone demonstrate how realistically to design a family-friendly autism performance for extant theater programs seeking to welcome autistic audiences.

Post-performance

After thanking the audience for their positive participation, the ensemble announces that they would like to transition from performance to a wider conversation with the following words: "We are of you. We are among you.

We are you. Do not be afraid." Post-performance, the audience members are prompted to turn to each other in pairs to share a moment that really spoke to them. This occasion allows them to revisit and validate what was meaningful for them individually and gives them a rehearsal in articulating their ideas for the wider conversation as the ensemble reassembles on stage. The ensemble members de-role, re-introduce themselves by name, and share a bit of personal information to move from the emphasis of performer to person. No stipulations are placed on the talk back. The auditorium and stage are still a "safe space." Lipkin emphasizes that "There are no stupid questions and nothing is off limits." The audience is invited to ask questions, share responses, and share personal stories evoked by the performance. In one sense, this repartee between the audience and ensemble is part of the authentic performance, except that the roles are reversed; ensemble members can observe what the audience makes visible.

The Scripts

As a professional playwright with a strong bent toward socially relevant themes and underserved populations, Lipkin has worked extensively not only with disability populations, but with women facing cancer, LGBTQ youth and adults, people with early-stage dementia and Alzheimer's, vulnerable youth, women who have been sexually trafficked, survivors of torture, people recovering from substance abuse, communities of faith, and college students. She regularly builds on a foundation of difficult tasks about inequity, justice, and the material conditions for marginalized people.

Since the performances are interactive, the scripts include specific points for audience engagement. As each audience is different, the scripts are often adapted and re-written for a particular audience, so there are several versions of each script. These adjustments are based on notes and observations of the engagement of the audience. At a recent performance in an art museum, for instance, Lipkin asked the audience, "Who here likes rap?" One autistic boy said he liked to rap and wanted to, so he was spontaneously invited on stage. He ran up and joined the ensemble, but once on stage, he didn't know what to do. What became apparent was that he simply wanted to participate. When asked if he had a rapper whose work he could perform, he said yes. Provided with a beat, he performed the piece and was affirmed by the audience with an enthusiastic ovation.

By making space for these spontaneous interactions, Lipkin generates ideas on how to modify scripts that invite audience engagement and explore new directions for future work. In this fashion, the scripts stay relevant as the project grows. It is worth noting, as well, that the creation of a short play from a script attributes a powerful form of authorship. When the script continues on in the repertory of the DisAbility Project, the experience and authority of the people who created that work are perpetuated as well.

The DisAbility Project relies on a repertoire of about 20 short plays written by Lipkin and other project members, from which roughly 8–12 comprise any given performance. These plays are based on themes related to daily life, including any issue that surrounds people considered disabled and has an impact on their ability to enter into the flow of cultural practice (see Chap. 2). Tangible issues help the company to push the envelope on the cultural ignorance and exclusion of disability. In addition, some scripts include attention to disability history (see Appendix 2). The group also performs works that are primarily visual in nature, featuring innovative movement and stage images created by performers with disabilities as another form for meaning making. By using verbal and non-verbal language, Lipkin adds to the artistic experience while supporting visual learning styles.

Rather than performing one lengthy play interwoven with multiple complex themes, the ensemble performs relatively short plays that do not strain the attention spans of the young audience members. The large repertoire allows the ensemble to select plays appropriate for the composition of the audience, which may range from second graders to adults and may be heavily populated by people embodying particular forms of difference. Some of the cast members also have brain-processing differences that work against remembering long scripts, and the shorter pieces are better adapted to their memory capabilities. Neuro-atypical experience may well produce some unexpected results, not the least of which is the art "imprint" that is created by working on the quality of communication and expression by participants on the autism spectrum. Scripting will have new challenges but also even more richness, as the ensemble's collective recall of these scripts comes to be. With a repertoire of short pieces, different people in the company can take on a variety of characters, which offers more opportunities for actors to expand their versatility and to do what is asked of any artist: to explore and connect.

As the selection of scripts is customized for each audience and sequenced thematically for exploration of the ideas throughout the entire series, careful consideration to which scripts to use for which performances is an on-going part of the process. Lipkin explained this sequence: "The experience of any performance is an emotional, spiritual, intellectual, and visceral journey. The arc of that journey is crafted carefully." In this sense, the stories, rather than having a discrete role in the repertoire, are elements of an overarching narrative whose storylines are tied together within the possibilities of related themes, and positioned dialogically within the broader conversation.

Audience members learn how difference has been portrayed historically, such as when they learn that "Freak shows exhibiting the bodies of disabled men and women were common entertainment in the Victorian period." They further learn that these debilitating conceptions of difference refer to a great number of people in modern society, such as when they learn that "People with disabilities are the largest minority in the United States." These issues of physical disability are often tied with other assumptions of deficiency, such as when the script informs them that "During witch trials, many of the women who were tried for witchcraft had disabilities," linking disability theater with historical feminist concerns.

To demonstrate, there is a sequence of scenes that address the harshness faced by disabled people who work, and they are presented so as to affect the cultural prejudice, followed by attention to how these biases affect a disabled woman and those around her, after which there are interludes and postscripts that involve a broadening of why this discrimination must change, designed to provoke the audience into action. *Facts and Figures* (see Appendix 2) and *Employment* (see Appendix 3) are often performed early in the sequence to inform the audience of the effects of language. This feminist critique of history undermines the tendency toward conceiving of disability only as a pejorative, in which people of difference are depicted as being of lesser humanity, such as when people refer to a weak excuse as "lame" or a foolish act as "retarded." In these short plays, the ensemble seeks to awaken the audience to attend to language differently and have their experience of the performance be grounded in a sense of history as a past form of what the ensemble is developing in the present.[3]

As the title suggests, *Facts and Figures*, the most informational of the three plays, is written to help able-bodied audience members understand that differences cannot be simply ignored, while also helping anomalous people to cohere emotionally and politically around their shared, perceived disabilities. The play helps to contest the notion of the normate, the optimal human condition realized in the able-bodied. In essence, this script takes on a feminist theme of being "othered," that is, being constructed as an outsider and a threat (see Chap. 2). Othering is used to amplify the presumed weaknesses of those in marginalized groups in order to assert the superior strength and value of those in power. *Facts and Figures* helps audience members recognize that figures of speech such as "You are so ADD" and the common phrase thrown at children on the autism spectrum, "you are so weird," are laden with deficit assumptions about whole classes of people, and that terms often used casually may reify the notion that difference is deficit; one trait of microaggressions—the everyday affronts, rejections, or insults that communicate hostility, disrespect, and condescension toward people based on their marginalized status—is that they are often unintentional (Sue 2010).

In contrast, *Employment* (see Appendix 3), the next script in the sequence, involves a young woman in a wheelchair applying for a job at a mall during a heavy shopping season. The manager of the business becomes very anxious because of his discomfort in dealing with, and his preconceptions about, her disability. Rather than dealing with his discomfort, the manager begins making excuses about why she won't be hired or is not hirable. The woman responds with options and solutions that the manager isn't ready to accept. The employer assumes that having a worker in a wheelchair might "turn off the customers," that the applicant might have little capacity for performing "a pretty demanding job," and that she can only find work in "sheltered workshop." The job hunter in exasperation addresses the audience directly, "Can this situation be saved?" The audience is vested with the responsibility of the outcome by generating the ending to the scene. Lipkin stops the scene and assists by explaining that often adults don't understand or are uptight about different experiences in life. She asks the student audiences for suggestions to help the young woman in the wheelchair explain how she would fill this position and its duties well. This invitation typically produces a great deal of advice from the audience, with some children and youth coming up on stage to share their recommendations. In this way the performance serves as a stimulus for reflection and discussion, rather than didactically depicting proper solutions to societal misunderstandings and misperceptions about those who are different.

Employment challenges assumptions about what people are capable of, further emphasized by using the term *ableist attitudes*, which fundamentally discriminate by the exclusion of the contributions of the disabled. This piece especially links these themes to the emphasis in feminist theater on economic inequities, with the special twist here on how assumptions are compounded when disability intersects with to gender issues. The challenges are made public when the audience is asked to participate in how the action might be different, using activist methods of involvement. This approach to generating ideas requires audience members to abandon the spectator role and become scriptwriters themselves. By asking the audience members to connect their own experience and language with those of the job seeker, the script helps to validate the feeling of rejection while building empathy and promoting collaboration as a problem-solving tool.

A final, less tangible and important result comes from script sequences. The ordering of content connects into extra-theatrical contexts long after the performance is over. As autism-specific theater is explored for the general public, its place within the schema of difference may prove radical. Just as actors in the DisAbility Project rework the effects of new sequences for their scripts, autism creatives are facing their own place in disability culture and difference. An autism-specific theater may revolutionize the sequencing of scenes and plays.

One dimension of the spectrum experience is the use of repetition for control. This tendency is not a universal trait of people on the autism spectrum, but the design of how ideas and expression unfold in disability theaters is highly energized toward the representation of differences like repetition (indeed to a degree, most performances are repetitions). The specific choices of language and material also may be framed and formed in ways that enhance the art in disability theater as well. An autism-friendly theater asks what language and what material may be framed in productive ways. Crutchfield and Epstein (2000) see the experience of autism as exposing and indicting a culture more invested in a *status quo* of trauma than in its healing.[4] To the autistic person, this world is always scary, rarely safe, and often damaging, particularly to one's senses. The repetition and safety needed to generate autism narrative and reconstruction tells the immediate environment of disability that this spectrum of neurodiversity is not just part of a rainbow. The content of autism creativity is enormous, so ornate as to require a return, again and again, to the point of disconnection. Yet still, the autistic creative is required constantly to do what is most traumatic, in the theater: to connect through a dangerous fourth wall.[5] The DisAbility Project ponders this connection, its tenuousness, and the edification found when connection is done truly humanely.

Audience Survey and Participant Testimonials

At this stage of autistic representation—contrary to typical disability depiction—the goal is to begin learning about autism and advocating for it as the community finds its own voice. Advocacy is central to The DisAbility Project's core mission: to approach everyone as is, safely, and to make communication the beginning of community change. Each DisAbility Project performance thus concludes with a survey (see Fig. 7.1) distributed to those in attendance. This survey serves three purposes. First, it allows participants to think about their attitudes and beliefs following the performances. Second, it informs the project directors about how the performances have functioned and the effects it has had on the audience,

---

The DisAbility Project theater response

YOUR NAME: _____ GRADE: ___ SCHOOL:

_____

Please circle Yes or No to the questions below. THIS IS NOT A TEST AND IS NOT GRADED!

Your response will help our actors and our ability to reach out to other new audiences.

1) YES / NO .... I am now more likely to say "Hello" to someone with a disability.

2) YES / NO .... I am less likely to use words that people might find hurtful.

3) YES / NO .... I am more likely to make friends with people with disabilities.

4) YES / NO .... I am more likely to stand up for someone who is being disrespected.

5) YES / NO .... I am less likely to be quiet if someone able-bodied parks in a disabled spot.

6) YES / NO .... I am more likely to agree that people with disabilities can sing, dance, and act.

7) YES / NO .... Today I have seen people with disabilities do things I didn't know they could do.

Any other comments for us:

_____

Fig. 7.1 Survey

to gather and learn from its own work. As noted, Lipkin and colleagues revise their scripts over time, in part based on how the audience evaluates them in these surveys, and how the ensemble reflects on them. Finally, it provides data to report back to sponsors and donors.[6]

The perspective-changing impact of the DisAbility Project is not limited to audience members. Because of the collaboration between audience and actors, ensemble members report major changes in their own orientation to issues of cognitive, neurological, and bodily difference. Ensemble member Rich Scharf, for instance, testified,

> Originally, it meant just an opportunity to create some theater with a woman who was nationally known in performance art circles. I wasn't necessarily attracted to or repulsed by the subject matter of the theater we would be creating, just interested in getting some acting experience. Of course, it has come to mean much more to me. It has raised my consciousness in a way that I was not aware needed raising. It has helped me to lose my fear of disability. It has made me realize that we can handle whatever God has given us. It's taught me that we can not only survive calamity but thrive as well. I hope it's made me a more sympathetic and empathetic human being. And it's given me lots of theater acting and writing experience!

This sort of reflection is typical of the ensemble's able-bodied performers who sign up for the acting and sign on to the notion of disability: the idea that being different is not a sign of deficiency, disorder, abnormality, diminishment, or other societal misconceptions. Scarf derives his theatrical experience via validation of disability culture rather than despite it. Through engagement with other performers who have a disability classification, and by means of interaction with audience members from across the various disability spectra, the experience of interrogating difference through dramatic art may influence these performers to become disability advocates for the 20 % of the US population whose makeup does not follow the evolutionary norm.

Similarly, members of the ensemble who themselves are classified as having a disability report personal changes through their engagement with the plays. The late cast member Thea de Luna, for instance, stated that

> Four years ago, I joined The DisAbility Project. Since I became a member of the ensemble, I've developed a great deal more self-respect with the knowledge that I'm making a difference in how people look at disability. My own

perspective on disability has also changed. I used to feel very self-conscious about my disability. Now, I find myself motivated to find new ways to adapt. The DisAbility Project is a great support system. I've made new friendships, and feel far less isolated than I used to. Acting on stage has helped me improve my speech, too.

This testimony is corroborated by other statements by cast members whose lives have been characterized by some form of difference. Significantly, the developmental mission of The DisAbility Project is realized across the range of participants, from actors to audience members to observers. In contrast to conventional theater, The DisAbility Project is designed to go beyond an afternoon's entertainment by affecting and challenging beliefs and attitudes about a large, often neglected part of the population whose lives have often been termed defective and worthless to society.

Discussion

In some senses, this chapter relies on some traditional theater values: a community of players, the creation of alternative worlds and new adventures, and the demonstration of the broadest and deepest human experience. Like participants in the autism-specific programs described throughout this section of the book, those in The DisAbility Project are given ample opportunity to play with their beliefs and to hypothesize about how they would act in situations similar to those depicted on the stage. The opportunity to take the stage during interludes allows for audience members to participate in the performances in ways that take advantage of their assets, often through opportunities to explore their emerging identities as people of difference. The mix of observation and participation allows for both (1) modeling and exemplification, and (2) a deeper understanding and empathy for the issues intersecting with disability.

As the curtain comes down metaphorically, the ensemble moves on and audience members are left with new ideas and beliefs of what it means to live life differently with a physical or cognitive disability. The palpability of the performance, paired with the intellectual intones of the interludes, complements the way many human brains function. Further, audience members may develop new ways of challenging obstructions to their personal potential, allowing them to participate in the construction of new social scripts outside the theater in which the greatest diversity of people enjoy the same opportunities for happiness and success as those for whom the world is already a comfortable, seemingly natural, and empowering place.

Specific to autism, removing obstacles to realizing potential will likely bring a wide range of results to theatergoers and creatives. Performances and scripts are built on the notion of dramatic tension such that ambivalence is brought to the foreground of relationships that teeter on the edge between acceptance and rejection, confidence and insecurity, self-awareness and other-awareness, and other emotions that arise when comfortable worldviews are contested. The DisAbility project continues to research techniques for supportive inclusion, including autism self-representation as promoted by the Autism Theater Initiative (see Viswanathan 2015). Harry Smolit, a 16-year-old consultant with ATI, says that

> My experience with TDF has shown me that I can use my autism to help people enjoy the theater as much as I do. One of the biggest problems I have is that I don't like the unexpected. The more information you give me ahead [of time], the less likely it is that anything will upset me.... If the show is going to start five or more minutes late, you should make an announcement and tell the people not to worry. (cited by Viswanathan; n. p.)

During and following successful performances at the DisAbility Project, we now aim toward a greater response to autism contexts nationally, improving the quality of representation, access, and creativity for autistic people with other disabled and able-bodied people, thus bringing the autism experience back into a more general but also more culturally rich theater. The participants who experiment with social rules and assumptions through this kind of autism-engagement with storylines may stand "a head taller" than before, to use Vygotsky's (2002/1933) phrase: not just children and youth on the autism spectrum, but neurotypicals whose growth into more aware and other-centered people helps to create more integrative environments for a greater range of people. If self-regulation is a consequence of play-oriented performance that tests boundaries and questions assumptions, then new rules will emerge to guide future behavior.

An ideal outcome of the performances is that some blend of adaptive behaviors emerges and oppressed people rise. Rejoining the reality of difference, typical and atypical participants alike become motivated to achieve the social goal of acceptance, using tools made available through the performances. These tools help make deliberate adjustments to how each individual presents to others who do not yet understand diverse ways of navigating the world. Typicals who pay attention to their own specificity would adapt to those adjustments by how they relate on a more visceral, humane level to the expression of ability and dignity of all societal members. When The DisAbility Project's performances meet these goals, they help each audience to return to their origins, committed to reconstructing their home settings to accommodate the full range of people who populate their places of work, play, and leisure, making for a better, richer public.

The wonder of theater and the wonder of autism are similar; their vision of a better world is not limited to the perceived norm. Autism, situated among the wealth of disability experience and culture, is normal for some people and expansive of normality itself. The transcribed words of Naoko Higashida[7] (2013), a non-verbal 13-year-old autistic boy who learned to communicate through the use of an alphabet grid, ask readers to look closely at what they consider normal:

> Well, I bet the people around us—our parents and teachers—would be ecstatic with joy and say, "Hallelujah! We'll change them back to normal right now!" And for ages and ages I badly wanted to be normal, too. Living with special needs is so depressing and so relentless; I used to think it'd be the best thing if I could just live my life like a normal person.
>
> But no, even if somebody developed a medicine to cure autism, I might well choose to stay as I am. Why have I come to think this way?
>
> To give the short version, I've learned that every human being, with or without disabilities, needs to strive to do their best, and by striving for happiness you will arrive at happiness. For us, you see, having autism is normal—so we can't know for sure what your "normal" is even like. But so long as we learn to love ourselves, I'm not sure how much it matters whether we're normal or autistic. (p. 45)

Higashida's uncertainty regarding how much normality, disability, and autism *matter* is exactly what our theaters should strive for, as well.

Appendix 1: You Going to the Show?

PERSON 1: You going to the show?
PERSON 2: Don't know. Are you going?
PERSON 1: Don't know. It's kind of weird.

PERSON 3: No kidding. I heard they're in wheelchairs. What are they going to do, feed them their lines?

PERSON 1: How else are they going to remember them? There's no other way.

PERSON 2: How would you remember your lines? You would memorize them. They memorize them, dummy.

PERSON 3: I still don't know. I feel weird sitting there, staring at a bunch of people. Doesn't it freak them out?

PERSON 2: Why would it freak them out? They're used to being stared at.

PERSON 1: 'Cuz they're, you know, different.

PERSON 3: And weak.

PERSON 1: Yeah, and come on. They can't even walk.

PERSON 2: Hey! My grandma can't walk!

PERSON 3: Yeah, but that's your grandma and she's old.

PERSON 1: And you don't HAVE to go see your grandma perform on stage.

PERSON 3: That's right. I kind of resent having to be here. What's it supposed to be? The politically correct thing to do? Watch a bunch of handicapped people try to act.

PERSON 2: Whoa, whoa, whoa!!! Wait a minute—

PERSON 1: Aren't they calling them, disabled these days?

PERSON 3: WHATEVER!!!!!!

PERSON 1: I wouldn't be here if I didn't HAVE to come for credit. That is so lame.

PERSON 2: Actually, my class (or department-customize so it fits the venue) doesn't HAVE to be here.

PERSON 1: They don't? Why are you goin' then?

PERSON 2: I thought it might be interesting and I kinda felt sorry for them. I didn't want no one to show up.

PERSON 3: I guess I do kinda feel sorry for them, too. But I always feel so guilty around people like them.

PERSON 2: Why?

PERSON 3: Because I can walk and they can't.

PERSON 2: So what? They use a wheelchair. Big deal. You get around usin' a car and no one feels sorry for you.

PERSON 3: Hey! You're talking about my ride! Don't dis the wheels! My wheels are sacred. Plus, I don't even know anyone who uses a wheelchair.

PERSON 2: I do. My grandma.

PERSON 1: But that's not the same. That's family!

PERSON 2: They're people just like us. They have families, eat, sleep, and go to the bathroom just like we do.

PERSON 1: Whoa! I know they go to the bathroom, but I know they don't go like we do.

PERSON 3: That's gross! I don't even want to think about it!

PERSON 1: You think that's gross. What if they have sex?

PERSON 3: They don't have sex! They can't!

PERSON 2: They're not the only ones not having sex. Look at your sex life.

PERSON 3: Let's leave my sex life out of it.

PERSON 2: I think we already have! (*Chairs circle*)

PERSON 1: Hey audience, we're not what you expected, are we?

PERSON 2: Welcome to a guilt-free zone. Sit back, relax, and enjoy yourselves. We are here to educate and entertain.

PERSON 3: If you don't have a good time, then we don't have a good time, deal?

PERSON 1 & 3: And we wanna have a good time

ALL: So, let the show begin!!

Appendix 2: Facts and Figures

Version #1: For Young Audience, 15 Items

ONE: That is so retarded.

TWO: A long, long time ago, they thought people got disabilities because they were bad and deserved them.

THREE: It would be horrible to be confined to a wheelchair.

FOUR: During witch trials, many of the women who were tried for witchcraft had disabilities.

FIVE: Man, you are so lame.

SIX: Court jesters (like the hunchback) with physical disabilities were common entertainment through much of European history.

SEVEN: Those kids are such freaks.

EIGHT: They used to sell tickets at carnivals to see people with disabilities, saying they were freaks or monsters.

NINE: Hey, why don't you look where you're going?! Are you blind?

TEN: People with disabilities are the largest minority in the United States.

ELEVEN: Hey, four eyes!

TWELVE: He/she/ze[8] is psycho.

THIRTEEN: Many people with disabilities have a hard time working because it is hard for them to get a ride to work or employers won't give them a job.

FOURTEEN: You are so ADD.

FIFTEEN: Most people with disabilities live below the poverty line.

Version #2: For Adult Audience, 16 Items

ONE: That is so retarded.

TWO: In medieval times, they thought people got disabilities because they were bad and deserved them.

THREE: The industry has been crippled.

FOUR: During witch trials, many of the women who were tried for witchcraft had disabilities.

FIVE: He's a lame duck.

SIX: Court jesters with physical disabilities were common entertainment through much of European history.

SEVEN: Those kids are such freaks.

EIGHT: Freak shows exhibiting the bodies of disabled men and women were common entertainment in the Victorian period.

NINE: Hey, why don't you look where you're going?! Are you blind?

TEN: People with disabilities are the largest minority in the United States.

ELEVEN: Hey, four eyes!

TWELVE: In many places in the world, children with physical disabilities are killed or abandoned at birth.

THIRTEEN: He/she/ze is psycho.

FOURTEEN: People with disabilities are the most underemployed population in the country. Mostly because our transportation systems make it difficult for them to get jobs, or employers won't hire them.

FIFTEEN: You are so ADD.

SIXTEEN: Most people with disabilities live below the poverty line.

Appendix 3: Employment

[*Depending on the audience (age, background, etc.), there are two possible endings to this play, to allow for maximal audience participation and creativity.*]

Characters: Sales Person, Manager, Job Seeker, Wild Shopper #1, Wild Shopper #2, Wild Shopper #3, Wild Shopper Crowd

(*Sales Person is found amidst the Wild Shoppers. The roar of the shoppers compels the Sales Person to run to the front of the store, excited and flustered.*)

SALES PERSON: It's a jungle out there! I'm putting in for combat pay.

MANAGER: You're just a little tired.

SALES PERSON: I won't go back in there.

(*Wild Shoppers roar and improvise comments again. Items of clothing go flying.*)

I won't. (*Starts to sob.*)

MANAGER: There, there—

SALES PERSON: Have you ever worked the post-Christmas sale?

(*More frenzy from the Wild Shoppers. Perhaps more roar. Sales Person sobs.*)

Post-Christmas. Pre-Christmas. Columbus Day?!!! I need more help.

MANAGER: We're doing all we can. But good help is hard to find.

(*Sales Person continues to sob. In rolls Job Seeker who is using a wheelchair.*)

JOB SEEKER: Excuse me. I'm here about the job.

MANAGER: Oh, you must be looking for the sheltered workshop. It's at the other end of the mall.

JOB SEEKER: No, I meant the job here. The one that was listed in the newspaper.

MANAGER: Oh. There must be some mistake. You see, we. Sell. Clothes.

JOB SEEKER: Yes, I can see that. And I wear clothes. That's why I'm here. I live to accessorize.

SALES PERSON: Fantastic! I love what you're wearing.

(*Manager pulls Sales Person aside to talk with her privately.*)

MANAGER: Excuse me. We can't hire her. It'll turn off the customers.

SALES PERSON: Oh, I don't know. She's more enthusiastic than most of the people we have working on the floor. And perky. You did say that perky was part of the job description. And she obviously loves clothes.

JOB SEEKER (*To audience*): I do love clothes. I get my inspiration from Project Runway—only the best designs.

MANAGER: It's not just that. The aisles are too crowded. She couldn't get through.

(*Wild Shoppers roar.*)

JOB SEEKER: I'd really like to work here. If you'd just take a look at my resume you could see I'm qualified.

SALES PERSON: And I'd like to do something but my hands are tied.

JOB SEEKER: Can this situation be saved?

(*Everyone hums theme song from Jeopardy. A Wild Shopper breaks away from the group to offer an alternative scenario.*)

WILD SHOPPER #1: Excuse me. I have an idea. Could we roll this scene back a little?

(*The Wild Shopper, Sales Person and Manager mime rolling back of time. The scene resumes.*)

JOB SEEKER: I'd really like to work here. If you'd just—

SALES PERSON: And I'd like to do something but my hands are tied.

WILD SHOPPER #1: (*Approaching Sales Person*) I have been here for an hour and a half and no one has offered to help. Or even said hello. What you need around here is a little more friendliness. Why couldn't she work as a greeter?

JOB SEEKER: (*To audience*) Hi. Hi. How ya doing? Thank you for coming. I love those shoes.

WILD SHOPPER #1: See? She's a natural.

MANAGER: I don't know. I'm not sure that something like that is in our budget.

WILD SHOPPER #1: Sheesh. Even Wal-Mart has a greeter. I'm not shopping here any more!

(*Wild Shopper #1 goes back to crowd. Everyone hums the Jeopardy song again, this time a little faster. Wild Shopper #2 interrupts before it ends*).

WILD SHOPPER #2: You say the aisles are too crowded? I agree. It's way too crowded in here. (*To audience*) How about if she were a cashier?

JOB SEEKER: (*To audience*) Cha-ching! Cha-ching!

(*The Wild Shoppers roar*)

SALES PERSON: We do need to open up another register.

MANAGER: I don't know. It's a pretty demanding job. How do I know that she is responsible?

JOB SEEKER: Oh, I'm very good with money. You have to be when you love clothes as much as I do.

MANAGER: I'm sure you are. (*To Sales Person*) But we'd have to make special arrangements for her. You know with the equipment and all. It could be expensive.

WILD SHOPPER #2: How expensive could it be? She already has her own chair! Good luck, lady.

[THERE ARE TWO POSSIBLE ENDINGS THAT BEGIN HERE]

Ending #1

(*Manager is clearly non-committal, so Wild Shopper #2 goes back to crowd. Wild Shopper #3 approaches.*)

WILD SHOPPER #3: You know anyone who loves clothes as much as she does—and I must say, you look mahvelous—

JOB SEEKER: Thank you, dahling.

WILD SHOPPER #3: Any one who loves clothes as much as she does should be a personal buyer.

JOB SEEKER: Oh, yes. I'd love it! And I would love to spend somebody else's money for them.

MANAGER: How would she get around?

JOB SEEKER: Hey, I got here, didn't I?

MANAGER: I don't know.

WILD SHOPPER #3: Well, I do. (*To Job Seeker*) Here's my card. (*To Manager*) I'm with that little department store down the street.

MANAGER: Not Le Blah Blah Blah?!

WILD SHOPPER #3: The very one.

SALES PERSON: And are you Monsieur/Madame Blee Blee Blee?!

WILD SHOPPER #3: Indeed, I am.

MANAGER and **SALES PERSON:** Oh no!

WILD SHOPPER #3: And I know talent when I see it. (*To Job Seeker*) Shall we discuss the details over lunch? (*He leaves, and she follows.*)

JOB SEEKER: Cha-Ching, Cha-Ching, Cha-Ching!

(*Wild shoppers roar, Sales Person and Manager look at each other in disbelief. Sales Person begins to sob and is absorbed into the crowd of Wild Shoppers.*)

(End Scene)

Ending #2

(*At this point, Sales Person could ask the audience if they have any ideas and then bring them up to discuss them. Improv is involved. Job Seeker remains enthusiastic and Manager is uncomfortable and unconvinced. After the audience has come up to propose several endings, the ensemble needs to bring the scene to a strong close.*)

SALES PERSON: (*To Manager*) So, what do you think?

MANAGER: I'm not sure.

JOB SEEKER: Look, I could be a greeter, a cashier. (*Job Seeker, and perhaps Sales Person, mentions the other possibilities that have been raised.*) Maybe you've just never worked with someone like me before. Please think about it. You know, open your mind.

MANAGER: You're right. And I really will.

SALES PERSON: Just do it soon, please?! (*The Salesperson returns to pack of Wild Shoppers who roar*). I need help fast!

(End Scene)

Notes

1. We use this term reluctantly in this context as part of the lingua franca of how human difference is discursively constructed in society and even among academics who challenge the notion of disability.
2. This value appears to be in place for the majority of autism-specific theatrical programs around the country, a prime example being the "theatrical intervention research program" called SENSE ("Social Emotional NeuroScience Endocrinology") begun by Blythe Corbett of Vanderbilt University (see http://www.sensetheatre.com/staff.html). Interestingly, several Autism-specific programs combine person-first language with a more abstract reference to the condition and/or experience of autism itself, for example, Theater Horizon's Autism Drama Program and the Autism Theater Initiative of the NY Theater Development Fund.
3. *Facts and Figures* was created by Joan Lipkin in conjunction with a class when she was an artist in Residence at Davidson College in North Carolina in March 2001. Lipkin instructed the group of students she was working with to create an original piece, and to research historical facts about the attitude and treatment of disabled people, as well as figures of speech concerning disabilities. Together they created *Facts and Figures*, which was originally done in performance at Davidson and then became part of the project's repertoire. *Employment* was developed in rehearsal through conversations and improvisations by participants of the DisAbility Project and has undergone revisions over time, as suggested by the availability of different endings to the drama.

4. Epstein's work in narration and trauma has led her to a home community of autism spectrum, to exploring what an autism-specific experience entails.
5. The *fourth wall* is the imaginary "wall" at the front of the stage in a traditional theater through which the audience views the drama. Speaking to the audience is known as "breaking the fourth wall." It is distinct from soliloquys and asides, which are not necessarily dialogues with the audience.
6. The DisAbility Project carries a 501(c)(3) classification from the Internal Revenue Service and is primarily funded through grants and donations. The company does not charge for individual attendance, and so it relies on sponsors to fund its performances and on-going activities.
7. All of 12-year-old Naoki's thoughts and expressions are ventriloquated through his editor, who may have taken liberties to produce such articulate observations.
8. "Ze" is an ungendered pronoun applied to those who do not identify with either masculine or feminine pronouns.

References

Bailey, S. (2009). Performance in drama therapy. In D. R. Johnson & R. Emunah (Eds.), *Current approaches in drama therapy* (2nd ed., pp. 374–392). Springfield: Charles C. Thomas.

Crutchfield, S., & Epstein, M. (Eds.). (2000). *Points of contact: Disability, art, and culture.* Ann Arbor: University of Michigan Press.

Dunn, D. S., & Andrews, E. E. (2015). Person-first and identity-first language: Developing psychologists' cultural competence using disability language. *American Psychologist, 70*(3), 255–264.

Fox, A. M., & Lipkin, J. (2002). Res(crip)ting feminist theater through disability theater: Selections from The DisAbility Project. *NWSA Journal, 14*(3), 77–98. Retrieved October 7, 2015, from http://www.madehereproject.org/uploads/files/disability_theater_1.pdf

Gardner, H. (1983). *Frames of mind: The theory of multiple intelligences.* New York: Basic Books.

Gerrig, R. J. (1993). *Experiencing narrative worlds: On the psychological activities of reading.* New Haven: Yale University Press.

Greenspan, S. I., & Greenspan, N. T. (2010). *The learning tree: Overcoming learning disabilities from the ground up.* Cambridge, MA: Da Capo Press.

Higashida, N. (2013). *The reason I jump: One boy's voice from the silence of autism* (trans: Mitchell, D. & Yoshida, K.). London: Spectre.

Mitchell, D. T., & Snyder, S. L. (2001). *Narrative prosthesis: Disability and the dependencies of discourse.* Ann Arbor: University of Michigan Press.

Sandahl, C., & Auslander, P. (Eds.) (2005). *Bodies in commotion: Disability & performance.* Ann Arbor: University of Michigan Press.

Siegel, D. (2011). *Mindsight: The new science of personal transformation.* New York: Bantam Books.

Smagorinsky, P. (1995). Constructing meaning in the disciplines: Reconceptualizing writing across the curriculum as composing across the curriculum. *American Journal of Education, 103,* 160–184. Available at http://www.petersmagorinsky.net/About/PDF/AJE/AJE1995.pdf

Smagorinsky, P., McCann, T., & Kern, S. (1987). *Explorations: Introductory activities for literature and composition, grades 7–12.* Urbana: National Council of Teachers of English. Retrieved November 12, 2015, from http://smago.coe.uga.edu/Books/Explorations.pdf

Sue, D. W. (2010). *Microaggressions in everyday life: Race, gender and sexual orientation.* Hoboken: Wiley.

Thomson, R. G. (1997). *Extraordinary bodies: Figuring physical disability in American culture and literature.* New York: Columbia University Press.

United States Census Bureau. (2012). *Statistical abstract of the United States: 2012.* Washington, DC: Author. Retrieved November 12, 2015, from https://www.census.gov/library/publications/2011/compendia/statab/131ed.html

Viswanathan, V. (2015). Making theater autism-friendly. *The Atlantic.* Retrieved November 12, 2015, from http://www.theatlantic.com/health/archive/2015/04/making-theater-autism-friendly/388348/

Vygotsky, L. S. (2002/1933). *Play and its role in the mental development of the child* (trans: Mulholland, C.). Retrieved October 7, 2014, from https://www.marxists.org/archive/vygotsky/works/1933/play.htm

Woodruff, P. (2010). *The necessity of theater: The art of watching and being watched.* New York: Oxford University Press.

CHAPTER 8

Curious Incidents: Pretend Play, Presence, and Performance Pedagogies in Encounters with Autism

Nicola Shaughnessy

Setting the Scene:

Autism Project Diary: 24 April 2012, Week 1, School 2, Group 1

Environment 1: Outer Space.

Note

[The "Space" environment is located within the "pod," a portable tent structure containing the interactive performance installations that are the settings for the workshop program. Outer Space features a launch pad where the lighting and sound board are housed. This small enclosure is decorated with stars, a hanging moon, a translucent space ball, and practitioner astronauts who teach the brace position and moon walking as the participants prepare for lift off. On landing, they are invited

---

This phrase is borrowed from Mark Haddon's (2003) novel *The Curious Incident of the Dog in the Night-Time*, which is narrated by a 15-year-old autistic boy who seeks to understand the death of a dog, and which has been adapted to the Broadway stage by the National Theatre. Haddon borrowed the phrase from Sherlock Holmes, who spoke it in Sir Arthur Conan Doyle's 1892 short story "Silver Blaze."

N. Shaughnessy (✉)
School of Arts, University of Kent, Canterbury, UK

Fig. 8.1 The alien puppet

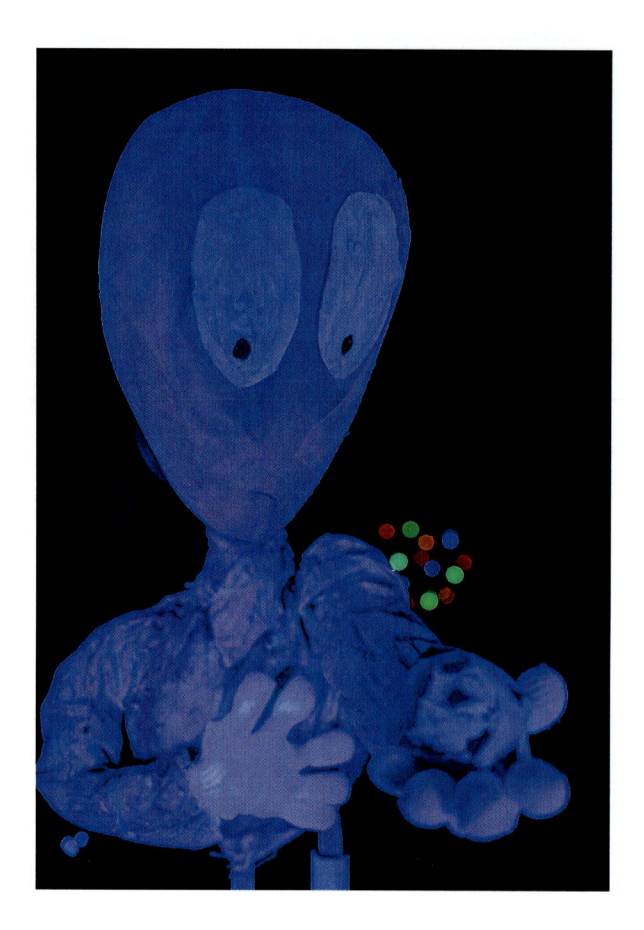

to enter an imaginary planet with stars, moon rocks, an alien creature (a puppet from the Japanese Bunraku theater tradition; see Fig. 8.1), and Professor Nucleus, a stereotypical eccentric professor who is undertaking space research and whose Asperger's-type behavior is modeled on high functioning autism. The three participants all have a diagnosis of autism and are identified as high functioning, but not on the Asperger's spectrum.]

> Ronnie: reluctant to participate. "It's all a fake." Concerned with not wanting to be tricked? We reassure him, agreeing that it is all pretence and that we have nothing to hide. He is invited into the pod to see the set and how it works. He is very engaged in this preview activity and seems more willing to participate, proudly telling his peers "I know how it works."

Archy: Very energetic. Volunteers to be the pilot. Then shows reticence on entering the space craft [enclosed space with projection and lighting/sound board where take off begins the journey]. "I don't know how to do this" and then questions the activity, "Oh this is ridiculous," but he's also intrigued.
Greg: Stays close to Archy and copies him. Withdrawn in waiting area, observing others. Change of energy on entering the space-craft; becomes animated and engaged, willingly entering the game and copying the shaking during lift off.
Eleanor: Shy but compliant. Very passive and overshadowed (perhaps overwhelmed) by the boys. Yet she seems curious. No resistance to the activities, but seems to be on auto pilot.
After "take off," the participants are invited to enter the space environment.
Greg: "Archy, It's creepy."
Interaction between Greg and Ronnie
Ronnie discovers Professor Nucleus: "He's there." [shared communication]
Locates a space rock and says, "I've found it."[showing others]
Archy interacts with a practitioner, waving silver foil that is one of the found materials in the space environment and says, "Anti gravity."
Greg joins Archy to play with silver foil and a practitioner (in space suit), facilitates peer interaction.
Eleanor discovers the alien (a Bunraku puppet): "He's upset."
Ronnie: "Ah" (sympathetically, on seeing alien. Eleanor attracts his attention through eye contact and pointing).
Archy: "Is this a person?"
Eleanor responds to alien's gestures by offering it moon rocks, which it accepts (mmm) or rejects (Yuk!), depending upon the colors. Turn taking games with Eleanor.
Greg is becoming distracted by foil and is "stimming.¹"
Professor Nucleus engages Ronnie, Archy, and Greg in his "experiment."
Ronnie: "It's vinegar and baking powder." [standing, hands on hips] "I think you're lying. I know what that is."
Eleanor joins group and wants to smell it.
Ronnie "It's glue."
Eleanor laughs at alien's noises.
Archy wanders around the environment.
Greg is absorbed with practitioner making a puppet from silver foil.
Archy: "Hey, Greg," directs G's attention to Robin. All three engaged in interaction with PN as he makes his experiment. All three respond sensually seeking to smell, taste, and touch the materials.
Eleanor takes space umbrella.
Eleanor to Greg: "Hello Greg. Look at me."
Archy: [to Professor Nucleus] "How about your mom has made a gigantic apple pie, bigger than the universe?"
They are very immersed in their play and interact with each other far more readily than at the start. When PN tells Eleanor it's time to say goodbye, she waves spontaneously.
Archy: "Bye, Alien," [to PN] "we're going to look after you."
Ronnie: [to me] "You were lying."

This transcript and narrative came from a workshop run in the context of a practice-based research project called "Imagining Autism: Drama, Performance, and Intermediality as Interventions for Autism." (See Appendix for information about the program and its research component.) The program involved three schools: In School 1, the pupils had a diagnosis of severe autism, and several were non-verbal. In School 2 (featured in this account), pupils were located at the higher-functioning end of the spectrum with much higher levels of verbal ability. In the third school, the participants were mixed.

Having worked with deeply symptomatic autistic children in School 1, the project team needed to adapt the workshop material to cater to children at a higher level of social acceptance on the spectrum. While the immersive environments and practical techniques remained the same in each school (improvisation with puppetry and interactive media), the project team worked within flexible narrative structures to shape the material according to the children's different abilities and interests. This form of structured play, which we refer to as *guided improvisation*, is informed by the "Drama Structures" approach of Dorothy Heathcote (Heathcote and Bolton 1994). We also drew upon our experience of teaching contemporary performance, referring to the Ting "Theatre of Mistakes" and the associated manual, *Elements of Performance Art* (Howell and Templeton 1977). The approach also has synergies with Phoebe Caldwell's (2008, 2015) work on intensive interaction and sensory integration, which assumes that for autistic people, "the brain is like a kaleidoscope where the pattern never settles. I use body language to tune into people on the spectrum. It's easy to learn."[2]

Practitioners were trained to follow the children's cues, rather than requiring them to follow ours (Shaughnessy 2014, Trimingham 2016), a practice adhered to by other theater-based autism programs described in Part 2 of this volume. This approach requires adaptations from the adults in the setting as well as the children and youth enrolled in the program (see Chap. 3). A training program was developed to facilitate perspective-taking on the part of the practitioners, helping them to engage imaginatively with the autistic experience. For example, the principle of *walking in the shoes of the other* was evident in a simple exercise of walking around a room with shoes on the "wrong" feet. Some autistic children don't appear to register whether or not shoes are on the right feet and will walk around unperturbed with shoes reversed (left on right).

When training to work with autistic youth, it can be very beneficial to find a means of experiencing perceptual and sensory difference, to develop embodied engagement with the perspectives of those on the spectrum. In this chapter, I discuss the principles and practices of the project's holistic methodology, the ways in which the adaptable and "enactive" approach recognized and responded to each individual as a spectrum (of abilities and difficulties), and the implications for training. I begin with an analysis of the notes above as an illustration of participatory performance practice and the *enactive mind* theoretical paradigm that informs our approach.

Is It for Real?

Klin, Jones, Schultz, and Volkmar (2003) discuss one of the key paradoxes of autism through a study of the discrepancy between what they describe as "social functioning in explicit versus naturalistic" situations, with "naturalistic" defined by the authors as "when they need to spontaneously apply their social reasoning abilities to meet the moment-by-moment demands of their daily social life" (p. 345). This situated perspective means that "normative IQ" autistic individuals are capable of successfully performing structured tasks (e.g., solving complex social reasoning tasks when all the elements of a problem are verbally given to them), yet do not in turn employ these skills in real-life social situations.

This discrepancy can be regarded as a disjunction between theoretical principles and practical applications. Pretend play in childhood serves a critical role in establishing the foundations for symbolization and hence the ability to translate the conceptual understanding emerging from fictional contexts into real-life social encounters. As pretend play is identified as an area of "deficit" in a diagnosis of autism, drama-based practices might be a means of addressing this misconception, offering a space in which social skills can be rehearsed. More to the point of this volume, treating what is considered a deficit as a talent to be nourished upsets the conventional wisdom about deficiencies and disorders that characterizes how most people view autism. There is some evidence of the potential of these approaches in the work of, for example, Matthew Lerner's Spotlight Program (Guli et al. 2013; Lerner and Levine 2007), Blythe Corbett's SENSE Theater (Corbett et al. 2014), Jacqueline Russell's work with Red Kite (Shaughnessy 2012), and Kelly Hunter's Heartbeat method (2014; see Chap. 7).

In the extract that opens this chapter, Ronnie's questioning of the fictional context and its artifice is to some extent symptomatic of the difficulties and differences autistic youth experience in activities that engage the imagination. "It's not real," he tells us, expressing a reluctance to participate in the pretense of being "other" to himself and the social world he inhabits. His relationship to the world around him has engaged him differently in contrast with the processes available to neurotypical children, so that he is drawn to the detail of what he is experiencing in the here and now through what he sees, hears, touches, and smells. Indeed, for autistic individuals, according to Pellicano and Burrs (2012), the world becomes "too real," creating hyper and hypo sensitivities, as I discuss below. Insights from cognitive neuroscience have established the importance of the earliest interactions with the physical and social environments that people inhabit to the development of cognition and language (Clark 1999; Damasio 1999; Gallagher 2001, 2005, 2008, 2015; Varela et al. 1993).

In autism, the neural pathways develop differently than they do for neurotypicals, as Klin and Jones (2007) encapsulate: "their play is typically devoid of representational elements or symbolic themes.... They go from 'parts to whole,' missing the overall meaning or context of what they experience, be it in learning, in communication, or in social interaction. Their thinking often becomes entangled in leaves while missing the forests" (p. 15). For example, in a psychological task using a Navon figure (Navon 1977), an image such as the following is presented to people who are asked which letter they see:

```
EEEE          EEEE
EEEE          EEEE
EEEE          EEEE
EEEE          EEEE
EEEEEEEEEEEEE
EEEEEEEEEEEEE
EEEE          EEEE
EEEE          EEEE
EEEE          EEEE
EEEE          EEEE
```

The typical respondent reports seeing an H, while autistic people are more likely to report seeing an E, because their focus goes first to the minutiae rather than the whole.

This concrete and detail-oriented tendency creates "preferential attention to physical contingencies over social ones in [the autist's[3]] naturalistic viewing of the world around her" (Klin et al. 2003, p. 345). Thus, autists watching films are reported to fixate on the mouth of characters and on physical objects, as these sources provide "the physical contingencies between sound and movement" (Fonagy 2003, p. 41). For Klin and Jones, moreover, "It is not that [autists] are impaired in their ability to integrate information into coherent wholes ... but that this integration occurs in the physical rather than the social domain" (p. 24). Most crucially, they suggest, in a hypothesis that goes to the heart (and mind) of the autism project (as exemplified in Ronnie's responses), autistic people

> are capable of learning *about* but may not be able to translate either implicit or explicit knowledge about people into real-life competence. They are able to learn *about* the world by acquiring factual information that can be acquired as a set of explicit symbols, but they are not capable of learning *in* the world—in action, as it were—by accumulating experiences in an immersive social environment, which, in turn, leads to the emergence of social capacities such as entertaining other people's beliefs and one's own, as well as desires, intentions, and predispositions. (p. 24; emphasis in original)

Could it be the case that by creating an artificial immersive social environment, one in which lights, sounds, objects, and action are self-reflexive and objectified as "not real," Imagining Autism is creating the conditions for learning within the performative world of theater? And in doing so, does it provide the sort of positive social updraft through which neuro-atypical children and youth can undertake development toward a valued social future in a setting in which their anomalies are not viewed as deficits?

The non-naturalistic practices that are the basis of the project are crucial to Ronnie's acceptance of and engagement with the methods. There is no pretense that the environments are real, so Ronnie is shown the set and how the different elements work to create the fictional framework. From this point, he is *pretending to pretend* in his encounters with the practitioners and peers. This concept of "not acting" is one of the core principles for the project's methods. Similar preoccupations are evident in Archy's engagement with the environment ("This is ridiculous") and then his query, "Is this a person?" on discovering the alien, a Bunraku puppet operated by a practitioner.

The puppet resembles an animated stick man with a large oval head (polystyrene), large eyes, and a tiny mouth that turns slightly down, creating an expression of sadness or curiosity, depending upon the angle of the head and the expressive noises made by the practitioner operator. It can demonstrate excitement, sadness, and fear through its vocalizations and movement. Its string limbs are linked to large white-gloved hands and feet, creating a fetus-type figure that seems strange yet familiar in its appearance. Indeed, its features draw attention to its eyes and mouth in ways that may mean they become a focus for the participants who would not normally respond to eyes in facial features.

Various eye-tracking studies have indicated how autistic people tend to be attracted to sensory detail such as color, shape, or objects, focusing on mouths in preference to eyes, rather than engaging in "normative face scanning patterns" (Klin et al. 2003, p. 346). This anomalous attentive practice means that in the everyday context of dynamic social interactions, autists often miss rapidly occurring social cues so that meaning-making is problematized. Imagining Autism environments, however, are appropriate for the "detail focussed processing style" that is associated with autism (Frith and Frith 1999; Frith et al. 2001; Happé 2010) and the "preferential orientation to inanimate objects" (Klin and Jones 2003, p. 351).

The environments objectify the social world, transforming people into larger-than-life personas, while working with puppets affords opportunities to engage with object versions of the human (or animal), thereby providing a more accessible and easier-to-read range of emotional expression. Whereas drama has been used in other educational and therapeutic contexts as a means of simulating social encounters and behaviors, in this project the non-naturalistic features are a means of working *with* autistic children (rather than an application to the condition as in a clinical model). Starting with the child rather than with an idealized notion of normality allows adults working in the project to explore attention, perception, and imagination in creative environments that are in tune with autistic perception. This adaptation of setting to autist is a key aspect of the program's approach.

So, the question about the alien's humanity is entirely appropriate as well as profound. The puppet contains some details that are human and is operated by someone real, but is also very evidently make believe, an alien indeed and clearly not real, as a puppet has no life without the practitioner operating it. When the site-based teachers encounter its lifeless body as we move our materials into the school settings, they will often express concern at the alien being "frightening" for the children, but this concern is rarely realized.

However, the space creature provokes curiosity and compassion, conveying a timidity that invites care, as evident in the notes above. It is non-verbal, but elicits communication through noises that convey its needs and responses. It gestures for the colored polystyrene moon rocks, and the participants describe it as hungry and try to feed it (demonstrating empathy). A repeated game investigates which color moon rocks it prefers (via an appreciative "mmmm" noise or rejecting "yuck" vocalization). Participants repeat this interaction in a delighted exchange that will often involve two or three children sharing attention. Ronnie's insistence on realism is also evident in his response to the larger-than-life persona of Professor Nucleus and his experiments: "It's vinegar and baking powder" (standing, hands on hips). "I think you're lying. I know what that is."

Presence

A further core principle underpinning the project's methods is the concept of *presence*. This stance involves being in the moment with participants, engaging in the theatrical temporality (and rhythm) of a continuous present, and allowing for a suspension of the time and space of the school environment to experience 45 minutes of being in the now and here (or the nowhere) of immersive performance. Participants enter the pod, aware that there will be a beginning and end to this experiential learning activity (with the lunch period generally designating its start or end). But what happens in between is determined to some extent by the participants, as co-producers with agency and authorship over what happens next.

We conceive of these events as "becomings" whereby the media[4] contained in the pod (puppets, objects, costumes, masks, microphones, props, lighting, and sound) are transformed into something other, imbued with meaning through the creative responses of the participants. The pod affords them an opportunity to explore a sensory environment in a space beyond the school routine. Visual schedules are often used in autism settings to ensure that children have a structured routine, reducing the anxiety of not knowing (or imagining) their immediate future. Structured routine is considered important for many autistic people whose difficulties with sensory integration cause anxieties around the concept of surprise. The potential for sensory confusion in autism is powerfully evoked by Naoki Higashida (2013) in *The Reason I Jump*, who describes[5] the overwhelming cacophony of sensory assaults that contribute to his experience of perceiving differently:

> The thirteen-year-old author of this book invites you, his reader, to imagine a daily life in which your faculty of speech is taken away. Explaining that you're hungry, or tired, or in pain, is now as beyond your powers as a chat with a friend.... Now imagine that after you lose your ability to communicate, the editor-in-residence who orders your thoughts walks out without notice.... A dam-burst of ideas, memories, impulses and thoughts is cascading over you instopably.... Now your mind is a room where twenty

radios, all tuned to different stations are blaring out voices and music ... your head feels trapped inside a motorbike helmet three sizes too small which may or may not explain why the air conditioner is as deafening as an electric drill, but your father—who's right here in front of you—sounds as if he's speaking to you from a cell-phone, on a train going through lots of short tunnels, in fluent Cantonese. You are no longer able to comprehend your mother-tongue, or any tongue: from now on all your languages will be foreign languages. (pp. 1–3)

In such a state of perceptual cacophony, it is understandable that "low arousal" learning environments are advocated. In such settings, structured routines and visual timetables may well reduce anxiety about the immediate future and provide stability for autistic children who benefit from knowing what is happening next, where it will take place, and whom they will be with. Familiarity can help to normalize the sensational world they inhabit, reducing its sensory features. This reduction in stimulus can, however, eliminate or radically reduce spontaneity and surprise from everyday encounters, or what has been described in educational discourse as "possibility thinking" (Craft et al. 2013). In Imagining Autism, surprise (shock even) provokes delight and curiosity as participants discover a strange world as if it is real, knowing they are in a safe and supported environment, where everything is predicated on pretense and the willing suspension of disbelief.

Difficulties in processing and adapting to social situations are also explained in relation to *priors theory*, in which, according to Pellicano and Burr (2012), autistic people

> see the world more accurately—as it really is—as a consequence of being less biased by prior experiences. Perceptual experience is influenced both by incoming sensory information and prior knowledge about the world, a concept recently formalised within Bayesian decision theory. We propose that Bayesian models can be applied to autism—a neurodevelopmental condition with atypicalities in sensation and perception—to pinpoint fundamental differences in perceptual mechanisms. We suggest specifically that attenuated Bayesian priors—"hypo-priors"—may be responsible for the unique perceptual experience of autistic people, leading to a tendency to perceive the world more accurately rather than modulated by prior experience.... Hypo-priors might explain key features of autism—the broad range of sensory and other non-social atypicalities—in addition to the phenomenological differences in autistic perception. (p. 504)

In the excerpt that opens this chapter, the activity does not promote insincerity or lying, to respond to Ronnie's concerns about fakery, as there is no deception. The participants know that the puppets are made of cardboard, the lighting and sound-board are visible in the space, and they are invited to create the imaginary scenes with the practitioners. The temporal quality of presence is a key to the curiosity that breeds creativity and discovery. The environment returns the participants to a mode of playful exploration that is fundamental to development of language and awareness of self, but is suppressed by autism's concrete orientation. These fictional environments are a world apart from the order (or disorder) of the social world. They offer the "curiouser and curiouser" that Alice noted after going down the rabbit-hole in Wonderland, inviting exploration of a multisensory playground and its specially designed scenes containing loose materials chosen for their textures, colors, sounds, smells, and even tastes.

Presence is important to the concept of intermediality (Bay-Cheng 2010; cf. Boenisch 2003) and to the pedagogical principles underpinning the project's methods. Intermediality, according to Rippl (2015),

> refers to the relationships between media and is hence used to describe a huge range of cultural phenomena which involve more than one medium. One of the reasons why it is impossible to develop one definition of intermediality is that it has become a central theoretical concept in many disciplines such as literary, cultural and theatre studies as well as art history, musicology, philosophy, sociology, film, media and comic studies—and these disciplines all deal with different intermedial constellations which ask for specific approaches and definitions. (p. 1)

The opportunity to engage with a variety of media provides the participants with a creative zone where flow—the feeling of engrossment in activity with an appropriately pitched degree of difficulty, with immersion so deep that time appears to pass quickly—is important to the creative and cognitive processes (Csikszentmihalyi 1996/2013). Each 45-minute workshop involves a transitional opening in that the journey into the environment frames the start of each workshop: an entrance on a boat, the sledge, the lift down to the under city environment, and the rocket that takes the participants to space. Time is suspended. There will often be a climax, a storm, a change of atmosphere as day changes to night. This dramatic tension affords the students opportunities to respond to what is happening around them. Sometimes they create repetition, using the lighting board to return to daylight or wanting to repeat the excitement of the storm at sea by finding the appropriate key on the sound-board.

The example that opens this chapter involves an elaborate scenario developed as the participants constructed the narrative around the apple pie fantasy. It includes the invention of Professor Nucleus's dog, who was lost in space and needed to be found on the return visit. In developing narratives, the participants bring previous experiences and references to their improvisations, creating *configurational acts* (Ricoeur 1983), as illustrated by Suskind's (2014) memoir of life with his autistic son and how his engagement with Disney films helped him bring order and meaning to his experiences (see Chap. 11).

For practitioners, being in the moment with participants involves leaving their habitual responses behind in order to be open to developing and discovering a relationship with the experience of autism. This orientation requires a particular approach to training and a process of self-abnegation as practitioners need to suspend their "priors" to be able to discover and bring genuine curiosity to their encounters with the "extraordinary." Time is suspended, but rhythm and a strong sense of ensemble become important. In the example above, the practitioner who works with Greg, Archy, and Ronnie responds to their interest in silver foil and uses this focus as a means of interaction in a mode of physical play. This activity doesn't engage Eleanor, however, whose preference is to play with the alien (and the puppeteer operating it), feeding it rocks and enjoying its responses.

The practitioners are in tune with the children, following their cues. Such interactions are also revealing in terms of current research on gender difference in autism and its different manifestations in boys and girls (Halladay et al. 2015). Recent research suggests that girls may be escaping diagnosis because they develop coping and masking strategies (Gould and Ashton-Smith 2011). Girls will observe and copy other children to develop skills in socialization and communication. They will be led by their peers, however, and will often have one or two special friends. They can have highly developed imaginations, and their special interests will often involve fantasy worlds and characters. They may appear quirky, may daydream, or simply seem shy so that their difficulties are regarded as personality traits rather than symptoms of autism. Girls who are diagnosed in early childhood tend to be more severely affected than their male counterparts, but it is now thought that girls who exhibit less extreme traits remain undiagnosed or receive a diagnosis as adults, when they may experience associated conditions such as depression or eating disorders.

One in four autists is a girl, and we worked with this ratio in two of the three participating schools (as there were no female participants in School 3). There were similarities noted in the engagement of the autistic girls, even though they were at very different points on the spectrum. One of the similarities was an interest in the tactile qualities of costume, particularly the heavy fur coat worn by the foxy character in the forest environment.

In Eleanor's case, a sustained interaction with the practitioner playing Foxy brought about a transformation in a sequence that we discuss as a demonstration of embodied cognition through performance practice (Trimingham 2016).[6] Eleanor has been observing the fox's movements in the forest environment. When the practitioner removes the fox mask (attending to another participant), Eleanor seizes the opportunity, moving behind the practitioner to try it on. Having placed it on her face for few seconds, she removes it, as if uncertain about the experience of the mask over her face, but then replaces it, leaving it on for longer before removing it again. The practitioner playing the fox has her attention drawn to Eleanor and responds to her cue, inviting Eleanor (silently) to wear the long fur coat by taking it off and gesturing to Eleanor to put it on. Eleanor consents with a slight smile and is helped into the costume and mask as she becomes "Little Foxy."

The practitioner moves alongside Eleanor to demonstrate the foxy movements, performing the swaying body (swagger) and moving hand gestures that characterize this persona. As Eleanor adopts the heavy costume and mask, her body shifts as she feels its weight and, carefully observing the practitioner who is scaffolding the movement, she copies precisely, carefully imitating the gestures and rhythm of the stealthy fox. Eleanor's preference for physical detail means that this sequence plays to her strengths as she executes a perfect copy of the fox.

What ensues is an example of Vygotsky's (1987/1934) discussion of imitation as involving copying, repetition, and extension as an insightful and intellectual, rather than mimetic, form of learning. Eleanor develops the movement, becoming her own version of Foxy as she travels beyond the practitioner modeling the action, dancing toward a small tent in which the "forester" practitioner is slumbering. In an encounter that is spontaneous and unrehearsed, the forester character is startled from his slumber and feigns irritation at having his naughty nap disturbed. Eleanor responds with an impish facial expression, delighting in her impersonation of Foxy's sly maneuvering. She responds with an utterance, making a noise (from the mask) that sounds like an excited squeak, thereby giving the fox a voice before moving out of the den and back into the forest, still executing the fox's dancing swagger. Ronnie (the cynic) is enjoying swinging on a hammock as Eleanor approaches him. "You're my friend, Foxy" he greets her, in an interaction that demonstrates his willingness to participate in this willing suspension of disbelief, pretending to pretend.[7]

In this instance, the autistic participants are playing in the shoes of another, while the practitioners, likewise, improvise in a style that is akin to pantomime or slapstick in what we refer to as "not acting" (see below). I see this as an example of Vygotsky's (1987/1934) "insightful imitation" whereby Eleanor is able to learn something new through a process that demonstrates embodied cognition through physical and social action and interaction. This process represents Vygotsky's zone of proximal development (ZPD) in a sequence that involves imitation, agency, and adaptation. This capacity for mindful imitation is illustrated by the role of play as a way of helping to create a ZPD such that upper thresholds are extended through "the active imitation of a model through play" (Vygotsky 1987/1934, p. 345). Both instruction and play can push and extend one's threshold for learning toward something fundamentally new, revealing the dynamic, flexible, and teleological nature of the ZPD.

IMPLICATIONS FOR TRAINING

Working with autism requires highly developed skills in what Baron-Cohen et al. (1997) call *mind-reading*. This area is generally defined as a deficit due to the difficulties autistic individuals often experience in reading and interpreting nonverbal cues (e.g., facial expression, gesture, body language, tone of voice). While there is continuing controversy concerning the causes of these difficulties and extent to which this tendency defines and/or determines the autistic experience, it is generally accepted that for individuals on the spectrum, understanding and engaging with the perspectives of others can be challenging.

Asking a question that has become central to our research on autism— "How could we enter their perceptual world and bring them into ours?"— Bogdashina (2003) reflects that "it requires an enormous effort of imagination" (p. 15). In short, what is required from the research practitioners in imagining autism (and the experience of autism) is a form of *kinesthetic empathy*, an embodied engagement with and understanding of the performances of the autistic participants within the interactive immersive and intermedial environments we create (Shaughnessy 2011).

Practitioners thus need to have a developed understanding of both autism and performance in order to be able to work responsively and intuitively to facilitate communication, social interaction, and creativity.

Imagining Autism is predicated on principles of difference, rather than deficit, and as the research has developed, we have become increasingly aware of the distinctiveness of the imagination in autism. In order to fully engage with neurodiversity, the practitioners involved have needed to work in particular ways as a company and as individuals. As teachers and practitioners of contemporary performance, we draw upon devising methodologies as the principle means of making each interactive performance environment. The skills developed here, as indicated in the example above, involve an understanding of ensemble, presence, being in the moment with the participant, and being able to respond flexibly, creatively, and spontaneously to the unpredictable and changing conditions of production. While the environments and methodologies needed to be consistent in keeping with the need to identify the specific components of the intervention (safeguarding against too many variables in the interests of testing efficacy), there was a need for structures that are sufficiently open and flexible to facilitate responsiveness to the imagination in autism. As our understanding developed and deepened, the need to devise special approaches to training emerged as one of the outcomes of our work.

In this project, we were working with a company we had selected and recruited for the different skills and expertise they brought to the research (as dramaturgs, puppeteers, technicians, performers) and with varying levels of experience working in special needs contexts. From the outset, it was evident that a shared vocabulary needed to be developed. Terms such as presence, persona, framing, and self-reflexive needed to be explored and interrogated in relation to role-play, scene, narrative, and acting. Our task was to engage participants as players, which involved doing more than entertain. We were not teaching skills, as such, but endeavoring to facilitate and extend communicative intent and shared attention and to develop and sustain imagination and creativity. We quickly learned to reduce language, to resist the urge to cue responses or to comment, and to become self-abnegating as performers, relinquishing as much control over the creative process as we could (safely) while preserving the integrity of what was defined as an "intervention," but which for us involved developing a means of engaging with autism. Although there were moments we celebrated as high creativity in rehearsal, it was the children who functioned increasingly as makers and performers.

Developing the collaborative understanding of an ensemble, in conjunction with an embodied and conceptual understanding of and engagement with autistic experience and our capacities for deep play with participants and with only an afternoon a week for rehearsal, presented considerable challenges. What has emerged over the course of the project is now being developed into a systems approach to training informed by the principles of distributed cognition, complex systems theory, and cognitive models of embodied communication.

The model of distributed cognition is useful as means of conceptualizing our work on a number of levels. First, it is appropriate to the company structure and its activities as an "expert group" (Hutchins 1995) of skilled practitioners (Grasseni 2004), a community involved in co-participation within an ecology of practice whereby training involved processes analogous to the apprenticeship models of learning discussed by Grasseni (2004) and Tribble (2011). Our weekly activities and performance environments functioned like Ingold's (1993) "taskscapes" (p. 158), which, as Grasseni explains, are "typically accessed by apprenticeship, through a process of education of attention" (p. 45).

Second, distributed cognition is an appropriate paradigm for the practical methodologies we developed and the system of training arising from this approach, involving iterative interaction and collaboration between the constituent elements in the performance environments. These elements include the material environment (the playing space); the technologies within it (sound, lighting, projection); the props, puppets, and personas (the human and material artifacts); and other aspects of the setting.

Third, the installations we created functioned as participant learning environments for the autistic communities we worked with, serving as a complex pedagogic system involving modes of co-participation and methods that drew upon Heathcote's notion of the "mantle of the expert" and that map neatly onto the notion of the expert in distributed cognition theory and the cognitive ecology discussed by Tribble (2011), whereby the social structures of the company "worked to induct younger players into the theatrical system" (p. 22).

Although the system has emerged organically, a starting point for developing a shared vocabulary was derived from The Ting "Theatre of Mistakes" exercises adapted from *Elements of Performance Art* (Howell and Templeton 1977). Divided into seven sections (Conditions, Body, Aural, Space, Time, Equipment, Manifestation), this approach has been a vital pedagogic resource and stimulus for our teaching of contemporary performance practice over the last ten years. It facilitates an engagement with performance as a series of interrelated elements, developing a holistic understanding of performance as, to use Tribble's (2011) terms, "a dynamic playing system that relies upon the complex interaction of its component parts and is regulated neither by master-text nor by master-director" (p. 20). Tribble's systems-based analysis of early modern company processes contains some important insights and parallels with the company practices we developed. Tribble draws on Salomon's (1993) iterative "spiral-like" model of cognition, which Salomon describes as follows: "to study a system assumed to entail more than the sum of its components, one needs to assume neither (a) that its components are *fully* determined by the whole system, not having existence of their own, nor (b) that they are totally independent of the system affecting one another without being changed themselves in *some* but not all of their characteristics through the interaction" (p. 121, emphasis in original; cf. Wilson and Clark 2009).[8]

Our approach to making the performance environments involved devising methodologies akin to improvisational jazz (see Tribble 2011, in relation to the Globe structures).[9] The various elements or components of performance functioned somewhat like the jazz "licks" Sawyer (2000) describes that contribute to rehearsed moments, or "nebulus" to use our dramaturgs' terms. These elements serve as building blocks and as structuring stimuli, which were the framework for what Sawyer refers to as "collaborative emergence" in musical improvisation. These performance elements are plastic and flexible, facilitating both individual and collective creativity as well as enabling us to be responsive and spontaneous in relation to the participants' cues and calls. The company's code of practice here (which developed intuitively through the working process) involved a shared understanding akin to the "jazz etiquette" Sawyer refers to, which, he explains, "is paradoxical—although 'etiquette' implies constraint, limitation and lack of individual freedom, in jazz it can sometimes work to encourage novelty" (p. 181).

Communication within the environment was often non-verbal. As Howell and Templeton (1977) describe such interactions, it was "generated and interpreted almost exclusively from the body," and required us to be simultaneously aware of everyone in the room as well as to be focused on our individual interactions: "think of the other performers, where they are, what they may be about to do. If in doubt, stand still. In an open situation like this, with no 'plot' for anyone to hang onto, every action you make may be read as significant. Listen and look as much as you do anything" (p. 15). This approach was critical to creating the appropriate conditions for creative production, as borne out by the Eleanor and Foxy sequence discussed above.

The pod structure (essentially a black or white tent) was fundamental to the conditions of the performance environments we created. Although the metal poles and drapes could be constructed in various configurations to create different spaces within the larger structure, the pod functioned as a frame, a container for the action. Although the participants were free to leave and return, the performance elements were dependent upon and confined to the spatial conditions we created. This arena provided our playing space, a liminal and intermedial environment, which we conceived as being spanning the range of neurodiversity. Within the room of performance, we were co-creators and co-investigators, playing by some loose rules but open to variation and development.

Howell and Templeton (1977) refer to the principles of theater in the round, and although the immersive environments we created involved various spatial configurations (e.g., participants on a boat, watching UV fish puppets as they journeyed under the sea prior to their entry into an open interactive space), the performance conditions are precisely those articulated by Howell and Templeton: "a performance where the point of view of the spectator is an integral part of the drama, an integral part of the dance" (p. 9). Within the pod (in rehearsal and in performance), we were "in the room" engaging in modes of playing within which, like jazz,

> we can't identify the creativity of the performance with any single performer; the performance is collaboratively created. Although each member of the group contributes creative material ... contributions only make sense in terms of the way they are heard, absorbed, and elaborated on by the other [performers]. The performance that results *emerges* from the interactions of the group rather than being associated with the virtuosity of individuals. (Sawyer 2000, p. 182; emphasis in original).

In our work, however, the emerging performance is for the benefit of the participants, rather than being created for an audience, although observers of the process and the documentation engage with the aesthetics of the work, appreciating and responding to its choreography, scenography, and inter/action. Thus, the place of performance, the immersive, multisensory playing space contained within the pod, functions as a participant learning environment. In this respect, there are further analogies with jazz improvisation and Sawyer's (2000) discussion of emergent, improvised behavior. We have speculated that the autistic participants engage in forms of play that are overlooked post-diagnosis, at approximately 18 months of age when play skills are often identified as part of the "disordered" profile as autistic children diverge from typically developing norms. Thus the child may be observed spinning the wheels of a car, exploring and enjoying its different parts, appreciating its shape, colors, textures, and physicality rather than using it functionally to create imaginative scenarios modeled on the social structures of everyday life (e.g., using cars in races, on a journey, and with human figures in role play).

This behavior is considered as a symptom of the child's retreat into the world of autism, and the emphasis of pre-school intervention and the ensuing special needs curriculum will be on socialization through a skills-based approach to develop language and communication and to encourage norms of behavior and social interaction. Learning to speak, read, write, and count are valued over creative play in order to help the autistic child to function as independently as possible and to be able to participate in inclusive classroom environments.

For Happé (2010), however, autistic people's differently developing imagination is capable of true originality. Our work recognizes, responds to, and nurtures this facility. By returning to play, moreover, the autistic children within our environments are engaging in sensory and experiential encounters that are fundamental to cognitive development, that precede speech, and that may explain why language and communication emerge with and through imaginative engagement in these processes. Indeed, there were lessons from autism for the project as a whole. In his commentary on improvisation in everyday life (drawing upon his studies of informal social learning in pre-school play) Sawyer (2000) refers to "the tension between pre-existing structure and interactional creativity" being "at the core of many contemporary social theories," suggesting that "improvisation is a critical issue for the social sciences" (p. 184). The interdisciplinary nature of Imagining Autism involved social scientists and drama specialists endeavoring in an improvisatory manner to work across and between disciplinary approaches and boundaries, negotiating different languages, research paradigms, and values. Qualitative and quantitative methods were used as we navigated the complexities of working within a living laboratory to engage with autistic children through participatory performance practices. Interactional creativity was needed throughout the project as we explored our relationships with the performance environments and the project participants, while the pre-existing structures pertaining to each discipline were tested for their rigor, flexibility, and the plasticity required for interdisciplinary collaboration.

In their explanation of "action" versus "acting as if," Howell and Templeton (1977) provided a key to the exercises we developed as a means of engaging with the "otherness" of autism: "let the performer attempt to repeat the behavior of another performer—being and attempting to 'be each other' rather than acting and pretending to enact a character" (p. 14). In working through and adapting the elements of performance art, the practitioners imagined themselves being one of the autistic children we were working with. While this role risked clichés (analogous to the clichés that can arise from "licks" in jazz improvisation where musicians fall back on the familiar and predictable), the exercises were undertaken at a point in the process where our relationships with and understanding of the autistic participants were sufficiently developed to ensure that we didn't resort to stereotypes.

What emerged was an embodied exploration of autism through exercises that involved us physically and conceptually *imagining autism*. In an exercise that we also used with teachers and care workers in the Imagining Autism workshop program, we invite participants to select an everyday object to work with, preferably something worn or contained in a bag: jewelry, watches, glasses, mobile phones, and other accessories. The object is explored for its sensory qualities, beginning with touch (shape, texture, temperature) by bringing the object into contact with the fingers, palms of hands, and face, with the invitation to smell and taste it and then to explore any sound qualities (holding it the ear, tapping it, etc.). Finally, the object is held to a light to explore its reflection before a short period of play to continue to pursue whatever has been found pleasurable or curious in the exercise.

Within a short period, a room full of professionals (often self-conscious) find themselves enjoying the experience of perceiving differently, happily engaging in what we refer to as "stimming" in autistic people and understanding why they engage with objects in the environment in this way and why repetition of such behavior becomes a source of sensual pleasure. In a related exercise exploring the aural element, the practitioners selected familiar songs (e.g., nursery rhymes, hymns) and varied the delivery to emphasize tone, pitch, sound, and rhythm (e.g., exaggerating/elongating vowels, changing pitch, volume, and pace in accordance with rules.[10])

A fascinating orchestration ensued, beginning as a cacophony and eventually becoming entrained as the performers became aware of each other.

In these exercises, the copying itself was less important than the endeavor to imagine the autistic experience and to be creatively engaged in action that required the performers to think differently. Many autistic children respond in these ways to aural stimuli, experimenting with intonation and the sounds of words, enjoying word play, repetition, nonsense rhymes, and Dr. Seuss. Exercises with equipment similarly involved us in exploring furniture from an alternative perspective, making the familiar strange as the practitioners played with chairs in different configurations and transformed objects, exploring the spatial and tactile qualities of "found" materials in the studio environment. Working with found sound and props, identifying triggers to simulate action (e.g., freezing in response to a lighting change), and responding to "happy accidents" became a key to making and sustaining performance. Sabotage, a technique derived from Ting and also used in speech therapy, involves setting up situations so that a child is more likely to communicate. Contrary to its sinister-sounding name, sabotage in this context refers to ways of intervening creatively when we felt we were stuck or in stasis.

Through these exercises, we are developing a system of training appropriate to working in these contexts, and which might be adapted for working with in related settings. Logic was abandoned and we began to conceptually and creatively engage in the art of perceiving differently.

Imagination in Autism

Differences in perceptual processing have also been linked to areas of ability and special talent in autism. Ockleford (2013) advances the convincing thesis that autistic children are affected by what he defines as "an Exceptional Early Cognitive Environment, similar to that experienced by blind children, and with the same potential to promote high levels of musical interest and development" (p. 20). Citing the relatively high proportion of autistic children with perfect or absolute pitch (1 in 20), he suggests that variances in sensory input during early childhood development create different neural networks. This acculturation may well lead to higher levels of sensory awareness, which might then be nurtured as abilities in conjunction with support for areas of deficit

The controversial "intense world theory," proposed by Markram and Markram (2010), also challenges the deficit model to conceive of autism in terms of enhanced abilities as well as difficulties engaging with the normate world. The progression of the condition is proposed to be driven by "overly strong reactions to experiences that drive the brain to a hyper-preference and overly selective state," leading to both "feats of talent" and states of over-arousal. The result is described as a constant state of feeling "hungover and jetlagged." The proposed treatment has provoked considerable debate and concern as it involves limiting the child's experience through the radical reduction of sensory stimuli: "if you could develop a filtered environment in the early phase of life," they suggest, "you could end up with an incredible genius child without many of the sensory challenges" (p. 224).

Concerns have been raised, however, that depriving children of sensory stimulation in early development could have a detrimental effect on their social, cognitive, and emotional functioning.[11] Imagining Autism, conversely, offers rich, high arousal environments, provoking questions about the risk of overstimulation. The comments from teachers and parents on how children recollected the environments indicate the strength of its sensory impact and its potential for generalization. One parent, for instance, reported that his child

> said things like "car was taking alien eyes off," "bell was ringing the alien was crying"; and he started to make expressions on his face. He commented on feelings which he has never said about.... For the first time in his life when he plays figures are talking to each other and he is making up a story.

Our hypothesis is that a short exposure to a high intensity, multisensory environment creates the conditions for experiential learning and, potentially, "the 4E's" that are increasingly cited in cognitive theory (and practice): embodied, embedded, extended, and enacted cognition (Ward and Stapleton 2011). The benefits recorded by the psychologists in terms of emotion recognition, peer interaction, and socialization, and the changes to imaginative play reported by parents, are evidence of its "uplift," similar to the notion of "updraft" in this volume. As well as having a positive impact on communication and social interaction, moreover, the project's approach cast new light on the imagination in autism. Diagnostic definitions of autism refer to the "social imagination" rather than the imagination *per se*, and prevailing representations of autism characterize the condition in terms of creative and imaginative deficit (Craig and Baron-Cohen 1999). Studies of autistic children's drawing, writing, and storytelling observe difficulties in creating and engaging with fantasy (e.g., drawing a fantastical creature) and creative imagination (e.g., adapting a toy and transforming objects). Evaluations of impairments in pretend play focus on role-playing in social contexts: whether or not a child will engage in symbolic play, pretend actions with objects, create improvised scenarios, and so on. As Roth (2007) has argued, while there is an abundance of evidence that autistic children have different developmental patterns compared to their typical counterparts, defining imagination as a core deficit in autism raises questions about how diagnosticians define imagination, not to mention normality, and whether this conception might be differently inflected in autism.

Roth (2007) also questions definitions of imagination and autism, making observations on the characteristics of autistic art and poetry. Autistic visual artists are "atypical in that their sophisticated drawing skills emerge early, apparently spontaneously, and completing bypassing the usual stages in the development of neurotypical children's art" (p. 285). Roth (2010) further challenges the dualisms associated with imagination and creativity:

> Imagination is *par excellence* the conceptual cluster that straddles the divide represented by Neisser's distinctions. It embraces forms of thought which can be both rational and intuitive, both logical and prelogical, though not necessarily at the same time.... The challenge, then, is to approach the imagination within a framework sufficiently broad in its theoretical scope and eclectic in its methodological perspectives to transcend this conceptual and empirical divide. (xxv–xxvi)

Imagining Autism's methods can be seen to respond to this challenge, enabling Ronnie to be both rational (it's not real) and intuitive (responding to Eleanor as Foxy).

Discussion

Imagining Autism can thus be seen as contributing positive social updraft for autistic youth, engaging imagination, emotion, and empathy through play-based participatory performance methods. Predicated on the principles of embodied cognition, the project offers evidence that supports the enactivist view of perception and cognition, depending upon individuals' interactions with their environment. In this case, the specially designed environments afforded opportunities for learning (through action) within immersive physical and social contexts. The project's methods facilitate communication (verbal and physical), social interaction (with practitioners and peers), social imagination (exploring "otherness" through self-reflexive fictional frameworks, that is, "pretending to pretend"), and creativity (through improvisation). Our approach emphasizes the importance of presence and being (rather than acting) as a means to work intuitively and creatively.

Within our environments, we create possibilities for play, turn-taking, liveness, open space, physicality, improvisation, shared attention, responding to the other, reading nonverbal cues, and working as an ensemble. The methods used complement the skills-based emphasis of traditional interventions and challenge assumptions about low-arousal spaces being required for learning in autism. Our multisensory environments are highly stimulating, while our participatory and process-based approaches emphasize autonomy and authorship, and offer a license to play creatively (often overlooked post-diagnosis). The research is leading to new understandings of the imagination in autistic children: how it is differently inflected and how it might be shaped by environmental and cultural contexts, as Mills (2008) observes in a discussion of autism: "The nature of play—and its symbolic and imaginative dimensions—might vary in relation to the particular manner in which the 'player' processes the world" (p. 118).

The promotional caption for the National Theatre's production of Haddon's (2003) novel *The Curious Incident of the Dog in the Night-Time* invites us to "see the world differently." In Imagining Autism, curiosity is fundamental to the imagining of our title and to the project's pedagogical principles. Practitioners and participants bring genuine curiosity to their encounters with the environments and each other, unfettered by priors. This state of imaginative curiosity facilitates the affective encounter with a nonillusionist world that is both familiar and strange. The cognition that emerges from interactions within these environments is enacted, embodied, extended, embedded, and, ultimately, affective.[12] Positioned in the now and here of the temporality of presence (where past and future coalesce), we create possibilities for seeing, understanding, and experiencing autism differently.

Appendix

Funded by the UK's Arts and Humanities Research Council, this three-year interdisciplinary collaboration between the fields of Drama and Psychology explored the potential of drama to address what is known as the "triad of impairments" in autism: language and communication, social interaction and emotional regulation, and social imagination (imaginative play, theory of mind, flexibility of thought).[13] The results indicated statistically significant improvements in key areas to include peer interaction, emotion recognition, and empathy.[14] The project was trialed in three schools, over 3 terms (1 term in each school). Participants (22 children aged 7–12 with a diagnosis of autism) were exposed to a weekly program of 45-minute drama workshops over a school term (ten weeks). The workshops took place in one of five scenic environments (space, forest, underwater, arctic, under the city) on a rotation basis with each environment being featured twice. The project recruited students across the autism spectrum (selected by teachers).

Notes

1. *Stimming* refers to acts of self-stimulation that are common in autism and involve repetitive movements one's body or of objects, for example, tapping, rocking, licking, and flapping. Grandin (2011) describes them as follows: "These behaviors self-soothe a child and help him regain emotional balance. Unfortunately, if children are allowed to stim all day, no learning will take place because the child's brain is shut off from the outside world. It is perfectly fine to give a child some time to stim but the rest of the day, a young two to five-year-old should be getting three to four hours a day of one-to-one contact with a good teacher to keep the child's brain open to receiving information and learning" (n. p.).
2. This citation is taken from the Phoebe Caldwell foundation website, which contains further information on intensive interaction and the extensive resources she has developed for educators and careers. http://www.PhoebeCaldwell.com
3. Editor's note: *Autist* is synonymous with the noun form of *autistic*. Usage of many terms in this field appears to follow personal preferences rather than established norms.
4. The intermediality of the project's title is the focus of discussion in "Material Voices: Intermediality and Autism" (Trimingham and Shaughnessy 2015). I use the term media to encompass the range of interactive materials and technologies that we work with. The media do not stand *between* the child and their experience but are integral to that experience.
5. As the quote demonstrates, all of 12-year-old Naoki's thoughts and expressions are ventriloquated through his editor, who may have taken liberties to produce such articulate observations.

6. The sequence is discussed in the present tense with reference to published extracts from the project's documentation. These can be found at www.imaginingautism.org
7. See Trimingham (2016) for a detailed analysis of this sequence in her discussion of the project's scenography, drawing upon theories of situated cognition and new materialism.
8. See Trimingham (2016) for discussion of the environments (particularly the Forest) in relation to the gestalt model of action and progress and with reference to dynamic systems theory.
9. See Shaughnessy (2016) for further discussion of the training program in the context of artistic citizenship.
10. This training is featured in the Imagining Autism DVD (2014) with particular reference to the aural exercise.
11. See Remington and Frith (2014).
12. For discussion of the relations between cognition and affect, see Shaughnessy (2013) and Ward and Stapleton (2011). For detailed analysis of Imagining Autism's practice in terms of situated cognition, see Trimingham (2016).
13. For further information on Imagining Autism, see www.Imaginingautism.org. A film documentary arising from the project is featured in the Routledge Performance Archives series (http://www.routledgeperformancearchive.com/search/video/1554).

    Imagining Autism was based at the University of Kent in the United Kingdom (October 2011-March 2014). Investigators were Professor Nicola Shaughnessy (Drama), Dr. Melissa Trimingham (Drama), Dr. Julie Beadle-Brown (Tizard), and Dr. David Wilkinson (Psychology). Participating Schools were St Nicholas School Canterbury (Spring term 2012), Laleham Gap, Broadstairs (Summer Term 2012), and Helen Allison School, Meopham (Autumn Term 2012).
14. The project results were initially reported in *The New Scientist* (April, 2014). See https://www.newscientist.com/article/dn25419-drama-helps-kids-with-autism-communicate-better

References

Baron-Cohen, S., Jolliffe, T., Mortimore, C., & Robinson, M. (1997). Another advanced test of theory of mind: Evidence from very high-functioning adults with autism or Asperger syndrome. *Journal of Child Psychology and Psychiatry, 38*, 813–822.

Bay-Cheng, S. (2010). *Mapping intermediality in performance*. Amsterdam: Amsterdam University Press.
Boenisch, P. (2003). coMEDIA electronica: Performing intermediality in contemporary theatre. *Theatre Research International, 28*(1), 34–45.
Bogdashina, O. (2003). *Sensory perceptual issues in autism and Asperger syndrome: Different sensory experiences—Different perceptual worlds*. London: Jessica Kingsley.
Caldwell, P. (2008). *Using intensive interaction and sensory integration*. London: Jessica Kingsley.
Caldwell, P. (2015). *Phoebe Caldwell*. Carmarthen: Caldwell Autism Foundation. Retrieved October 31, 2015, from http://thecaldwellfoundation.org.uk/phoebe-caldwell/
Clark, A. (1999). An embodied cognitive science? *Trends in Cognitive Sciences, 3*(9), 345–351.
Corbett, B. A., Quals, L. R., Valencia, B., Fecteau, S. M., & Swain, D. M. (2014). Peer-mediated theatrical engagement for improving reciprocal social interaction in autism spectrum disorder. *Frontiers in Pediatrics, 2*, 110.
Craft, A., Cremin, T., Burnard, P., Dragovic, T., & Chappell, K. (2013). Possibility thinking: Culminative studies of an evidence-based concept driving creativity? *Education 3–13: International Journal of Primary, Elementary and Early Years Education, 41*(5), 538–556.
Craig, J., & Baron-Cohen, S. (1999). Creativity and imagination in autism and Asperger syndrome. *Journal of Autism and Developmental Disorders, 29*, 319–326.
Csikszentmihalyi, M. (1996/2013). *Creativity: The psychology of discovery and invention*. New York: Harper Collins.
Damasio, A. (1999). *The feeling of what happens: Body, emotion and the making of consciousness*. London: Vintage.
Frith, C. D., & Frith, U. (1999). Interacting minds: A biological basis. *Science, 286*(5445), 1692–1695.
Frith, U., Happé, F., & Briskman, J. (2001). Exploring the cognitive phenotype of autism: Weak central coherence in parents and siblings of children with autism: I. Experimental tests. *Journal of Child Psychology and Psychiatry, 42*(3), 299–307.
Gallagher, S. (2001). The practice of mind: Theory, simulation or interaction? In E. Thompson (Ed.), *Between ourselves: Second-person issues in the study of consciousness* (pp. 83–108). Thoverton: Imprint Academic.
Gallagher, S. (2005). *How the body shapes the mind*. Oxford: Oxford University Press.
Gallagher, S. (2008). *Brainstorming: Views and interviews on the mind*. Thoverton: Imprint Academic.
Gallagher, S. (2015). The invasion of the body snatchers: How embodied cognition is being disembodied. *The Philosophers' Magazine*, pp. 96–102. Retrieved

October 30, 2015, from https://www.researchgate.net/publication/276474146_How_embodied_cognition_is_being_disembodied#full-text

Gould, J., & Ashton-Smith, J. (2011). Missed diagnosis or misdiagnosis: Girls and women on the autism spectrum. *Good Autism Practice, 12*(1), 34–41.

Grandin, T. (2011). *Why do kids with autism stim?* Arlington: Autism Asperger's Digest. Retrieved November 2, 2015, from http://autismdigest.com/why-do-kids-with-autism-stim/

Grasseni, C. (2004). Skilled vision: An apprenticeship in breeding aesthetics. *Social Anthropology, 12*(1), 45–55.

Guli, L., Semrud-Clikeman, M., Lerner, M., & Britton, N. (2013). Social Competence Intervention Program (SCIP): A pilot study of a creative drama program for youth with social difficulties. *The Arts in Psychotherapy, 40*(1), 37–44. Retrieved October 30, 2015, from https://www.researchgate.net/publication/257053742_Social_Competence_Intervention_Program_(SCIP)_A_pilot_study_of_a_creative_drama_program_for_youth_with_social_difficulties#full-text

Haddon, M. (2003). *The curious incident of the dog in the night-time*. New York: Doubleday.

Halladay, A. K., Bishop, S., Constantino, J. N., Daniels, A. M., Koenig, K., Palmer, K., Messinger, D., Pelphrey, K., Sanders, S. J., Singer, A. T., Taylor, J. L., & Szatmari, P. (2015). Sex and gender differences in autism spectrum disorder: Summarizing evidence gaps and identifying emerging areas of priority. *Molecular Autism, 6*(36), 1–5. Retrieved October 30, 1915, from http://www.molecularautism.com/content/pdf/s13229-015-0019-y.pdf

Happé, F. (2010). *Autism and talent*. Oxford: Oxford University Press.

Heathcote, D., & Bolton, G. (1994). *Drama for learning: Dorothy Heathcote's mantle of the expert approach to education*. London: Pearson.

Higashida, N. (2013). *The reason I jump: One boy's voice from the silence of autism* (trans: Mitchell, D. & Yoshida, K.). London: Spectre.

Howell, A., & Templeton, F. (1977). *Elements of performance art*. London: The Ting Theatre of Mistakes.

Hunter, K. (2014). *Shakespeare's heartbeat: Drama games for children with autism*. New York: Routledge.

Hutchins, E. (1995). *Cognition in the wild*. Cambridge, MA: MIT Press.

Ingold, T. (1993). The temporality of the landscape. *World Archaeology, 25*(2), 152–174.

Klin, A., & Jones, W. (2007). Embodied psychoanalysis? Or, on the confluence of psychodynamic theory and developmental science. In L. C. Mayes, D. P. Fonagy, & M. Target (Eds.), *Developmental science and psychoanalysis: Integration and innovation* (pp. 5–38). London: Karnac Books.

Klin, A., Jones, W., Schultz, R., & Volkmar, F. (2003). The enactive mind, or from actions to cognition: Lessons from autism. *Philosophical Transactions of the Royal Society B: Biological Sciences, 358*, 345–360. Retrieved October 30, 2015, from http://rstb.royalsocietypublishing.org/content/royptb/358/1430/345.full.pdf

Lerner, M. D., & Levine, K. (2007). The Spotlight method: An integrative approach to teaching social pragmatics using dramatic principles. *Journal of Developmental Processes*, 2(2), 91–102. Retrieved October 30, 2015, from http://www.psych.utah.edu/people/people/fogel/jdp/journals/3/journal03-05.pdf

Markram, K., & Markram, H. (2010). The intense world theory: A unifying theory of the neurobiology of autism. *Frontiers in Human Neuroscience*, 4, 224–253. Retrieved October 30, 2015, from http://journal.frontiersin.org/article/10.3389/fnhum.2010.00224/full

Mills, B. (2008). Autism and the imagination. In M. Osteen (Ed.), *Autism and representation* (pp. 118–132). New York: Routledge.

Navon, D. (1977). Forest before trees: The precedence of global features in visual perception. *Cognitive Psychology*, 9(3), 353–383.

Ockleford, A. (2013). *Music, language and autism: Exceptional strategies for exceptional minds*. London: Jessica Kingsley.

Pellicano, E., & Burrs, G. (2012). When the world becomes too real. *Trends in Cognitive Sciences*, 16(10), 504–510.

Remington, A., & Frith, U. (2014). Intense world theory raises intense worries. *Spectrum*. Retrieved November 1, 2015, from https://spectrumnews.org/opinion/viewpoint/intense-world-theory-raises-intense-worries/

Ricoeur, P. (1983). *Time and narrative* (Vol. 1; trans: McLaughlin, K. & Pellauer, D.). Chicago: University of Chicago Press.

Rippl, G. (2015). Introduction. In G. Rippl (Ed.), *Handbook of intermediality: Literature–image–sound–music* (pp. 1–31). Berlin: de Gruyter.

Roth, I. (2007). Autism and the imaginative mind. In I. Roth (Ed.), *Proceedings of the British Academy: Imaginative minds. Proceedings of the British Academy, 147* (pp. 277–306). Oxford: Oxford University Press.

Salomon, G. (Ed.) (1993). *Distributed cognitions: Psychological and educational considerations*. New York: Cambridge University Press.

Sawyer, R. K. (2000). Improvisational cultures: Collaborative emergence and creativity in improvisation. *Mind, Culture and Activity*, 7(3), 180–185.

Shaughnessy, N. (2011). Knowing me, knowing you: Autism, kinesthetic empathy and applied performance. In D. Reynolds & M. Reason (Eds.), *Kinesthetic empathy in creative and cultural practices* (pp. 33–50). Bristol: Intellect.

Shaughnessy, N. (2012). *Applying performance: Live art, socially engaged theatre and affective practice*. Basingstoke: Palgrave Macmillan.

Shaughnessy, N. (Ed.) (2013). *Affective performance and cognitive science: Body, brain and being*. London: Methuen.

Shaughnessy, N. (2014). *Imagining autism: Now I see the world*. DVD. New York: Routledge Performance Archive & Digital Theatre.

Shaughnessy, N. (2016). Valuing performance: Purposes at play in participatory theatre practice. In D. J. Elliott & M. Silverman (Eds.), *The Oxford*

handbook of artistic citizenship (pp. forthcoming). Oxford: Oxford University Press.
Suskind, R. (2014). *Life animated: A story of sidekicks, heroes, and autism.* New York: Kingswell.
Tribble, L. (2011). *Cognition in the globe.* Basingstoke: Palgrave Macmillan.
Trimingham, M. (2016). Intra-active, transactional space in Imagining Autism. In J. McKinney & S. Palmer (Eds.), *Scenography expanded: An introduction to contemporary performance design.* London: Bloomsbury Academic, [details forthcoming].
Shaughnessy, N., & M. Trimingham, M. (2016). Material voices: Intermediality and autism. *Research in Drama Education: The Journal of Applied Theatre and Performance, 21*(3), 293–308.
Varela, F., Thompson, E., & Rosch, E. (1993). *The embodied mind: Cognitive science and human experience.* Cambridge, MA: MIT Press.
Vygotsky, L. S. (1987/1934). Thinking and speech. In L. S. Vygotsky, *Collected works* (Vol. 1, pp. 39–285) (R. Rieber & A. Carton, Eds.; trans: Minick, N.). New York: Plenum.
Ward, D., & Stapleton, M. (2011). E's are good: Cognition as enacted, embodied, embedded, affective and extended. In P. Fabio (Ed.), *Consciousness and interaction: The role of the natural and social environment in shaping consciousness* (pp. 89–104). New York: John Benjamins.
Wilson, R., & Clark, A. (2009). How to situate cognition, letting nature take its course. In P. Robbins & M. Aydede (Eds.), *The Cambridge handbook of situated cognition* (pp. 55–77). New York: Cambridge University Press.

PART III

Mainstream Activity Niches

CHAPTER 9

The Collaborative Online Anime Community as Positive Social Updraft

Leslie S. Cook and Peter Smagorinsky

In this chapter we present a case study of a young woman, Chloe,[1] whose disruptive conduct at home led to a set of related diagnoses for chronic depression and anxiety, Asperger's syndrome, Tourette's syndrome, oppositional-defiance, and obsessive-compulsiveness, each presented to her and her family as a set of disabilities and disorders. Considered to be an outsider to the mainstream youth of her social surroundings due to the different orientation to the world that these conditions afforded her, she found an affirmational social setting through her engagement with the online anime community. When online with virtual, and eventually material friends she met through this medium, she was no longer constructed as odd and ill-fitting. Rather, her differences were understood by her peers as strengths, and she was recognized as a key contributor to the artistic and narrative worlds available online. This high degree of support provided Chloe with the positive social updraft that was largely unavailable to her in her daily life in school and at home.

L.S. Cook (✉)
Department of English, Appalachian State University, Boone, NC, USA

P. Smagorinsky
Department of Language and Literacy Education, The University of Georgia, USA

© The Author(s) 2016
P. Smagorinsky (ed.), *Creativity and Community among Autism-Spectrum Youth*, DOI 10.1057/978-1-137-54797-2_9

In contrast to her parents' concerns that excessive computer time would delay her social development, her online involvement provided her with her primary peer cohort and means of social support. Further, in contrast to the concerns of many who cared about her, her intensive participation in a narrow field of interest enabled her Asperger's and obsessive-compulsive tendencies toward highly focused topics and projects, those requiring meticulous attention to detail, served her developmental needs well. Within the parameters of the anime genre, her work involved the production of both art and collaborative narrative composing in the medium of "fanfiction," in which popular fictional book series are subjected to new treatments by groups of fans producing new stories based on the series' characters (see Black 2008).

In presenting Chloe's case, we consider the inappropriateness of forcing people with dispositions that are oriented to pursuing narrow interests in a highly concentrated manner to try to develop broader interests. As Chloe's case indicates, attempting to do so increases the anxiety that is already chronic and creates, rather than solves, problems of social engagement. Much as society forces left-handers to abandon their natural tendencies and requires right-handedness so that they appear to fit in better, regardless of the psychological damage done in service requiring conventional conduct of unconventional people, those on the Asperger's spectrum are often urged to develop wider interests. As we will detail, the denial of computer time in the interests of expanding her horizons only elevated her systemic anxiety and led to disruptions to her home.

Introducing Chloe

A 9th grader at an academically rigorous private school in the first year of the two-year data collection, Chloe was the older of two children in an upper-middle-class family. Her father was a university professor and her mother stayed at home with children upon Chloe's birth, leaving a job in the financial sector of the economy to be a fulltime parent. At the beginning of the study, Chloe and her brother attended the same school (he in Middle School, she in the Upper School) and were both identified as intellectually gifted. Her computer was the focal point of her life outside school. She maintained several websites where she uploaded her art and engaged with other youth in collaborative artwork and story writing. Her immersion in anime culture was most apparent on her own *Deviantart.com* site, where she had regular subscribers and commenters.

Chloe's interest in anime led her to further explore Asian culture, even motivating her to learn Japanese in an adult education class in the evenings. Her intense focus on anime began as early as 4th grade when she and her brother began to collect and watch Pokémon, a phenomenon created by a media company in the mid-1990s. In this genre, players use cute, fictional characters to train and fight for sport. As both Chloe and her brother grew older, they continued to participate in anime culture, though their interests took them down different paths. Her brother, a student and practitioner of the martial arts, followed *Gundam Wing* and *Dragon BallZ*, two mainstream anime shows popular with boys. Anime was one among many interests for him, and not one that he followed with passion over time. Chloe began to seek out anime with more complex plots and characters like *Fushigi Yuugi* (Watase 1992), a Japanese manga series based loosely on the four mythical creatures of China that told the story of two teenaged girls, Miaka and Yui. With her parents' economic support, if not always their emotional support, Chloe was eventually able to claim the status of an "otaku," a formal, honorific form of the Japanese pronoun "you" coined in 1983 for those with an obsessive interest in anime culture.

Chloe's gravitation to the anime culture was well aligned with her growing understanding of herself as different from her peers. Okabe and Ishida (2012) describe this phenomenon as common among youth who enter this culture: "While fujoshi develop their identities in opposition to the mainstream [as] many other subcultures do, they do as much work to erase, or make invisible, their fujoshi identity as they do in making it selectively visible. These processes of visualization and erasure work in tandem to create a unique subcultural identity" (p. 209). The US environment, in which anime was less pervasive than in Japan, undoubtedly intensified the outsider status of those who considered themselves among the *cognoscenti* of this medium. This status came in contrast to the social rejection that these same youth often met with in their everyday lives. Chloe's involvement in the otaku subculture was not, however, what her family or community expected of her, even as it provided her with her most satisfying social and artistic experiences in life.

At the time of the interviews, Chloe had not been officially diagnosed on the autism spectrum, even though her frame of mind was not that of the neurotypical. Her mother noted concerning behaviors in her daughter by age two; and in 2nd grade, she began presenting symptoms of anxiety by engaging in trichotillomania, that is, continually pulling out her hair.

By 5th grade she had begun seeing a therapist who specialized in autism using play therapy, but Chloe's diagnosis on the autism spectrum did not occur until she was 18. From the time she entered in to the mental health system, she had been diagnosed with Tourette's syndrome, depression, chronic anxiety, obsessive-compulsiveness, oppositional-defiance, and mild psychosis.[2]

The interviews with her parents before her diagnosis of Pervasive Developmental Disorder-Not Otherwise Specified (PDD-NOS) all point to her place on the autism spectrum, yet she was being treated both medically and therapeutically for a multitude of the other diagnoses. Her behavior and relationship were characterized by many of the traits typical of the Asperger's population: unusually intense or focused interests such as her obsession with anime and its virtual community, repetitive body movements such as continuous finger snapping that others found distracting, repetitive use of objects such as repeatedly switching lights on and off or lining up toys, and sensory sensitivities including avoidance of everyday sounds and textures such being hugged by family members. She also presented cognitive traits typical of the diagnosis, in particular difficulties with organization and cleanliness as indicated by the messy manner in which she kept her room at home. Finally, she displayed emotional and social atypicality such as an apparent lack of empathy, difficulties forming and sustaining friendships, and giving unrelated answers to questions.

CHLOE AND THE ACTIVITY SYSTEM OF AN ANIME OTAKU

In Japan and in the USA, otaku culture is seen as fringe. The coining of the term otaku came from an article in an erotic anime magazine, *Manga Burikko*. The writer, Nakamori Akio, described otaku as "[a]lways sitting off in a corner of the class, virtually invisible, with a gloomy expression, without a single friend" (cited in Morikawa 2012). Despite the term's derogatory beginning, the otaku subculture, which had "achieved group consciousness and [was] simply waiting for an identifying name" (Morikawa, p. 4), adopted the term and has used it in a range of self-deprecating and self-aggrandizing manners.

Chloe's understanding of and interaction with the discourse conventions of anime was complex and multilayered. There were those who dabbled in it, "the LOWER class" as she called them, and those who truly understood its intricacies, the *otaku*. She considered herself among the latter. Though in some anime communities otaku is a derogatory term for those overly focused on technology and anime, Chloe expressed high regard for this term and those who earned it. In a similar way, she proudly referred to herself as a "geek" because of her relatively obscure computer-based obsession. In this manner, she participated in the otaku "culture of resistance" (Eng 2012a, p. 99). Okabe and Ishida (2012) recognize that with *fugoshi*, or female otaku, "identity construction represents an example of a subcultural and oppositional feminine identity constructed in a self- deprecating and 'undercover' mode" (p. 209). In Chloe's familial and social spheres, being an otaku, one who was highly focused on drawing and sharing *yaoi*, that is, male–male partnership anime, required her to resist other people's preferred pathways for her. In her own mind, becoming part of the otaku culture better suited her personal and social needs.

Anime itself began as a Japanese countercultural movement in film and art. Anime videos first appeared in the USA in the 1960s with titles such *Astro Boy* and *Speed Racer*, and with the advent of the VCR and subsequent recording devices, a robust anime video trade took hold. In the 1970s, anime films gained a following, and early anime fans formed clubs where they would often exchange hard-to-get videos. Anime otaku emerged as a distinct subculture out of Japan during the period from the mid-1980s to late 1990s (Eng 2012a), making its way into the USA primarily through films and manga, that is, anime graphic novels, with Hawaii serving as the US portal to the Asian market.

Technology in the 1980s enabled fans to write their own subtitles onto the video screen instead of relying on printed scripts. *Fansubs*—that is, foreign videos for which fans provide subtitles in translation—helped spread anime to more people outside Japan. Through the late 1980s and early 1990s, before the Internet became widely available, anime made its way through college anime clubs, who formed tape-trading networks and expanded anime's availability and popularity.

Additionally, US military personnel would bring anime tapes from Japan to the States. A few distribution companies provided anime from Japan, but often these videos were more focused on sexual and violent content than plot and were not popular with the otaku on US college campuses. With the more widespread use of the Internet beginning in the mid-1990s, anime fans shared information and videos by means of newsgroups, File Transfer Protocol (FTP) software, and Gopher, a predecessor of the World Wide Web that was designed for distributing, searching, and retrieving documents online. Eng notes that an article in a mid-1990s *Fortune Magazine* was one of many that credited early otaku as "a subculture on the cutting edge of technology, especially the Internet" (2012a, p. 91). The early otaku were "some of the earliest, most prolific, and most sophisticated video-file sharers on the Internet" (2012b, p. 165).

Chloe's early interactions with anime culture, both virtually and materially, reflect the historical development and spread of anime across the USA. Throughout her high school years, she became well versed in the specific discourse, commerce, and literacy practices of anime, and was a global producer and consumer in the early subculture through the use of her computer. Eng (2012b) discusses how, contrary to popular belief that anime culture is solely an online phenomenon, "most anime fans actually get their start in fandom via face-to-face interactions" (p. 166). Like many other youth in the USA during the early 2000s, after initial exposure through television, Chloe entered the culture of anime through a club, which met at a community art space. Cartoon Club, as it was called, was where Chloe met Katie, with whom she had an arts-based friendship that eventually was affected by Chloe's tendency to suffocate friends with demands for attention. Similarly, she met her other friend Jason at a Pokémon trading and gaming session that met every Saturday morning in a bookstore in town. Although she met her best friend Casey through a young woman she'd gotten to know during her first hospitalization following extensive, violent outbreaks in her home, their friendship grew on the basis of their shared interest in anime. Chloe's and Casey's mutual friend's more severe challenges in life led Chloe's parents to be wary of this friendship, but Casey soon became a welcome visitor to the home in spite of her own unstable family background.

Chloe noted several times that her life online was more exciting than her life offline. Her mother, Joan, stated that she wished the whole Internet arena did not exist, even as she herself used it daily in her own life. Caught in the rapidly changing technology landscape of the early 2000s, Joan recognized how quickly the social networking tools Chloe used grew beyond Joan's ability to monitor them. Chloe learned to navigate the Internet to suit her interests, but her parents' concern for their daughter's safety led them to try to stop what they could not control. Arguments and fights occurred over Chloe's use of the computer, the one tool that connected her to the stimulating online world where she found belonging.

Joan's fears were not unfounded. An incident did occur where a young man Chloe had met online showed up at her school to see her, an incident that greatly alarmed the school administration, not to mention Chloe and her parents. Subsequent restrictions on Chloe's ability to give out any information online stifled her trading. She had often purchased drawings she saw online and had them sent to her. To protect Chloe from potential harassment, her parents required her to get a post office box rather than use her home address to receive all Internet-bought materials, causing additional anxiety in awaiting their arrival and constant badgering of her parents to drive her to the inconveniently located post office to pick them up.

Because of the financial resources necessary to participate as an otaku in the anime culture of the early 2000s, this culture was predominantly available to the middle and upper class, though the class divide is changing with the sharing culture enabled through the Internet. Chloe collected *fansubs* that could cost up to $100, and later made her own contributions as a *scanlation* producer: Using knowledge of Japanese that she learned in taking classes outside her school curriculum, she would scan manga and translate them into English for online sharing. She also engaged in *cosplay*, a mash of the terms *costume* and *play*, in which the participants, known as *cosplayers*, wear a pop culture character's costumes and other fashion accessories and perform scenes.

Chloe also played online group video games and attended anime conventions, all of which cost money. Conventions allowed Chloe to build online and offline networks and gave her access to material items not available elsewhere in the USA. Eng (2012b) notes that "for otaku who cosplay, run their own panels, organize and staff the conventions, anime conventions are a place where… becoming well connected or well known within otaku circles allows one to engage with the community at a high level" (pp. 176–177). Chloe participated in cosplay as her favorite character both at home and when she attended the conventions. Cosplayers reference the cross-dressing model constructed by the cosplay community, and they express the idealized masculinity and femininity that the community has created (Okabe 2012). These interests separated Chloe from most of her peers and also her family members, whose interests, aside from her brother's less intense interest in a subset of anime programs, were more embedded in mainstream US culture, of which anime was not yet a part. As one who distanced herself from mainstream interests, Chloe found the cultural stream provided by the anime community of practice to be one in which the traits found to be odd and ill-fitting to many in her surroundings were valued and affirmed.

Developing in Contrast to Expectations

Chloe's involvement in anime seemed to run counter to her parents' expectations for her well-being, partially because the burgeoning subculture with which their daughter was engaging was completely foreign to them and because Internet predators were becoming better publicized to families concerned with their children's safety. Interviews with Chloe's parents were essential to understanding what they expected of her. They had aspirations and concerns for her social life, her academic performance, her various diagnoses and what they portended for both present and future, and her ability to sustain herself once she turned 18. Bodovski's (2014) work on the influence of parental expectations affirms that "parental educational expectations represent to a certain extent parental habitus ('given who we are, what is possible for my child to achieve?')" (p. 393). Chloe persistently defied the expectations that adults and her mainstream peers had for her interests, appearance, and life direction.

Often as parents become aware of their child's extranormative behavior, so do the schools. A clash of expectations between and among the child, parents, and school begins. Parents, in particular, feel forced to readjust their hopes for their child. Broomhead (2014) reports that "many children with BESD [behavior emotional and social disorders] are perceived to experience complex home lives, where parenting is deemed to be ineffective and blameworthy due to social disadvantage and family pressures" (p. 137). Chloe's parents, who both held advanced degrees and highly valued education and social interaction, underwent a long process of readjusting their expectations for their daughter, undertaking adaptations to a child who consistently defied their anticipated sense of whom their children should turn out to be. During her childhood and adolescence, Chloe had participated in a wide range of conventional extracurricular and community activities designed for young people: T-ball, softball, basketball chorus, orchestra (in which she played the viola), art classes, horseback riding, and others, often finding them enjoyable and fulfilling. She gradually discarded them, however, as her interest in and focus on anime grew.

Her parents supported her in each of these relatively mainstream activities, and also in her anime obsession, although often with misgivings. Even as they adapted to their daughter, however, Chloe felt that they didn't adapt nearly enough to accommodate her need for complete immersion in an arcane interest, including open access to the family computer whenever she was home, a demand that conflicted with her mother's and brother's interests in getting online (her father's career provided him with a separate computer). Both felt their parenting skills were called into question by the schools, by the psychotherapeutic community, by each other, and by Chloe.

Their responses to Chloe's rapid immersion into the otaku subculture and her ongoing issues stemming from her neurodivergent makeup were both supportive and authoritarian. Because parental influence has a great deal to do with a child's self-construction, looking at key narratives Chloe's parents told about their daughter within the context of Chloe's own self-narration serves as an empirical portal to view her development within two social channels: the positive social updraft afforded by her immersion in the anime culture and its online access, and the less supportive teleological direction envisioned for her by those in authority who surrounded her.

Concerns Over Peer Relationships

Both of Chloe's parents expressed concern over Chloe's friendships. Because Chloe had moved to new states in different parts of the country twice in her 14 years, she had to make friends in each new place. Since she was not interested in what she said most girls at her school talked about—boys, makeup, and parties—Chloe accepted her outsider status in school settings. She talked during the research about a close friend she'd had in each of the places she had lived in and how much she missed these friends. Her latest, recent move to a small southern university town forced her to yet again meet new friends, a difficult experience for her given her limited range of interests and her tendency to consume friends with her attention and often alienate them. Establishing friendships produced anxieties around the household as it exacerbated her own anxiousness and contributed to concerns her parents had over her ability to find happiness in her new home. What allowed her to develop relationships was her quick gravitation to the community's nascent anime culture that was getting established among its youth.

Joan described Chloe's off-putting tendency to become obsessed with her friendships as a behavior that often drove off potential friends rather than allowing her to get closer to them. The friendships that Chloe described as close and special were at times only available away from the gaze of classmates. One such friend from her second city of residence even told Chloe she could not talk to her in school, saving their friendship for when they played together at their houses. Joan was pleased with the way

Chloe's face-to-face friendships progressed; she noted that the friendships Chloe had developed since moving to their current town were "much more equitable" than what she'd had in previous stops, in part because of Chloe's growing expertise in anime art and culture and the manner in which such authority positioned her in friendships based on this shared interest.

Casey and Katie were two of Chloe's closest friends at the time of the research. Both young women loved anime and drawing, which was often the center of their social interactions. Casey was Chloe's best friend. Casey's mother, a single mom whose own bipolar diagnosis provided her with a disability classification, described the relationship as occasionally strained by "social economic issues," but allowed that they had ridden out the rough times together.

Casey recognized Chloe is a needy friend who became enmeshed in relationships to the point of obsession, a tendency that Joan believed to be a problem in Chloe's online friendships. Joan also recognized that Chloe's shunning of social norms was a double-edged sword. She was conflicted over Chloe's view of herself as an outsider and reasoned that she would need to "let go of" a lot of her expectations for Chloe's external appearance, which was affected by her inattention to hygiene and her gravitation to anime fashion that was unique among her local teen community and a source of embarrassment to her brother. Joan admired her daughter's rejection of trying to fit in with the girls who talked about makeup and boys all the time; she was glad that her daughter had not gone to the extreme of scrutinizing every pore on her face as a way to appear attractive to her peers.

Because some of Chloe's parents' biggest concerns surrounded her social development, it is important to reiterate the social nature of the anime community Chloe was engaged in. Chloe's first exposure to anime drawing and films came through Casey and Jason, her closest friends throughout high school. Once exposed to anime culture through her face-to-face friends, Chloe was able to use the Internet to connect with others who shared her new-found interest. Anime became her social activity.

Joan commented that Chloe had a strong sense of who she was and recognized that her daughter saw herself as "an outsider"; therefore, her "I don't care what people think of me" attitude toward her external appearance represented a "healthy attitude." In her parental role, Joan worried about Chloe's health and hygiene. In this realm, Chloe shattered her mother's expectations of how a typical 15-year-old should mature. From Joan's perspective, either her daughter was socially delayed or she had skipped a crucial step in the process most girls go through in maturing into self-supporting adults.

Chloe's father Phil described Chloe as "hard to be friends with," sedentary, "a computer geek," volatile, unpredictable, lacking in relational reciprocity, and a "demanding friend." He also described her as "a normal teenager just waiting to make the right friends." Yet in the same interview, he discussed how Chloe had been on suicide watch for several years. Phil's own perception of what "normal" teenagers did was well informed. Previously a high school teacher himself, Phil had both a professional and personal perspective on adolescent development based on his teaching of thousands of students over his teaching career, couple with his own graduate education focused on adolescent literacies. His own parents' expectations had encouraged him to succeed academically, with college and graduate school assumed for him in prepubescence. Phil was raised in a family that accepted no excuses for failure and viewed any lowering of performance standards as a character flaw. Seeing his daughter veer away from standard pathways to success via school and college and into the anime community's foreign trajectory created additional tensions in their relationship. These expectations were exacerbated by Chloe's angry, often violent response to any intervention that took her off the computer in the evenings.

Phil's expectation that Chloe would find friendship among the 25 girls from her class in the private school she attended—one she soon chose to leave because of the monoculture that excluded her interests and fashion style—clashed with what Chloe herself wanted. She saw herself as an outcast there and described the girls at school as shallow and concerned with superficial things. When she decided to go to the homecoming dance with her friend, Jason, Phil saw it as a potentially transforming experience for her, but unfortunately that social event helped to precipitate Chloe's first of two stays at mental health facilities. According to Phil:

> She had gone to a homecoming football game at [the private school]. And we'd been hoping and hoping and hoping that she would kind of buy into the school as a kind of psychological anchor for herself. But she really resisted it. Certainly at the beginning she was resisting the school because we thought she'd like it. And it was part of her rebellion against moving. I thought, "Well you know, she's going to the homecoming game with

all the other girls in the class, and then there's this big sleepover at a kid's house," and I just thought, maybe that's the kind of thing that'll finally help her bond with people. And [the dance was] followed by the overnight. But when I picked her up the next day, her mood instantly changed to angry. And she had a day that was like all these nights that we've had, of just being so hostile. You couldn't engage with her. And then if you tried to disengage, she'd become angrier. And this went on and on and on, and at the end of the day we talked to her. At the end of the day we took her to [the mental health facility in town]. We just said, "We can't do this anymore." And she agreed that something that was out of control, and she needed to go somewhere. And we drove her up, and checked her that evening, late that afternoon. She did residential program for a week, and then, 2 weeks of day treatment—outpatient. So that was the first time.

Phil felt that Chloe's breakdown after the sleepover was part of an ongoing problem, not something triggered by the events of the night before or their own actions as parents. Joan, however, recounted that Chloe had had an experience during a school trip to Washington when, with four girls assigned to one room with two beds, three of these same girls slept in one bed in order to avoid sharing the space with Chloe. Although the specifics of the overnight party never came out, it could possibly have been precipitated by the sort of rejection she had so often experienced from mainstream peers. Chloe, in ultimately deciding to transfer from the private school to the nearby public high school, allowed that the girls were never mean to her, and some were quite nice, but that at best, they "humored" her by including her. Feeling outcast in a setting that her parents had fervently hoped would provide the best educational and social environment for her possibly contributed to the rage that she expressed upon being picked up from an event that had been accompanied by such high hopes from her parents.

And yet, Chloe's online friendships spanned the globe and provided her with the relational interactions that were missing in much of her engagement with her flesh-and-blood surroundings. She described one such friendship as follows:

> I have one of my friends that I met about year ago. She goes online as Silvery. She's the one from Finland. . . . And she's really funny. She's one of the, I'll tell you about the two people who can crack me up, but she's really, she's 13. But she's, she's not, she's really good [at drawing anime art] for her age.... And she's really, really sweet. And I met her on my birthday.

And I had just met her, and I told her it was my birthday and so on her AOL instant messenger profile, she put, "Happy Birthday, Moon!" And it was really sweet cause we had just met. She's just a really, really nice person. And then one of my older on-line friends. She goes as Ia, and she's the other person. She's so funny. Um, I met, where did I meet her? I met her at this gallery. This on-line gallery, and she had just joined. And I had been there for a while. So I emailed her saying, "Hi, welcome to the Lost Artists. Do you want to do a trade?" So I remember right after I emailed her, the day after I had to leave on a two week trip so I got back, and she had replied and I'm like, "Ah, I'm sorry. I was gone. I'm sorry." And so I got her Yahoo screen and we just started talking. And I've been friends with her since. We've gone through a lot. Like we've gone through some really bad fights, but she's one of the people I'm closest to online.

In the absence of flesh-and-blood relationships that were sustainable and not worn thin by Chloe's tendency to overwhelm friends with intense demands for reciprocation, the online world provided her with friends who could choose how to manage their interactions to control their degree of involvement. Online, then, she was able to accomplish what her material relationships could not achieve: a degree of stability that enabled her to learn social propriety at a distance.

CONFLICTING NOTIONS OF AN APPROPRIATE LIFE TRAJECTORY

Phil recognized Chloe's differences from the time she was "2 or 3." He stated that her obsessiveness came through early in little acts, such as her need to line her vast collection of videotapes up in particular ways, but that he viewed this trait in the context of what he termed as the common parental perspective that "everything your kid does is a sign of genius." Phil repeatedly raised the expectation that Chloe was highly intelligent, that she had the "raw smarts to be a good student," but that she didn't have the "frame of mind" for it. Though he often related how he believed that he and Chloe were similar, academics was one area where he noted they had a difference, while also acknowledging that he himself hadn't become a serious student until after college. Phil believed that Chloe would find her own medium that would enable her to capitalize on their shared "product-oriented" personalities. He saw her finding a specialization in an interest she felt passionate about, and growing increasingly confident and independent in her "career network" once she had found her niche in life, presumably in something other than anime, which he regarded as a childish stage that could be cultivated into more mature interests he believed could sustain her through adulthood.

Phil was working on his doctorate when Chloe was born. He mentioned that for the previous 18 years he had been going "full throttle," having undergone the death of a spouse, a new marriage and two children, several job changes, and moving, which meant buying and selling houses and displacing those who had come to call each location home. All of these major stressors occurred while Phil was moving from teaching high school, to getting a PhD while teaching full time for five of his six years of doctoral work, to starting on the tenure track position at two state namesake universities.

His career trajectory and the moves it required did not sit well with Chloe, who did not like and had a difficult time adjusting to change. When she was four and a half, they moved to a new state to accommodate his first university position, and Chloe wanted to return to her state of origin for several years. Just as she was getting used to this move, his career took them to yet a new position in another faraway state. As is common among youth with Asperger's, these abrupt changes proved difficult for Chloe to adjust to and precipitated resistance and anger that, typical of those with her classification, she undertook with passion and full commitment that proved disruptive to a household already unsettled by family moves.

Phil's expectations shaped the way he took in information about Chloe's diagnoses. He did not trust the practices of the doctor in Chloe's second state of residence, who told him that Chloe should be hospitalized based on the outlier responses she gave on a Rorschach test. He felt that the doctor's reliance on a diagnostic script led him to misunderstand Chloe's reasoning behind her interpretation of the ambiguous text of the inkblot, and was further astonished to learn that the diagnostician believed that inkblots could be subject to correct interpretations based on typical responses. Phil found the doctor who conducted the diagnosis to be very odd in affect and, based on his professional interests in the interpretation of texts and the dynamics of researcher–participant interactions, was shocked that the doctor never considered that he himself might have contributed to the manner in which Chloe interpreted the inkblots. In sum, he was outraged at the manner in which the medical model epitomized by the doctor used diagnosis to pathologize his daughter (see Chap. 1). He was more inclined to trust the doctor in the next state in which they resided, who concluded that she could be classified on the Asperger's spectrum.

When Chloe was first hospitalized in this third of three communities that Chloe had lived in, Phil felt crushed by the diagnosis that she was "mentally ill," as her documentation described her. In terms of anticipated social trajectories, this characterization was far from how he anticipated his own family members would undertake their lives. This diagnosis summoned images of the mentally ill as confined to an "insane asylum" and as "weak" in character and awakened in him a "tough realization" that his daughter's life, and his and Joan's family, would not walk life's well worn, if illusory, pathways. What was less evident to him and Joan was that the area that they found so problematic in Chloe's life, her obsession with anime culture, provided her with one of the few gratifying and affirming updrafts in her life. Further, Phil's engagement with Chloe's diagnosis led to his understanding that he shared most of Chloe's neurodivergent conditions, at a lesser rate, and that he was genetically complicit in her makeup and how it affected her ability to find her niche in life.

This conflict between presumed life trajectories—the one anticipated by her parents and the one chosen and followed by Chloe—was never resolved while she lived at home. At the time, her parents believed that her anime obsession was symptomatic of what ailed her, rather than serving as the primary means of self-esteem she experienced as one of her immediate social world's outsiders and outcasts. When online, she became a highly regarded producer of art and narrative, frequently affirmed by her fellow community members. And yet when online, she was subject to continual, often abrasive criticism within her own home for not developing broader interests, not making more friends in her personal relationships, not engaging with schoolwork, and not exploring the natural world that provided the bucolic setting for their house. All of these problems were exacerbated by her growing conflicts with her younger brother, who felt embarrassed by her anime stylings and increasingly fought back against Chloe's tendency to impose her will on the only person in the house over whom she had advantages in size and age.

The relatively late diagnosis of PDD-NOS contributed to a number of problems within the family in understanding Chloe's refusal to fit in with her peers and her conflicts with those with whom she shared anime interests, largely due to the obsessive way in which she approached her friendships to the detriment of a reciprocal relationships. Chloe had been well diagnosed in terms of anxiety, depression, and Tourette's, and exhibited sufficient oppositional conduct to make the oppositional-defiant diagnosis easy to provide and relatively easy to digest for her parents.

The absence of an Asperger's classification, however, denied her parents, therapist, and school personnel the information needed to create a learning environment geared to her unique cognitive and neurological differences. Had her mother's keen research skills been put to use researching autism spectrum conditions, she would have found useful information, even at that time when Asperger's was relatively unheard of in the general population. These resources would have helped her see how independence from social convention was manifesting in her daughter.

Despite her mother's insistence that her daughter was not developing independence and was overly dependent on anime art for satisfaction and verification, Chloe demonstrated her independence online by establishing friendships across the world and engaging in trade with her art. She sought out and became a part of a community, both online and face to face, where she was able to turn these negatively framed diagnostic criteria into a positive force that would eventually shape her worldview and her daily life. Neuro-atypical minds require different ways of looking. The patterns produced by Chloe throughout her childhood and youth—repetitive movements, temper tantrums, rages, disassociation, and lack of personal hygiene—fit well into the autism spectrum range of behaviors and dispositions. Chloe, however, was verbally precocious and an advanced, voracious reader who had read entire chapter book series before beginning first grade, which is perhaps why so many professionals overlooked her as being on the autism spectrum and focused instead on addressing her anger and resistance to efforts to expand her horizons beyond the narrow realm of anime texts.

Validating Sexuality

Except for when Phil mentioned that Chloe's therapist let them know she identified as a lesbian, Chloe's parents did not discuss their daughter as a sexual being during interviews for the research, focusing more on her struggles and how they affected her ability to form and sustain relationships. Her pre-teen crush on Kimberly, the Pink Power Ranger from the popular TV show, was only in retrospect seen as an indicating of Chloe's sexual orientation; at the time it was viewed at home as a form of identification with the only White female in the Power Ranger group. Phil recognized the relationships in which Chloe was involved with Casey and Jason were complex. He revealed that Jason, Chloe's companion and date to her school's homecoming dance, shortly thereafter identified as gay and developed a same-sex romantic interest with a teen with whom Chloe was also friends.

Chloe's use of anime to explore gay love was evident in her and her friends' use of the characters they created to explore gender and sexuality roles. In the middle of the self-box interview, Chloe noted a drawing given to her by her friend Phoebe during a summer graphic arts program. She described Phoebe as "a big fan of *Yoai* but she hates girls. Her goal in life is to, as soon as it's completely possible, she's going to get a sex change and become a gay man." Phoebe's drawing was of Chloe's favorite characters, Akira and Hikaru. She mentioned that this picture was one of her favorites and discussed how anime artists play with "different pairings" such as "guy/guy sex," "guy/guy relationships with no sex, kissing yes," and similar "girl/girl" relationships.

Male/male pairings show up in *dojinshi* drawn by and for girls called *yaoi*. Chloe had preferences for which characters she liked to see together, though her parents did set limits on what she could view:

Chloe: Ok there's *Yaoi*, which is guy-guy sex. And then there's *shounen*, which is guy-guy just like relationships like kissing and stuff but no sex or there might be. I guess some people refer to sex with not showing anything as *shounen*, just like heavy *shounen ai*, so there's a gray area in between, and then there's the same thing, there's *Shoujo* for girls and the sex part is *Yuri*.

Q: And your parents are Ok now that you're older, looking at that?

Chloe: Yeah. They don't want me looking at sex. I watched a level C which is like a *Yaoi*. It was a PWP, which is a Plot, What Plot [fanfiction with no plot other than what occurs in graphic sexual scenes].

The term YAOI is an acronym of three Japanese words: *yamanashi* (without climax), *ochinashi* (without ending), and *iminashi* (without meaning). "*Yaoi*" was coined in the late 1970s by a group of young women whose *dojinshi* carried out the earlier stories appearing in commercial manga in which young men engaged in love affairs. The intricacies of this form of anime were reflected in Chloe's artwork: stories of incest such as brothers in love, a *seme* (dominant) and an *uke* (submissive) male pairing, and exquisite drafting of the characters. Wilson and Toku (2004) posit that yaoi "permits women to reconstruct themselves along masculine lines and to gain status" (p. 100). The male body, less known to most adolescent females, provides a blank slate on which to ascribe new forms of femininity. *Yaoi* provided the positive social updraft that was complex enough to satisfy Chloe's needs as a developing sexual being.

Sex is often what most parents fear their children are exploring online. Joan in particular had a fear for the kinds of people Chloe met via the computer. She was worried that the people who spent as much time as her daughter on the Internet were "emotionally fragile" and would tend to become enmeshed like Chloe herself. Her parents were particularly vigilant about Chloe not giving out her contact information online, even though Chloe did do a good deal of commerce with her online friends. She abided by her parents' rule as much as possible, but she felt their lack of knowledge about online environments was getting in the way of living the life she wanted for herself. Eventually she found ways to work within and around her parents' rules for computer usage. Her portfolio drawings were clear evidence that Chloe had played with defining the kind of "sex" she was allowed to view. She found the "grey area" and chose to explore it through online collaboration.

Validating Commercial Potential

The economy of anime is based both in trade and monetary exchange. Chloe's collection of manga and fansub was impressive. Chloe explained the manner in which she both produced and collected anime texts, saying

> We do sometimes we do gift pictures for each other. Which are just pictures where we don't do anything in return. Or we'll do what's called a trade picture, which is when I'll draw something for him or her, and he'll draw something for me, or she. Or there's things called commissions which is what that one was, which is paying someone to draw what you want. And usually how commissions go, is you'll tell them what you want, and they'll do the sketch. And they'll get it approved by you, and if you want something changed they'll go back and fix it and show it to you again. And once you're satisfied, you'll pay. And then they'll go and finish it.

At age 14, Chloe had also been commissioned by an online acquaintance for a drawing, but because her parents would not allow her to send people her home address for security reasons, her father came up with what she termed a "this bizarre idea....The person wouldn't pay me. Dad would pay me. So I was still getting paid, they were still getting their picture. I wouldn't give out my address, but they're not paying. But I'm getting paid for it." With her father's help, Chloe worked around the fears for safety to profit from her *otaku* obsessions. Though she recognized the seeming absurdity of establishing a separate address from which to do business, she was willing to play along with her parents' rules in order to participate more fully with her chosen community.

At anime conventions, Chloe and a friend set up a table to sell their work and also bought art from people she met in person. "The guy I was sitting next to on Sunday, I asked him how much he charged for commission and he said 15 dollars for a pencil sketch so I asked him to draw Armena, and since I had to leave in an hour or two, he didn't have time to like tighten up the pencil lines so he only charged me 5 dollars for that. Isn't that awesome? I love that picture." Chloe was both a consumer and producer in the anime economy that supported the online and offline exchange of goods and services. Economic interactions within the anime community allowed Chloe to gain status, clients, and a professional reputation.

Validating Creativity

Among the forms of validation that Chloe received through her online engagement with fellow anime enthusiasts was positive feedback from other artists and consumers. She said of one collaborative fanfiction story to which she contributed,

> I write as that person from that persons' point of view and other people write from their characters' point of view. And we have, tie together into one story, or more than one story. It's really fun. And then I'm on fan art mailing list where we all send in the art that we've done and we give comments and tips on it. It's a lot of fun. And then I update my web pages sometimes.

She uploaded her art as well to various online galleries such as her *fan art* web page, a medium in which an artist mimics the style of a popular program such as Gundam Wing and draws either characters from the series or characters of their own drawn according to the show's conventions.

Chloe drew and developed "a lot of characters of her own," many in an anime style. She created her own "furries," animal-based characters with a human form; "*Animorphs*," a book series that she and her online friends carried into their own novel; and her online persona, Moon, a character who changed over the course of time in relation to Chloe's own maturation (Cook and Smagorinsky 2014). Her broad interests within the anime community connected her with different groups who had different requests of her artistic skills. She was often commissioned to draw a character for an online friend or to color in a character someone else had drawn. Character creation for Chloe initiated the stories in which they were involved.

Through websites dedicated solely to fan fiction and fan art, Chloe wrote and drew several collaborative manga. Some of the characters in a manga she was working on while in high school included Tayato, the evil villain; Lena, his guardian the wolf-woman; Kati, a metal goddess; Kotakoza, the wind; Hirishi, his guardian and a bird of paradise; Kiane, a fire girl; Shikasi, her guardian; and Kokashi, the plague. These characters were adaptations of online characters with which she and her virtual and material friends interacted.

In talking about her persona Moon's collaborative creation through drawing with her friend Kate, Chloe illustrated both the role of collaboratively produced texts and the agentive role they had in her life:

> That was my birthday picture this year. That's my persona online. I go by Moon online and that's Moon's boyfriend in the story and he is my boyfriend-he would be if he were real. So kind of as a joke she put my persona and my boyfriend together, and she's wearing his outfit, and her boyfriend is going "ohh." That my character's boyfriend, Moon Anante, and that's Koshita. He was in the girls' picture too.

Chloe was adept in the literary act of creating characters. She spent a great deal of time in drawing fan fiction and in character creation through online and in-person collaborations with her friends. When asked to explain her online life as if she were trying to describe it to her mother, she said:

> I talk to friends, and I'm on a couple mailing lists, and I do RPGs, like role playing games where I role play as a character, and I write as that person from that person's point of view and other people write from their characters' point of view. And we have, tie together into one story, or more than one story. It's really fun. And then I'm on fan art mailing list where we all send in the art that we've done and we give comments and tips on it. It's a lot of fun.

Through collaborative character creation, Chloe and her friends played in the figured worlds of anime, which rely on artifacts, "by which figured worlds are evoked, collectively developed, individually learned, and made socially and personally powerful" (Holland et al. 1998, p. 61). Chloe's access to these worlds enabled her to try on roles in virtual and, eventually, material environments. The movement for Chloe was contingent on the artifacts, or mediational means available. Her online worlds and the community at the art school she attended provided her with an affinity space where sexual exploration was normative.

Discussion

Chloe's participation in the culture of the anime world was an integral part of her personal self-construction. Anime allowed her to escape from culturally valued social and sexual norms for a teenage girl in the USA, roles in which she felt out of sorts and unaccepted. For one whose neurodivergent profile suggested the need for a narrow range of interests, in spite of living within a social setting that pushed her toward a broadened scope of attention, Chloe participated in the anime world so that it provided her with a positive social updraft in which her strengths were validated, her personality was not viewed as weird and ill-fitting, her tendency toward intensely concentrated work found an outlet, and she was happy and affirmed as a person.

Her case illuminates the difficulties of adaptation required for those who occupy Chloe's place on the autism spectrum, as well as for those who surround them and try to direct them toward a satisfying and sustainable future. Chloe made adaptations reluctantly, often creating havoc around her household when denied computer access to engage with the primary focus of her attention, the online anime community and its practices. Her parents and brother adapted to some aspects of her personality, such as accommodating her insatiable need for more Pokémon cards, more videos, more computer time, and other demands, albeit in reluctant, resistant, and limited ways. Her parents, however, also subjected her to rules that became entrenched once Chloe's opposition began and both sides dug in to do battle. Lost in the daily commotion was her brother and his needs, which were often overlooked in Chloe's parents' efforts to normalize their household around conventional notions of family life and social interaction. Ironically, the effort to force Chloe into broader interests and more reciprocal material relationships appeared to exacerbate the very aspects of her makeup that made those adaptations so difficult for her to begin with.

Vygotsky's (1993) notion of the *secondary disability* (see Chap. 1) is illuminating in considering how Chloe's happiness varied, depending on her surroundings. When on computer or when with friends whom she didn't overwhelm, she was generally free of negative judgments about her personality makeup and was liberated to work on what she found important. As her own account suggests, she engaged in disputes with online and immediate friends, although in ways that she had begun developing means for resolution. On the computer, she was not subject to demands that other people felt were important for her, except the condition that she limit her computer time, which she fought heatedly. Off the computer and outside the anime world, she felt like an outcast, one subject to either the pity of those who found her disposition and interests to be weird and inappropriate, or the scorn of those who found her to be peculiar and abject. The positive social updraft afforded by her participation in anime resolved the secondary disability and provided her with daily respite from the negative judgments of others.

Her response to the imposition of rules corresponded to what Vygotsky (1993) called *moral insanity*, the lashing out by those of extranormal makeup at those who treat them as inferior, in need of rules and monitoring, and otherwise incapable of functioning in the world (cf. Smagorinsky 2012). Vygotsky's solution was not to cure the sick individual, but to educate those who surround her, to change the setting of her developmental trajectory to allow for greater understanding of what made her different and how those differences were manifested in her approach to the world and conduct in it (see Chap. 2).

Chloe made a cultural shift from her family and her peers, one that enabled her to enter a social updraft that gave her positive feedback instead of the criticism and regulation to which she found herself exposed elsewhere in life. Though at 14 she didn't have a sense that she could live her lifestyle in a way that would support her, she did understand that people around the world were as passionate and as focused on anime as she was. Through her skills and talents, hidden from most people who encountered her and available primarily online, she forged her way into being able to live the identity that she drew into existence through her art. Her character creation skills were admired by her online and offline friends. Attending the anime conferences helped her envision that adults were making a living doing what she loved the most. In her teens, Chloe was exerting more independence of will than she was given credit for. Her parents both recognized her hyperfocusing tendencies and their potential to be her source of happiness, but both initially rejected anime culture as a potential source.

Like the young men in the Beat generation followers who started growing their hair long and the young women who rejected traditional feminine roles, Chloe was a harbinger for a new cultural movement, one that relies on video streaming, file sharing, global communication, and blurred lines between binaries. Parents across generations who watch their children diverge from familial and social expectations have fought the departure from their anticipated norms. Perhaps a better understanding of what makes children and youth on the autism spectrum tick could produce more satisfying lives, both for those classified with this state and the people who love and surround them.

Notes

1. The data for this case study come from a larger narrative inquiry involving five young women, all of whom had been diagnosed with a mood disorder (Cook 2004). "Chloe" is a pseudonym, as are all names of people she referenced in her interviews and the names of her parents. At times, she is referred to by "Moon," a pseudonym for the name she used in her online world (see Cook and Smagorinsky 2014). Chloe was selected through purposeful random sampling (Patton 1990). Her parents shared some of Chloe's story with first author Leslie Cook, who then recruited her for the research with her parents' permission. Institutional Review Board permission was granted for the research.
2. Although these terms are typically accompanied by a condition such as "disorder," we avoid such phrasings in our own writing when possible.

References

Black, R. W. (2008). *Adolescents and online fan fiction*. New York: Peter Lang.

Bodovski, K. (2014). Adolescents' emerging habitus: The role of early parental expectations and practices. *British Journal of Sociology of Education, 35*(3), 389–412.

Broomhead, K. E. (2014). A clash of two worlds'; disjuncture between the norms and values held by educational practitioners and parents of children with behavioural, emotional and social difficulties. *British Journal of Special Education, 41*, 136–150.

Cook, L. S. (2004). *Authoring self: Framing identities of young women diagnosed with mood disorders*. Unpublished doctoral dissertation, The University of Georgia.

Cook, L. S., & Smagorinsky, P. (2014). Constructing positive social updrafts for extranormative personalities. *Learning, Culture and Social Interaction*, *3*(4), 296–308. Retrieved September 18, 2015, from http://www.petersmagorinsky.net/About/PDF/LCSI/LCSI_2014.pdf

Eng, L. (2012a). Strategies of engagement: Discovering, defining, and describing otaku culture in the United States (trans: Sato, E. & Ito, M.). In M. Ito, D. Okabe, & I. Tsuji (Eds.), *Fandom unbound: Otaku culture in a connected world* (pp. 85–106). New Haven: Yale University Press.

Eng, L. (2012b). Anime and manga fandom as networked culture (trans: Sato, E. & Ito, M.). In M. Ito, D. Okabe, & I. Tsuji (Eds.), *Fandom unbound: Otaku culture in a connected world* (pp. 158–178). New Haven: Yale University Press.

Holland, D., Lachicotte, W., Skinner, D., & Cain, C. (1998). *Identity and agency in cultural worlds*. Cambridge, MA: Harvard University Press. Retrieved September 25, 2015, from http://www.infoamerica.org/documentos_pdf/holland02.pdf

Morikawa, K. (2012). Otaku and the city: The rebirth of Akihabara (trans: Sato, E. & Ito, M.). In M. Ito, D. Okabe, & I. Tsuji (Eds.), *Fandom unbound: Otaku culture in a connected world* (pp. 133–157). New Haven: Yale University Press.

Okabe, D. (2012). Cosplay, learning, and cultural practice. (trans: Sato, E. & Ito, M.). In M. Ito, D. Okabe, & I. Tsuji (Eds.), *Fandom unbound: Otaku culture in a connected world* (pp. 225–248). New Haven: Yale University Press.

Okabe, D., & Ishida, K. (2012). Making Fujoshi identity visible and invisible (trans: Sato, E. & Ito, M.). In M. Ito, D. Okabe, & I. Tsuji (Eds.), *Fandom unbound: Otaku culture in a connected world* (pp. 207–224). New Haven: Yale University Press.

Patton, M. (1990). *Qualitative evaluation and research methods*. Thousand Oaks: Sage.

Smagorinsky, P. (2012). Every individual has his own insanity: Applying Vygotsky's work on defectology to the question of mental health as an issue of inclusion. *Learning, Culture and Social Interaction*, *1*(1), 67–77. Retrieved September 1, 2016, from http://www.petersmagorinsky.net/About/PDF/LCSI/LCSI_2012.pdf

Vygotsky, L. S. (1993). *The collected works of L. S. Vygotsky. Volume 2: The fundamentals of defectology (abnormal psychology and learning disabilities)* (R. W. Rieber & A. S. Carton, Eds.; J. E. Knox & C. B. Stevens, Trans.). New York: Plenum.

Watase, Y. (1992). *Fushigi Yuugi: The mysterious play*. Tokyo-to/Chiyoda-ku/Hitotsubashi: Shogakukan.

Wilson, B., & Toku, M. (2004). Boys' love, yaoi, and art education: Issues of power and pedagogy. In D. L. Smith-Shank (Ed.), *Semiotics and visual culture: Sights, signs, and significance* (pp. 94–103). Reston: The National Art Education Association.

CHAPTER 10

Composing Poetry and a Writer's Identity: Positive Social Updrafts in a Community of Writers

Christine M. Dawson

> Creative writing is a bridge for me in several important ways. It is a bridge of communication between myself and other people across the communication canyon of my autism. It is a bridge between my disability and my ability as a writer. It is a bridge between my isolation on the island of silence and the bustling and talkative city that the other students inhabit in their communicative world. It is a bridge between my imagination and the understanding of the rest of the world. It is a bridge to self-esteem as I am able to travel mentally to other people and influence their lives. ~Scott's[1] written reflection, produced during his senior year in high school

As a young man on the autism spectrum, Scott may have seemed to be silent, with a broad chasm separating him from his talkative peers. Scott's autism significantly limited his use of oral language, requiring him to type on a computer or handheld device as a primary communicative mode. Because Scott communicated primarily through the written word, it could be easy to focus overly on his "disability" and not see his many abilities. Yet through his creative writing, and perhaps especially his poetry, Scott has been able to

C.M. Dawson (✉)
Skidmore College, Saratoga Springs, NY, USA

build a bridge between himself and others, enabling him to influence their lives and to participate actively in the world around him.

Scott composed the above "bridge" metaphor as part of a reflective writing assignment during his senior year in high school, to account for the role of creative writing in his socially situated development as a writer and a person. This chapter follows Scott several years later when he was 23, as he participated in writing groups and online poetry workshops. For six months, Scott shared the poetry he wrote for his online poetry workshop and corresponded with me about his writing practices. What emerged from these communications was a rich description, authored by Scott, revealing whom he considered himself to be as a writer at that point in his development, as well as how his poetry and writing decisions reflected that sense of self-understanding. These self-descriptions and the ways Scott enacted them through his writing practices are at the heart of this chapter.

These personal accounts suggest that as Scott composed poetry and participated in a variety of writing communities, he also experienced, and contributed to creating, positive social updrafts that supported his ability to author his own writing identities. Across online and in-person writing groups, Scott was able to position himself as a writer, and the social context of these interactions involved other authors responding thoughtfully to his writing and sharing their own. Within these interactions the focus was rightfully on Scott as a poet and fellow writer, rather than as a young adult on the autism spectrum. His self-descriptions also opened empowering routes for his development as a poet, enabling him to interpret assignments and feedback in ways that were congruous with his strengths, interests, and areas for growth.

The research methods for this study are described in the Appendix. To move the reader directly into Scott's experiences within the social updraft of writing communities, I next describe Scott and his conception of his role and development within these supportive collectives.

Scott as Poet-Memoirist and Advanced Student of Writing

Across our conversations, Scott used variations of two primary terms to describe himself as a writer. He described himself as a "poet-memoirist," identifying his writing in terms of genre and purpose, and he described himself as an "advanced student of writing," identifying himself in terms of his perceived level of independence and his relation to other writers.

Scott wove his discussion of these identifying terms together, drawing on both concepts across his communications with me. His poetry and writing practices revealed ways in which Scott drew on each of these identities and the contexts in which he developed them through his composition of poetry.

Identifying Through Genre: "Primarily a Poet-Memoirist"

Although I have had opportunity to read Scott's work across several genres, much of his formally composed writing in recent years has been in poetry. As a result, when I sat down with Scott and his mother at the beginning of this study and asked him what genre he preferred writing within, I was not surprised that he responded, "poetry." He went on to explain that he preferred writing poetry because it allowed him to "distill the emotion"[2] in his writing. His mother agreed, commenting that writing group members and classmates often described even Scott's prose as "poetic."

Yet Scott did not simply describe himself as a poet. Rather, he described himself as a "poet of memoirs," and he stated in a later email that, regardless of how he may grow in coming years as a writer, the "one thing I expect to remain constant is my vision of myself as primarily a poet-memoirist." Through these statements, Scott deliberately located himself in terms of a hybrid genre, where he combined the form and "distillation" of poetry with some of the purpose and subject matter of memoir. He wrote, "I am most drawn to writing poetry that crystallizes the shards of my own life," implying an interest in taking small, discrete, and possibly fragmented pieces or experiences from his life and assembling them in his poetry. The notion of "memoir" thus did not necessarily refer to a conventional linear narrative, but rather his expression of whatever encapsulated his experiences, particularly images.

Scott observed that writing about his experiences enabled him to "be more dedicated in the writing," implying that he felt more invested in pieces that he wrote from personal experiences than he did in topics from which he was detached. Scott explained that he sought authenticity in his writing by avoiding "ease of generality," and that his online writing instructor encouraged him to "look for the affect of real experience." These comments not only further clarify Scott's concept of a "poet-memoirist," they also show ways that Scott drew on this self-identification to guide his poetic compositions. Drawing on the specificity of real life experiences in his poetry seemed to feel more genuine to Scott than writing about other topics, and this authenticity appeared to feed his sense of commitment and engagement with his writing.

Scott also explained that writing memoirist poetry enabled others to "enter into my womb," which he described as "where i truly find my spirit." His very language here is full of imagery and reminiscent of his bridge metaphor that opened this chapter, implying that this genre invited readers to share central and personal aspects of his experiences. Scott later commented that "no one knows my feelings from my outside," and that through sharing his writing he could "dream we communicate" such that "my feelings can be shared and not isolated and strange." Scott seemed to recognize a connective purpose associated with writing, and his statements demonstrated the positive social updraft he experienced, and hoped to continue experiencing, through composing memoirist poetry and sharing it with his writing communities. By distilling his experiences and feelings into poetic language, Scott allowed readers to cross into and share something of his life that would otherwise be hidden from them.

As our communications progressed, I wondered about the particular way Scott was using *experiences* and *feelings*, questioning if I was interpreting his use of these terms accurately. I had initially assumed that by "experiences" he was referring to specific occurrences or stories from his life, and by "feelings" he was referring to something like emotions, but Scott later clarified that he had a more specific intention for each of these terms. Although he drew on personal moments and events in writing his poetry, Scott used "experiences" to refer to *details and sensations he observed during those moments*, rather than the full occurrence or event. In this way Scott seemed to marry the nonfiction and experiential aspects of memoir with the imagery of poetry, drawing on his own experienced sensations in order to select particular images and evoke certain effects in a poem.

Toward the end of the study, Scott explained his commitment to being a poet-memoirist by writing, "I never want to stray too far away from the authenticity of my own experience in my poetry. I want to continue to generate my poetry out of my own center of understanding." When I asked him some questions about this statement, he ended up revising his language: "I decided that my phrase 'center of understanding' was not well-chosen because it makes it sound like I wish my poetry to be explanatory and I really find myself resistant to that." He went on to clarify that, although he often was "urged to be more explanatory," he felt that

> I am a weak poet when I try to explain. My strongest poetry recaptures a sensation I have felt. I truly mean sensation rather than emotion. To me emotion is a reaction to sensation that is moving toward explanation, putting the sensation into context. I want to capture the intense sensation before all this reacting and thinking kicks in. So what I should have said is "I want to continue to generate my poetry out of my own center of sensation." To my mind my writing is not emotional or intellectual. It is physical and based on sensory experience.

Here, Scott's revision of "center of understanding" to "center of sensation" further clarified his identification as a poet memoirist, within the community of practice in which such work is valued and through which his choices and identity were affirmed. Although both memoir and poetry often explore emotion, and although memoir often focuses on specific stories from a life, Scott wanted his poetry to capture sensations without the reflection. Scott clarified that, unlike many memoirists, he focused on the *sensation* he experienced, rather than the complete or narrativized experience itself. In making this move, he also situated his purpose in the "physical" rather than the "emotional or intellectual," and he distinguished himself not only as a certain kind of writer, but also as a certain kind of poet-memoirist.

Scott's language in the above quote shows that for him, being a poet and a memoirist were interwoven, and that these identities also connected to his sense of success and effectiveness as a writer. Scott identified himself as a stronger poet when he focused on experienced sensations and as a "weak poet" when he wrote to explain. In this way, Scott also linked his effectiveness as a poet with the extent to which he was true to his understanding of himself as a poet-memoirist.

Scott's clarification of terms here, and his ability to position his writing so specifically in terms of genre and purpose, provide evidence of the positive social updraft he experienced through his poetry and participation in his writing practices. This effort to locate his writing within the anticipated conventions of an established genre allowed his texts to be *in tune* (Nystrand 1986) with his readers' expectations and understandings. Scott was the author of his developing identity as a writer, and he was drawing on this emerging identity to describe his poetry and his writing choices. This identity gained substance and appreciation through the feedback that came from his readers, who comprised the sort of mutually supportive community that served as the medium of updraft. Rather than contributing to a secondary disability, which Vygotsky (1993) found to typify the experiences of those whose points of difference lead them to be treated as disabled or deficient, this writing community focused solely on Scott's craft decisions and assets as a writer, just as, one would imagine, they expected Scott to do for them and their writing. These assets and abilities, when foregrounded in others' views of him, provided Scott an earned sense of status among fellow expressive writers.

Writing as a Poet-Memoirist

Not surprisingly, Scott's identification of himself as a poet-memoirist also aligned with evidence from his poetry and writing processes. It appeared that Scott drew on his interest in memoirist poetry most significantly as he selected topics and interpreted assignments.

Of the 11 poems Scott wrote during the six focal months of this study, he described drawing on his own actual experiences or observations in some way in each piece. For example, when assigned to write an "ecstatic poem," Scott wrote, "It occurred to me that I should not need an exotic experience for the poem, that the first sensation of feeling your body come alive when you wake up should be ecstatic enough for anybody." This interpretation allowed Scott to approach a fairly open assignment by playing to his strengths and focusing on experienced sensations. Within that poem, Scott also drew inspiration from his observations of swallows nesting in his hedges, describing the way they "fly in circles in a panic and then return to the hedges." It reminded him "of how my heartbeat feels when I first wake up" (see Chap. 5 for attention to the role of the heartbeat in children on the autism spectrum). Scott thereby entered his assignment by capturing the sensation he associated with waking up, using his own observations of the birds to create the effect he wished to express. Because his overall focus was on emphasizing the sensation, he allowed himself to slightly idealize his observations in order to heighten the effect he sought in this poem: "Their wings do not bronze in the sunlight, but I wish they did, so that is the way I described them." The final version of his poem reads:

> Waking
>
> A crescent dream slips
> to the periphery
> then dissolves.
> Birds feet
> scratch eyelids open
> to the hum
> of blood in the ears
> the skid
> of a heartbeat
> in the sternum,
> a stutter
> of drab sparrows
> fleeting
> from the shadows
> of a skeletonized thicket,
> their wings bronzed
> by the brittle rays
> of a winter sun.

This assignment was fairly open-ended, allowing Scott to adapt it easily to his identified style. Some other assignments were more confining in their specificity. Still, Scott drew on his sense of self as poet-memoirist, explaining,

> Even with the assignments [my instructor] Michael gives to expand my range, I mostly try to bring those skills [of a poet-memoirist] to bear on what I feel I really know best, my own sphere. Even the war poem, "As Reported," was about my own understanding of what I had read in the paper. Even "Insomniac" drew from my interest in movies, although the voice was not my own.

Thus, even when his instructor assigned Scott to write about an unfamiliar topic or in a style or voice different from his own, Scott sought to enter these assignments in ways that aligned with his views of himself as a poet-memoirist. Instructor Michael's flexibility as Scott's reader helped to provide the sort of environmental adaptation that enabled Scott's own adaptation of the assignment to serve as a legitimate and well-appreciated text (see Chap. 3). For example, when writing the assigned war poem, Scott commented, "Since I only know about war from what I read in the paper, that is what my poem is about." As he incorporated key events from the newspaper, Scott focuses on the *sensations* and *images* associated with these moments, describing "GI's choking in a chlorine cloud" and the way "the force of a detonation in the open market … knocked a bag of tomatoes and onions from the arms of a 35 year old elementary school teacher." Scott did not write an emotional or reflective piece, which could have fit the assignment, but rather focused on crafting sensations based on what he had personally read in the newspaper. In this way, even though the poem was not memoirist in a traditional way, Scott remained true to his commitment to poetry that "crystalizes shards" of life.

The assignment for "Insomniac," the other poem Scott referenced above, targeted style rather than topic. His task was to use the poet Marianne Moore's work as a model for writing long lines. Scott commented that this assignment "was hard because I usually use a short line," adding, "usually I find myself dividing lines and making them shorter with more line breaks when I revise." This assignment challenged Scott to move beyond his identified style and comfort zone. Having full choice over topic, Scott chose to write about sensations he had experienced in movie theaters:

> The darkness comes in grained shades and shadows
> the dreams in flicker and stutter. The film's jammed,
> the celluloid's burning, a reel's missing in this avant-garde
> cinema verite black-and-white serial where the plot
> makes no sense

Indeed, across other assignments, from poems modeled after E. E. Cummings to a poem about plumbing, Scott seemed to draw on his identification as a poet-memoirist in foundational ways, shaping the topics and details he chose for his poetry. When he had open choice over topic, Scott wrote from his own experience, but across poems, he emphasized sensations and imagery that had their roots in his own lived moments. Scott's ability to draw deliberately upon his own sense of identity as a writer seemed to empower him to meet writing challenges, to interpret assignments in terms of his strengths, and to draw deliberately on these abilities as he expanded his craft. This asset-oriented approach met with approval from his peers and mentors, thus reinforcing to Scott that his stance as a writer granted him a legitimate role in the broader community of poetic authors.

Identifying in Relation to Other Writers: "An Advanced Student of Writing"

In addition to identifying himself in terms of genre and purpose, as he did when he described himself as a poet-memoirist, Scott also described his writing identity in terms of his perceived independence and relationship to other writers. When I asked Scott at the end of the study (via email) to describe how he thought of himself as a writer, he devoted three of his four paragraph response to elaborating on his opening lines: "I do not see myself as a mature writer yet. I see myself more as an advanced student of writing." Viewing himself developmentally suggests the presence of a positive social updraft through which his abilities might be cultivated, in that development must be headed toward a social sense of endpoint (see Wertsch's [2000] discussion of *telos*, that is, an ideal destination or outcome). As a poet, then, he was able to stand "a head taller" (Vygotsky 1978; cf. Holzman 2009), especially in relation to other labels, including the potentially debilitating label of being autistic that might characterize him, in some social channels, in terms of deficits rather than strengths and produce the secondary disability of feelings of inferiority that follow from adopting other people's beliefs of inadequacy (Vygotsky 1993; see Chap. 1).

Across that response and our subsequent emails, Scott provided two primary rationales for his identification as an advanced student of writing: his role as an actual student in writing courses and his comparison between himself and "mature writers." In his email response, Scott stated that the main reason he described himself as a student writer was "because I am still taking on-line independent study poetry writing classes." He felt he benefited, in that context, from assignments, feedback, and instruction from professors or mentors:

> I continue with these courses for three reasons. First, I still need the crutch of regular assignments to continue to write regularly. Second, I still do not feel confident in my editing skills and want the feedback of a professor who

knows my work well. Third, Michael exposes me to work very different from my own and gives me assignments that urge me to expand my themes and experiment with a variety of poetic voices and lines.

This combination of incentive, access to feedback and encouragement, exposure to varied poetry, and participation in the production of emerging genres led Scott to take courses where he could learn and deliberately improve his craft. The online poetry classes he took with Michael involved a weekly written "lecture," often discussing the style and features of several model poems, as well as an assignment to write a poem somehow connected to that lesson. Scott would read through the lecture and accompanying poems, draft and revise a poem that responded to the assignment, and submit it to Michael for feedback. After Michael's feedback, Scott would typically revise the poem once again. This structure positioned Scott as the learner and Michael as the teacher, a relationship reflected in Scott's identification as a student of writing. Yet this student role was not necessarily permanent or limiting. Scott qualified that he "still" needed these supports, indicating a possible future boundary of his student writing identification. Additionally, Scott's sense of himself as a *learner* contributed to his ability to grow toward greater social competence and acceptance through his participation in his relationship with Michael.

As a student, Scott privileged feedback he received from trusted instructors such as Michael, and he looked to them to help him target specific writing goals. He explained that he felt that he needed encouragement from courses and instructors like Michael, "because sometimes I feel the style of my poems is too similar from poem to poem." As evidence, he referenced feedback from a previous instructor, who had praised the originality and strength of his imagery but commented on occasional awkwardness in his lines. Scott noted,

> She advised me to work on the musicality and line of my poetry. I did work very hard on that. I shortened my lines and worked on enjambment. I tried to keep the originality of my imagery while simplifying the language so it would sound more natural. In pursuing these aims I think I developed a distinctive style that people seemed to recognize as specific to me.

For Scott, this intentional use of an instructor's assessment provided further proof that his growth as a writer (specifically his success in addressing feedback and thereby developing a "distinctive style") was related to his self-identification as a student writer, an identity not possible without the mentoring available from Michael and others in his community of writers. While Scott felt his "writing has markedly improved," he also commented that he felt "in danger of falling in a rut." He added, "That is why I am pleased with poems I did for Michael last spring.... I wish I knew how to vary my style like this on my own, but for now I still need a mentor/teacher to guide me." This statement links to Scott's earlier claims, where he said he "still" needed an instructor to provide feedback and to push him to continue to grow. In this way, Scott drew on evidence from his own poetry from the online course as indications of why he benefited from being a student writer.

Scott emphasized the role of learning in his student-writer mindset, stating, "Even if I always need a mentor and remain an advanced student of writing for the rest of my life, I would be content with that status. What is most important is that I find a way to get whatever support I need to have the confidence and focus to continue writing and continue developing and improving as a writer." Scott thereby seemed to embrace his identification as a learner, emphasizing that his goal was to develop as a writer. He went on to define his concept of a mature writer in terms of discipline, interpretation of feedback, and ways of relating to other writers:

> To me a mature writer would have the discipline to write each day without needing any outside assignments or incentives. Also, although mature writers like student writers need outside feedback, I do not think they consider the people giving them feedback to be mentors. To mature writers they would be peers. I do not always make the changes Michael suggests but most of the time I do, and when I decide that I do not wish to follow one of his suggestions, I wonder if my decision is right. This shows my student writer mindset. I do feel, however, more like a peer to the fellow members of my writing groups. Sometimes I will make changes according to their suggestions, especially if several of them back a suggestion. However, if I find myself internally disagreeing with a suggestion, I feel far less conflicted than I do when I disagree with one of Michael's suggestions for revision.

Because Scott felt that he needed incentives and feedback, and because he designated some of those people giving the feedback to be mentors whose comments he privileged, he again identified himself as an advanced student of writing rather than a mature writer.

It is interesting that Scott only explored the role of incentives and feedback in his above response. This focus may have been a result of Scott responding directly to my questions, where I inquired specifically about these elements and their significance. Still, it seems meaningful that Scott did not reference achievement (e.g., of publication) or overall mastery of technique/craft as indications of mature writing. Rather, he defined mature writers primarily *by how they interact with writing and with other writers*, suggesting a good understanding of the role of writing within the channels provided by a broader community of supportive writers. The bulk of his paragraph (seven of eight sentences) focused on the way a mature writer interprets and uses feedback; he defined a mature writer as one who views other writers as peers, rather than mentors, and who feels confident to trust his own judgment to take or leave suggestions without internal conflict. For Scott *maturity* as a writer seemed to link to his sense of *independence* rather than accomplishment.

Scott's description of himself as an advanced student of writing once again reflected his experience of a positive social updraft through his writing practices, and most especially through his relationship with other writers. His positioning of himself as student was positive and empowering overall, and he seemed to draw on this self-identification in deliberate ways as he formed and pursued goals for his writing, using these goals to guide his development both as a writer and as a person.

It is also noteworthy that Scott was once again the author of this identity, rather than allowing others to define him as a writer or in terms of his autism. Instead, he described relationships with peers from in-person and online writing groups, who provided feedback as fellow writers and as readers of his poetry. He also described interactions with mentors/teachers, who likewise focused their energy on his poetry and his development as a writer, thereby foregrounding his sense of self as *advanced student of writing*. By rejecting one set of labels and the associations that came with them (autistic poet) and embracing others (advanced student of writing), Scott shifted both his social identity and his personal trajectory within social channels that were more affirming and less debilitating than what some conventional outside views might allow for.

Writing as an Advanced Student of Writing

Whereas his identification as a poet-memoirist seemed primarily to shape the way Scott entered writing assignments and made choices related to content and style, his identification as an advanced student of writing seemed to shape the way he interpreted and used feedback to develop his poetry.

Thus, Scott's *poet-memoirist* identification seemed to be foregrounded as he began and drafted a poem, and his *advanced student of writing* identification appeared foregrounded as he sought and interpreted feedback and engaged in revision in his effort to "grow a head taller" through his social process of poetic composition.

As previously noted, Scott referenced examples of the poems he wrote in Michael's workshop as evidence of why he considered himself a student of writing and why, as he put it, "I still need a mentor/teacher to guide me." The poems Scott referenced were ones that required him to vary his style, and he pointed to these efforts as evidence of his growth as Michael's student. The table below shows three versions of one of these referenced poems, called "Yosemite Still Life," with the changes Scott made between drafts in boldface type. Drafts 1 and 2 were written before receiving feedback from Michael, and the final version was written in response to Michael's comments.

In our email conversations about this poem, Scott commented that his primary goal in revising his first drafts was to "find shorter words to tighten the sound in a couple of spots." This goal was reminiscent of the feedback he had recounted from his previous instructor, who had noted that his images were strong but that some lines seemed awkward, and who had advised him "to work on the musicality and line" of his poetry. He also noted, "I think the heartbeat and lulling images [in the final lines] are maybe too clichéd but I could not figure out a more accurate way of describing the feeling." Scott submitted the poem to Michael for feedback at the Draft 2 stage. He later reported that Michael "liked the poem a lot. He just wanted me to cut sheer because there were too many adjectives in that one line of description." Because Scott considered Michael a respected mentor, and because he considered himself a student writer, he attached significance to Michael's overall assessment of his poem.

Scott then drew on Michael's comments as he wrote his "final version" of the poem (third column in Fig. 10.1). In responding to Michael's feedback, Scott seemed to draw on both his own student writer identity and his poet-memoirist identity, showing how these identities overlapped and interacted at times. Scott explained that while Michael "wanted me to cut [the adjective] sheer," he chose a different revision move:

> I cut [the adjective] massive instead. I wanted the adjective describing steepness to stay because I wanted to keep the aspect of danger. Massive is already covered with looming and dominated. I then felt I had to change some of the line breaks because with the cut that line sounded too short and choppy.

Draft 1	Draft 2 (pre-feedback)	Final (post-feedback from Michael)
Yosemite Still Life	Yosemite Still Life	Yosemite Still Life
I have already lost the visions of Half Dome and El Capitan, their sheer massive granite facades that dominated the landscape within and without for those four days. Their looming presence is diminished by photos that capture all of their sculptured beauty and none of their stifling terror, as shrunk as the reflections wavering in the dwindling waters of Mirror Lake. All I can recall is the abiding pattern of the Merced ringing the rocks with froth, the river of mercy rhythmic as a heartbeat, lulling me with the slow relentless erosion of their memory.	I have already lost the visions of Half Dome and **El Cap**, their sheer massive granite facades that dominated the landscape within and without for those four days. Their looming presence is diminished by photos that capture all of their sculptured beauty and none of their stifling **dread**, as shrunk as the **wavering images reflected** in the dwindling waters of Mirror Lake. **All I can recall is the abiding** pattern of the Merced ringing the rocks with froth, that river of mercy rhythmic as a heartbeat, lulling me with the slow relentless erosion of memory.	**I have already lost the visions of Half Dome and El Cap, the sheer granite facades** that dominated the landscape within and without for those four days. Their looming presence is diminished by photos that capture all of their sculptured beauty and none of their stifling dread, as shrunk as the wavering images reflected in the dwindling waters of Mirror Lake. All I can recall is the abiding pattern of the Merced ringing the rocks with froth, that river of mercy rhythmic as a heartbeat, lulling me with the slow relentless erosion of memory.

Fig. 10.1 Three drafts of "Yosemite Still Life"

Rather than following Michael's feedback exactly and making the simple and minor change Michael had suggested, Scott stayed true to his vision for his poem and maintained that the word "sheer" needed to be in the poem. This targeting of a specific effect and sensation linked more to Scott's identification as a poet-memoirist than his identification as a student writer, emphasizing Scott's own vision and intention in the revision. Yet Scott seemed to agree with Michael's assessment that one of those adjectives needed to go, which was perhaps more in line with his identification as a student writer. Scott's subsequent revision of some line breaks again demonstrated his ownership of this poem, as he recognized additional changes that needed to be made beyond what Michael suggested.

This process of drafting and getting feedback involves a good degree of play in the use of drafts to try out ideas. Although not performing in the sense of theatrical drama, which is illustrated throughout Part 2 of this volume, Scott was nonetheless using playful performance to produce, over time, an evolving text that ultimately coalesced into a final draft, a final performance of this text. Even a poet's designation of a speaker or narrative voice may be viewed as a fundamentally performative act, in that the speaker represents a sort of "character" created by the author to voice a particular perspective.

Surprisingly, although Scott had mentioned struggling with clichés in the early drafts of "Yosemite Still Life," he did not reference the issue in his synopsis of Michael's feedback or his revision. I inquired, asking Scott to explain what his concerns had been. He replied:

> I just thought the river lulling me like a baby in the womb listening to my mother's heartbeat was an image I had heard before. But our room was right next to the river and its sound did put me to sleep and now I still think I hear it sometimes at night. Michael liked the sound of that part and the line breaks, so I guess that was a problem I made up in my head.

Scott's explanation of clichés as images that he "had heard before" aligned with comments he had made when he had revised a previous poem, where Scott had noted that "most of the revisions involved changing what sounded like clichés into fresher images." Indeed, when I met with Scott and his mother, Scott had indicated that he was most proud of his poetry that had an "originality of place and image and theme," explaining that by "originality" he meant "different from what everyone else I read ha[s] done." Despite his initial concern that he had strayed into clichés with this poem, Scott later defended his description of the river lulling him like a baby. While the image did seem familiar to him, Scott argued for the image's authenticity in creating his desired effect. Here Scott may be seen foregrounding his identification as a poet-memoirist again, as he defended the image for the way it represented the actual sensation he associated with an experience. When Michael apparently liked the sound and form of that part, despite Scott's initial misgivings about cliché, Scott was able to conclude, "I guess that this was a problem I made up in my head."

Once again, this example provides evidence of Scott experiencing a positive social updraft through his relationship with Michael and his engagement in writing practices. He displayed confidence in seeking out feedback that would support his growth as a writer. Across the poems Scott shared with me, as well as his descriptions of his writing processes and decisions, he seemed to draw on his identification as an advanced student of writing as he sought out feedback (such as on improving conclusions or avoiding clichés) and as he made use of feedback on his writing. Scott considered Michael as a mentor and therefore privileged his feedback, especially in areas where Scott felt less confident or independent as a writer. Still, Scott showed that he did not simply accept and apply everything Michael said. Rather, Scott was able to consider Michael's feedback in ways that helped him develop his poem according to his own purposes and intentions as a poet-memoirist, as he did in "Yosemite Still Life." Perhaps Scott designated himself as an *advanced* student of writing in part to explain how he navigated the overlap and potential conflicts between being a poet-memoirist and a student writer.

Identifying as a Writer: "The Lens that is My Autism"

I realized that throughout my many conversations with Scott during this study, he rarely directly referenced his autism. He and I had known each other for years, so it was not any secret between us. But being autistic was not at all central to the ways Scott chose to describe himself or his writing.

One of the only times that Scott directly mentioned autism in the context of describing his writing life was when we met for our initial in-person conversation. At the time Scott was taking an online university course in American literature in addition to his poetry workshop. When his mother asked if he liked the literature course, Scott replied "Yes," and when she asked why, he typed, "no one knows ... about my autism." The structure of that online class required that all communication occurred via written language, and there were no in-person interactions. Therefore Scott's participation in the class was much the same as other students', and his autism was not evident unless he chose to make it so.

During that same conversation, when Scott was explaining why he preferred writing from his own experience, he also referenced his experiences with autism less directly. It was at this point that Scott commented, "no one knows my feelings from my outside." When I asked him then if part of his purpose had been to share that inner self with others, he agreed, adding he "dream[ed] that we communicate," and that he hoped "that my feelings can be shared and not isolated and strange." As noted previously in this chapter, these comments are reminiscent of Scott's bridge metaphor, through which he observed that his ways of communicating were different and often isolated him from his peers. When I then asked him how he thought about the members of his writing groups, and whether these people figured into his audience or purpose for his writing, he replied, "I feel comfortable when I know the people in the groups because they know my writing is good [and are] expecting me to write well." He went on to describe the members of his writing group "as accepting me even though I am different."

These comments again highlight the ways Scott experienced a positive social updraft from writing and participating in his writing communities, wherein he could overcome some communicative challenges and participate as a fellow writer through the sort of "roundabout" means described by Vygotsky (1993; see Chap. 1). Being known by fellow writers, and having them expect him to write well, created a context that foregrounded Scott's identity as a poet and author. In his email explanation of why he considered himself to be an advanced student of writing, Scott described the way his writing groups were both comfortable and helpful. He referred to the "core of familiar faces of people who know me and my writing. They know the history of my writing the past three years and can not only discuss my writing in terms of a new piece but also in terms of my overall progress as a writer." In the context of these groups, the history of sharing writing over time mattered to Scott, so that members knew both him and his writing. They had a context for both. He added, "If a piece of [my] writing seems atypical to them, that leads to interesting discussions," again emphasizing the relationship he had with his fellow group members, who were able to contextualize Scott's writing in relation to his work over time.

Beyond these few moments, and including the email responses Scott composed to further describe himself as a writer, he did not otherwise directly reference his autism. I asked him about this omission, noting that he wrote and shared his writing in a variety of forums, some of which masked his autism (like online workshops) and some of which did not. I wondered how, if at all, he thought his autism played into his writing and the ways he thought about himself as a writer. I also asked him how he would like me, in my own writing, to represent his autism. Scott explained:

> I really do not want to be thought of as that poet with autism like some kind of exotic animal in a zoo. I don't want people reading my poems as some way to crack the mysterious code of autism. Of course, I write out of the lens that is my autism. I can only guess at how that makes my perceptions different from other people. I am fascinated with how shapes and colors and textures collide and the empty peacefulness of motion. Of course I am frustrated by my inability to speak the way everyone else takes for granted. But I hope people would still like my poems as much even if they did not know I had autism.

Scott's response highlights the challenge inherent in even writing this chapter. He was understandably opposed to a limited interpretation of his writing and himself that only focused on his autism, or that highlighted his autism over his writing. His comments are aligned with other authors who would not want their writing to be read as merely a window into their gender or race or ethnicity. Notably, Scott did not focus his response on how *he* defined himself or his writing. Instead he emphasized his hopes for how *other people* would interpret him and his poetry, thereby deliberately resisting others defining him and his writing primarily in terms of his autism. His first two sentences are written in the negative ("I do not want" and "I don't want") to reflect this resistance, and he ended the paragraph with a hope that readers would engage with his poems on their own merit.

Scott did, however, discuss possible relationships between his writing and his autism. These sentences are written as positive statements that focus on his actions ("I write") and interests ("I am fascinated with"). He wondered at the ways his perceptions may differ from other people's, implying that his fascination with shapes, colors, textures, and "the empty peacefulness of motion" may in some way be affordances of writing "out of the lens that is my autism." These statements also resonate with his earlier descriptions of his interest in capturing sensation through language.

Scott's response to my question once again highlights the positive social updraft he experienced in his varied writing communities, where he felt "known" and where fellow group members had high expectations for his poetry and foregrounded his identity as a strong writer. Scott's words here also may be read as his active resistance to taking on a secondary disability (Vygotsky 1993; see Chap. 1) associated with outsiders' negative or narrow interpretation of him and his writing. Being treated as and accepting the lower expectations for an "exotic animal in a zoo" would represent a manifestation of just such a secondary disability. Rather, Scott was deliberate in foregrounding his perspective as a writer, thereby further resisting the assignation of a secondary disability.

In that same email response, Scott commented that some of his poems were about being autistic, and he shared a poem (see below) that he wrote in response to an assignment "about locating a positive experience from a negative experience." He then concluded, "I guess my poetry does come out of my autism and is sometimes about my autism as well, but I also try to downplay my autism because I do not want people to just focus on that." These statements again demonstrate Scott's awareness of the potential of experiencing a secondary disability, and his interest in focusing his readers' attention on the qualities of his poetic ability. Even this poem, while referencing aspects of his experience and frustration at being silent, did not explicitly refer to autism as a topic.

Swing
By Scott

The boy never knew why
he could not speak.
Silent amid the babble
he would swing, pumping
his legs harder, still harder
leaning back into the wind
to swing higher, yet higher
only to fall behind, lungs
caving. He believed if only
he strained his arms hard
enough, kicked his legs high
enough, he would rocket
over that bar and free fall,
scraping his feet along

> the dried mud grooves,
> back where he began
> yet now somewhere
> else, a place where
> when he opened
> his mouth, out sprang
> the words, or at least
> a world where those
> who swung beside
> him stayed silent too.
> In dreams he would arc
> and plunge, the words
> swelling his throat.

Although Scott's autism may have silenced him in some ways, like the boy on the swing, his poetry and his use of written language did allow the "words swelling in his throat" to spring forth powerfully and move his readers. He was well justified in expecting his readers to interact with his poems on their own merit, with no allowances for or focus on any interactional limitations or difference.

Discussion

Across his poetry and our conversations about his writing, Scott articulated specialized writing identities according to genre, purpose, relationship with other writers, and his perceived level of independence as a writer. He drew on these self-descriptions in deliberate ways to seek out writing experiences (classes, writing groups), select topics and enter projects (favoring writing about sensations from life experiences), seek and interpret feedback, and craft his poetry. Many of his statements demonstrated the way Scott purposefully related his sense of himself as a poet-memoirist and/or as an advanced student writer to his writing decisions. Rather than allowing others to define him simply as autistic or deficient, Scott drew on his own poetry and past writing experiences, in the supportive environment of communities of writers, as evidence to fortify his own self-identifications. He noted that what was truly important for him was to continue to "find a way to get whatever support I need ... to continue writing and continue developing and improving as a writer."

Scott's example shows that identifying as a specific kind of writer, one with social value, can be empowering. When he was given a challenging assignment in his poetry class, Scott was able to draw on his sense of himself as a poet-memoirist to help him consider ways of entering that assignment successfully. Similarly, Scott was able to draw on his student writer identity in ways that allowed him to seek and use feedback as he set and pursued his own writing goals.

Perhaps most noteworthy in the context of this current book, Scott demonstrated the significance of articulating his own identity as a writer, and of challenging those who might define him in more limiting ways. As Scott deliberately asserted some of his qualities as a poet and resisted being defined in reductionist ways in terms of his autism, he may be seen as pushing back against the possibility of his adopting the societal beliefs that produce a secondary disability. His participation in long-term, face-to-face writing groups and online writing workshops provided contexts in which Scott's *writing* was foregrounded, enabling him to further craft his own identities and foreground his growth as a writer.

Overall, this chapter highlights the ways in which Scott's poetry and participation in committed writing communities provided him with positive social updrafts, which helped him develop a style of writing that capitalized on his extraordinary ability to isolate and describe sensations associated with lived experiences. By engaging in social contexts with other writers, where trust was built over time, Scott was able to feel comfortable and known. His peers and mentors were familiar with his writing and expected him to write well. His writing, rather than his autism, was the focus of his participation. And that focus, paired with the moving quality of Scott's poetry, is what helped him build the bridges that enabled him to communicate with, influence, and learn alongside other writers.

Notes

1. In his IRB consent form, Scott elected attribution over anonymity. For this publication, he and his parents asked that I use only his first name. Other names throughout the chapter are pseudonyms.
2. All quotations from Scott are verbatim and not corrected for fidelity to convention.

Appendix: Research Method

I first got to know Scott several years ago, when he was a student in two consecutive high school creative writing courses I taught. During Scott's Advanced Creative Writing class, he composed the reflection that opened this chapter. Even at that point, it was evident that Scott was a gifted writer. He won a number of poetry contests, and his work was consistently admired among peers in my classes. Scott and I stayed in touch after he graduated, and he continued to share his poetry with me via email when I moved out of state. When Scott was 23 years old, I invited him to participate in this study for several primary reasons: I knew him to be someone who thought purposefully about his writing, and I knew that he actively sought out multiple opportunities and contexts to develop his craft (e.g., classes, writing groups, workshops). I also was fascinated by the many ways Scott used writing in his life.

Because Scott communicated so significantly through written language, studying his *writing* and how he described himself *as a writer* involved recognizing the varied types and purposes of Scott's written texts. When involved in an in-person interaction, for example, Scott used a handheld computer to type his responses (so, when he participated in an in-person writing group, other people typically commented orally while Scott typed his feedback on his handheld computer). Scott's written comments during an in-person conversation were necessarily brief and more similar to text messages than lengthy composed replies. By contrast, Scott typically emailed me more formally composed messages, which were still conversational in tone but usually conformed to standard writing conventions. Finally, Scott's poetry represented formal, composed writing, in which he deliberately crafted his language, organization, form, sound, effect, and meaning. Thus, Scott's *writing* encompassed a wide variety of genres, contexts, and purposes that exceed limitations he may have experienced with spoken speech.

For the purposes of this chapter, however, I focus on the ways Scott described himself as a creative writer, highlighting his formally composed writing, usually his poetry. At the beginning of the study, I visited with Scott and his mother in their home, explaining my interest in learning more about Scott's writing practices. During that meeting, they shared with me a file of Scott's poetry. After that initial meeting, Scott and I corresponded via email, which worked particularly well because it placed us both in a situation where we were typing our responses. Through those email exchanges, I asked Scott many questions about his writing life and how he thought about himself as a writer. Finally, for the six months of this study, Scott shared the poetry he composed as part of an online poetry workshop he was taking, as well as his commentary on his composing processes.

As I read through Scott's poetry and our various email interactions, I considered each piece of Scott's writing as a "turn" in an ongoing dialogue, recognizing that there were always many overlapping conversations occurring (Bakhtin, 1981). Each written utterance, whether a poem or an email message, both responded to prior and predicted future utterances, like turns in a conversation. For example, when Scott wrote a poem in response to an online assignment, I considered the assignment itself as a conversational turn, to which Scott responded through his poetry. His online instructor then responded to Scott's draft, and Scott then took another conversational turn via his revisions and email comments. All of those turns occurred within the context of an ongoing, broader dialogue between Scott and his instructor. In this way, the varied written texts I collected served as connected, overlapping turns in a conversation that unfolded over time.

In my reading of Scott's texts, I considered "what texts do" in the social and interactional context in which they were produced (Bazerman and Prior 2004, p. 3), examining the ways in which Scott, through his use of written language, directed my attention, how he developed ideas within a text, and how he referenced other texts.

Because this chapter focuses on ways Scott described himself and his writing practices, I concentrated first on the conversations that Scott and I had in person and via email about his poetry and his writing life. In these conversations, which primarily occurred at the beginning (in-person) and toward the end (via email) of the six focal months, I asked Scott to describe himself as a writer and to explain some of his writing choices and commitments. Analyzing the in-person conversation required me to first braid together our varied communicative modes from that meeting (transcription from audiorecording the oral conversation, a print-out of Scott's written comments, and fieldnotes on our physical interactions). By contrast, our email communications involved clearly demarcated turn-taking. I used open coding to note Scott's explicit identifying statements (e.g., *I* statements in which Scott wrote "I am" or identified himself as a certain type of writer) and to identify descriptive statements (e.g., those comments in which Scott described what he does as a writer—often using action verbs to name his decisions or preferences). I then used refined coding to trace the appearance of these identifying and descriptive statements across both conversations (Miles and Huberman 1994). I considered each identifying statement that Scott made as a claim, and I coded his in-person and email responses for additional references to that claim, as well as for evidence he used to support these claims (e.g., clarifying or explanatory statements, examples from his own poetry).

I connected these conversational data to the poems Scott composed, where I looked for ways that Scott's poetry and writing decisions aligned with or reflected his self-descriptions. Over the six focal months of the data collection, Scott emailed me the poems he wrote for his online poetry workshop (11 total, many with multiple drafts), as well as a brief explanation of the context, purpose(s), feedback, and revision decisions for each piece. I often asked follow-up questions via email, to which Scott replied. Scott also shared a number of additional poems with me (13 total), which he referenced in our in-person and online conversations. In analyzing these poems, particularly the 11 that he composed during the study, I compiled a master file with all references to a given poem (including, if possible, a description of the assignment, Scott's draft poems, his reflection on his writing decisions, his final version, any feedback he wanted to share from his instructor, my clarifying questions, and his replies). I used these comprehensive poem files first to trace Scott's references from our conversations (e.g., where he referenced a poem as evidence to support an identifying/descriptive statement he made about himself or his writing). I also coded these poem files for alignment with Scott's self-descriptions as a writer, allowing me to trace ways that Scott's poems reflected his claims about his writing.

Because I was in contact with Scott throughout the initial data analysis, I was able to use email communications to clarify and check the interpretations I was making. Relevant to this chapter, for example, were a series of emails Scott and I exchanged shortly after he completed the poetry workshop, when I asked him about how he thought about his writing in relation to his autism, as well as how he wished me to represent his autism in my own writing.

References

Bakhtin, M. M. (1981). *The dialogic imagination: Four essays by M. M. Bakhtin* (M. Holquist, Ed.; C. Emerson & M. Holquist, Trans.). Austin: University of Texas Press.

Bazerman, C., & Prior, P. (2004). *What writing does and how it does it: An introduction to analyzing texts and textual practices.* Mahwah: Erlbaum.

Holzman, L. (2009). *Vygotsky at work and play.* New York: Routledge.

Miles, M. B., & Huberman, A. M. (1994). *Qualitative data analysis: An expanded sourcebook* (2nd ed.). Thousand Oaks: Sage.

Nystrand, M. (1986). *The structure of written communication: Studies in reciprocity between writers and readers.* Orlando: Academic.

Vygotsky, L. S. (1978). In M. Cole, V. John-Steiner, S. Scribner, & E. Souberman (Eds.), *Mind in society: The development of higher psychological processes.* Cambridge, MA: Harvard University Press.

Vygotsky, L. S. (1993). *The collected works of L. S. Vygotsky. Volume 2: The fundamentals of defectology (abnormal psychology and learning disabilities)* (R. W. Rieber & A. S. Carton, Eds.; trans: Knox, J. E. & Stevens, C. B.). New York: Plenum.

Wertsch, J. V. (2000). Vygotsky's two minds on the nature of meaning. In C. D. Lee & P. Smagorinsky (Eds.), *Vygotskian perspectives on literacy research: Constructing meaning through collaborative inquiry* (pp. 19–30). New York: Cambridge University Press.

An Autistic Life, Animated Through the World of Disney: A Loving Autoethnography

Peter Smagorinsky

In this chapter, I take the family memoir of journalist Ron Suskind (2014a) and reexamine it through the theoretical foundation provided in Part 1 of this volume. Suskind and his wife, Cornelia, raised two sons, Walt and Owen.[1] Owen's development appeared to be on the typical track until the age of two and a half when, suddenly and without apparent cause, he stopped talking, lost his physical bearings, and ceased interacting with others. Suskind's book details the next 20 years or so of the family's life, telling a powerful story of how he and his wife adapted their home by constructing an environment through which Owen's life found a trajectory that enabled him to animate his life with ideas, phrases, whole texts, and meaning, all appropriated and reconfigured through his incessant engagement with movies from the Disney catalogue.

If Suskind were an academic instead of a journalist, his book would be called an *autoethnography*: a form of narrative inquiry in which a person systematically describes and analyzes personal experience in order to come to a personal understanding of situated experience and sensitize readers to issues not available through conventional detached analysis and

P. Smagorinsky (✉)
Department of Language and Literacy Education, The University of Georgia, USA

interpretation. Given that Suskind and Cornelia undertook their inquiry out of love, I would call it a *loving ethnography*, one that produced a diagnosis quite different from what autism researchers and diagnosticians who look for pathology would arrive at. Although Suskind's *Life Animated* was written for a general rather than scholarly audience, I believe that the book and its excerpts (e.g., Suskind 2014b) do provide data, given Suskind's keen eye for detail and insights into Owen's social development, often surpassing those of the specialists brought in to diagnose and treat his differences.

In an autoethnography, readers must both trust the story and recognize that many parts of it must go untold, and for a variety of reasons: not all details are salient; some events may involve confidentiality; parts of the story are too personal to be made public. In my own autoethnographic account of my family's experiences with Asperger's syndrome (Smagorinsky 2011a), for instance, I asked family members to read it before publication and deleted parts that they felt were not appropriate to share outside the family. I also self-edited disagreements between my wife and me about our parenting, something I might have done differently had the essay been written after our divorce. All personal accounts of this sort must be taken as the best available story from the infinite possibilities that complex experiences allow, with attention to how revelations may affect those who are part of the narrative and who might see things quite differently.

The Suskind family story is thus partial, even as it occupies over 350 pages of text. I will attend to the aspects of it that I find relevant to my own interest in the role of mediating cultural settings in the social development of autistic youth, especially those functioning highly enough to engage to some degree with their human and material settings.

A Pair of Qualifiers

Before I begin, I must inject two caveats. First, I personally do not like what comes out of the Walt Disney studios. I've been to Disneyland and Disney World, and find them to be a gaudy, endless series of product placements and promotions. Suskind acknowledges Disney's problematic role in US culture early on, noting that his family's immersion in Disney films produced

> mild disdain of some of our graduate-degreed, baby boomer friends. They had a world-wise, right-minded riff: that Disney was a voracious, commercialized, myth-co-opting brainwasher, using primal tales to shape young

minds into noxious conclusions about everything from dead mothers (forget about step-mothers) to what happens to thrill-seeking boys (Pinocchio's Pleasure Island, as donkeys *forever*) to how a princess out to look (utterly unattainable!), all before the tykes knew what hit them.

On other occasions, Suskind registers wince-worthy responses to other aspects of the Disney films that Owen watched relentlessly, such as the racist stereotypes of Native American characters in *Peter Pan*. He thus provides some balance in explaining how Disney provided the script through which Owen joined the social stream, in spite of what critical adults find to be the studio's many and varied flaws.

The second caution concerns the resources that the Suskinds invested in their son. A close friend of mine with an autistic son once wrote me, "Hope is expensive." Ron Suskind has won two Pulitzer Prizes for his six books, and his writing has made things affordable for him that most of us can't imagine. Periodically, he reveals the costs of the interventions he and Cornelia invested in Owen's life, such as the $90,000 a year he estimated having spent over 17 years, which my calculator found to total over $1.5 million. One two-hour meeting with a team of specialists ran a tab of $1,500. The Suskinds were supported by "Team Owen": an innovative play therapist, an occupational therapist, swimming instructors, piano teachers, a psychiatrist, a psychologist, an educational specialist who provided tutoring, and others. Cornelia took time off to homeschool Owen in a room in a church basement, rented out at $500 per month. Owen had access to Prozac, and unnamed medications for his obsessive compulsiveness. Furthermore, Suskind is connected in ways most aren't, allowing him to arrange meetings between Owen and Disney animators, voiceover actors, and others. Pity that Dustin Hoffman was not available when Suskind called upon him for a favor. Suskind refers to friends who have spent $65,000 a year on special schools and programs, with no results. The Suskinds, financially and in terms of family stability, have had advantages that few parents can imagine investing in one child.

The availability of such expensive support from occupational therapists, speech therapists, and others might suggest that Suskind's story is only possible for those in the top 1% of the income distribution. But this chapter is not about how much money parents can spend to provide their children with the best possible life. Perhaps the least expensive, and most effective, means of mediation for Owen came through readily available DVDs of Disney films, watched in the family basement and usually purchased inexpensively, although occasionally requiring bigger fees, such as the copy of the discontinued (due to racist imagery) film *Song of the South* that was ordered from overseas and adapted to US technology—available through Suskind's work relationship with ABC television's Ted Koppel, who is not in the rolodex of the average person—to the tune of $500 for a playable copy.

Even though most of us don't have access to so much, I believe that the Suskind family story has much to tell us.

Owen's Diagnosis

After Owen experienced a seemingly sudden developmental regression in his third year of life, the Suskinds consulted with specialists to diagnose his condition. He was found to have a pervasive developmental disorder, one known as PDD-NOS, with NOS signifying "not otherwise specified." My daughter has this same diagnosis, as does my nephew; and if I had ever been diagnosed, I believe that I would be characterized in this way as well. It's a wide-ranging diagnosis applied to people who, in many ways, do not resemble one another in their autistic traits, yet who tend to be very narrowly focused on idiosyncratic interests, often in ways that isolate them from other people. They are often cognitively advanced and socially delayed, with the social immaturity often creating the appearance of cognitive limitations.

Suskind was initially relieved that his son was diagnosed with PDD-NOS rather than autism, but like others, including me, soon found that labels are what you get when you work with diagnosticians. I was quite taken aback, for instance, when my own daughter's diagnosis following a stay in a local facility was that she was "mentally ill," a name that conjured images of unkempt people ranting on city streets. What I've learned since is that such labeling reinforces the notion that people who are different are abnormal, deficient, and disordered, often because the diagnosis names them as such. What I now believe is that labeling of this sort emphasizes the "disordered" developmental paths they are on without attending to the assets that such an orientation provides for them, pathologizing them such that they and their families are more prone to accept the idea that they are lesser human beings. A whole family can thus be prone to the secondary disability described by Vygotsky, the feelings of inferiority that develop through incessant derogatory assumptions made by the people who surround them, based on a source of difference (see Chap. 1).

Like any parents who believe in their children, the Suskinds were determined to overcome Owen's diagnosis. Suskind concluded after one encouraging visit to a specialist that Owen "is 'atypical' ... and his problems are assorted delays. They can be corrected. We sleep that night in a wash of relief. We will save this boy, rebuild him—rebirth him!—every waking hour of every day. *Fools*," he concluded of those who had considered their son limited in his life's prospects; yet I read a sardonic message as well that he was speaking of himself for believing that his son's differences could be "rebuilt" into normality, simply through the power of parental good will and investment.

Suskind's own learning curve included a lot of informal education about the autism spectrum. His account includes references to Hans Asperger and the syndrome that bears his name, to Carl Jung and his idea of *the shadow*[2], to Lev Vygotsky and his notion of inner speech[3]. This knowledge helped him make sense of the new world of difference in which his life became embedded in seeking ways for young Owen to overcome his "pervasive developmental disorder" and grow into a normal person. What he found instead was that Owen's unique makeup, although ill-suited for much of conventional society, enabled him to grow in ways that ultimately indicated that, beneath the veneer of disorder, he had insights unavailable to the typical people around him, those who lacked his capacity for dedicated study of and inquiry into a narrow field of interest.

Echolalia and Ventriloquation

Like many kids of the 1990s, the Suskind boys were raised in an environment in which the television, especially its video-playing capability, played a major role. Coincidental with the availability of home videos and following a major downturn in the company's cultural impact, the Disney corporation began a commercial comeback with the release of *The Little Mermaid*, then *Beauty and the Beast*, then *Aladdin*, all available on video along with new releases of the studio's Golden Age animations of *Dumbo*, *Fantasia*, *Bambi*, and other classics. Although ambivalent about the messages conveyed through these films, the Suskinds, like other working parents, found them convenient means of occupying their sons in the spaces when their complex work commitments reduced their possibilities for hands-on parenting.

Watching videos is often considered "mindless" by critics of entertainment, and television in particular. And a superficial look at children "glued to the boob tube" suggests that this observation has merit. More careful observation, however, might yield a different interpretation. At one point, the family noticed that Owen would re-watch the same scenes over and over, using the rewind function on the remote control to focus in on particular scenes. At about the same time, they began to hear Owen repeating the same nonsense phrase, "juicervoce." While watching a scene from *The Little Mermaid*, however, Cornelia made a connection when Owen repeatedly watched a scene in which the character Ursula shouts:

> Go ahead—make your choice!
> I'm a very busy woman
> And I haven't got all day
> It won't cost much
> Just your voice!

Just your voice, juicervoce. Cornelia put it together that Owen was watching the excerpt very deliberately, focused on the theme of the scene. When Suskind asked Owen—who rarely engaged with other people—if he indeed was saying "just your voice," Owen made eye contact for the first time since shutting down at age two and confirmed that he was indeed. In an emotional moment, Cornelia began to cry and said, "Thank God ... he's in there."

But could it be that a child so disconnected from other people could begin to shape his thinking in relation to an animated film? Their speech therapist thought not, dismissing his repetition of the phrase as an instance of *echolalia*, the meaningless repetition of sounds without any associated meaning, a behavior often attributed to autistics. This early discouraging response, they ultimately learned through careful attention, was wrong; Owen was not simply repeating sounds. Rather, he was engaging in what Wertsch (1991), borrowing from Bakhtin (1981), calls *ventriloquation*: the appropriation of a voice and wordings, personalized and instantiated to express feelings and perspectives, through both direct phrasings and adaptations of words and their meanings to their expressive needs.

Nonetheless, the expert opinions of the specialists they consulted influenced the Suskinds to explain Owen's phrasings as echolalia, or as Suskind put it, "Parrot stuff. He's just repeating sounds." But Owen continued to speak in gibberish phrases that took on meaning in light of the Disney films currently on his watch list. After a period of incessantly watching *Beauty and the Beast*, he began repeating "bootylyzwitten," which

Cornelia ultimately deciphered as the line from the film, "Beauty lies within." The line was not random, but in fact encapsulated the primary theme of the story, and as they realized, of Owen's feelings about his own social relationships.

In a dramatic moment when Owen was six years old, on his brother's ninth birthday when Walt became emotional and tearful, Suskind and Cornelia walked into the kitchen. Owen followed, and as related by Suskind, "He looks intently as us, one, then the other. He seems to have something to say. 'Walter doesn't want to grow up,' he says, evenly, 'like Mowgli or Peter Pan.'" Suskind described the moment, saying that it had been as if

> a thunderbolt [had] just passed through the kitchen.... Beyond the language, it's interpretive thinking that he's not supposed to be able to do: that someone crying on their birthday may not want to grow up. Not only would such an insight be improbable for a typical six year old; it was an elegant connection that Cornelia and I had overlooked.

"Thank God ... he's in there," Cornelia had once said; this occasion suggested that he was not only in there, he was processing his world astutely, relying on Disney themes through which to classify and make sense of new experiences. Alone with his videos, Owen was living in a social world, filled with characters whose messages resonated with him and enabled him to express his own sense of self in the world, performed through the vehicle of Disney's scripts and storylines.

Recognizing Owen's ability to ventriloquate phrasings and themes through Disney characters, Suskind found an opportunity to connect with Owen on a level deeper than he had previously reached. One evening, with Owen looking intently at a Disney book, Suskind crept in and put on a hand puppet of the character Iago from *Aladdin*. Carefully and painstakingly positioned so that only Iago was evident to Owen, Suskind began speaking through the puppet in the voice of Gilbert Gottfried[4], who provided the voice for Iago in the film. "How does it feel to be you?" asked Suskind. Owen replied, "I'm not happy. I don't have friends. I can't understand what people say." What Suskind found so extraordinary was the naturalness of Owen's voice, something he hadn't heard since Owen's autistic break at age two.

This exchange then developed, with Owen taking on the voice of Jafar, a villain in the film, to talk about his feelings. This event[5] served as a turning point in the family's understanding of Owen and his use of Disney to account for his experiences. From that point on, dialogue in the Suskind household often became a form of performance, with parents and son talking through the voices of animated characters from various Disney films.

Suskind's use of the Iago puppet opened up a new possibility for the family: for the parents to conduct conversations with their son, in character and in roles that fit particular situations. A year later, following Owen's reprimand at school for not paying attention and voicing Disney characters under his breath, Suskind took the opportunity to initiate a conversation with him in the role of Merlin from *The Sword in the Stone*, adopting the vocalizations of British actor Karl Swenson, who voiced the part in the film. Owen's response, in Arthur's voice, resulted in an exchange that left Suskind reflecting as follows:

> Owen and I have never had a conversation like this. But as Merlin and Arthur we do. It has a knowing, sentient quality. The grammar is perfect, as is the word choice. Is this just a more complex, interactive version of echolalia, or are we really talking? Can't say for sure where to draw that line.
>
> But I'm certain about one thing: the warmth passing between the characters in the movie—one Owen has watched a hundred times—now passes between us. I can feel it.

As Suskind noted, there were two issues coming together in this vignette. First, Owen was able to ventriloquate appropriately in order to express his understanding of his situation. Second, Owen expressed himself with full emotional resonance, suggesting a quality well beyond echolalia, which involves the repitition of phrasings without an understanding of meaning. Rather, Owen phrased his perspective not only correctly from a syntactic point of view and in terms of his assessment of the situation, he did so invoking his feelings about himself, an aspect of development that the classification-oriented autism diagnostic research I have attempted to read—and generally that I have trouble engaging with because of its emphasis on technicality, pathology, and detachment—appears to overlook. Perhaps it takes a dedicated parent in a home setting to understand what is not available to the clinical diagnostician. For the Suskinds, the discovery of the role of emotion in Owen's Disney obsession led them to even more careful observation and understanding of their son, and engagement with his passions that validated rather than discouraged his obsessions.

Contextualizing Disney Narratives

A further realization came when Owen began rewinding tapes at the end of films and re-watching the credits, often for over a half hour. His parents ultimately realized that Owen, after others had left the room, was carefully studying the closing credits to understand the people behind the production. Watching Owen from a distance, Suskind found that he would

> Play, stop, rewind, play, stop, rewind, frame by frame. The methodology is logical and deliberate.... First he decodes the name of the character.... That's a warm-up for the tougher, fresher terrain of the actor who voices [the character].... We hear him say the name softly, almost reverently, repeating it a few times. And then other words, like *assistant* and *associate*, *lighting*, *director*, and *producer*. He seemed happy and focused, scrolling frames, calm and intensely engaged, with so many movies to choose from. Our only job is not to disturb him.

Along the way, Suskind's (1998) work on *A Hope in the Unseen*, a book focused on an African American male who defied cultural stereotypes to escape poverty, led to further insights. Suskind learned of *stereotype threats and boosts*: the manner in which other people's assumptions can either limit or enhance one's opportunities in life, with those assumptions drawn from superficial markers such as skin color or sex. He described the process that Vygotskian scholar Cole (1996) refers to as *prolepsis*, the subtle and unconscious means through which assumptions and expectations by others shape the pathways available to individuals subject to their influence. People like Owen are thus assumed to be abnormal and deficient, as pervasively developmentally disordered, and are treated as such; and as Owen's occasional allowances indicate, he accepted pathologizing judgments that limited his potential.

His immersion in the Disney world, however, with the support and understanding of his parents and brother, made his involvement in this play world less deviant and more accepted and affirmed, and thus more legitimate. Indeed, in a quite touching essay written by his brother at a summer camp, Walt said:

> I want to begin by telling you a little about the best teacher I have ever had. He is eighteen years old, sketches cartoon characters like there is no tomorrow, and every Friday we make our ritual trip to the video store. He is my brother, Owen.... When I wonder if life would have been easier if Owen was

"normal" kid, I always remember it is because of him that I am the person I am.... [It] is in the face of the seemingly insurmountable challenges that you have your greatest victories and learn things about yourself you'd never thought possible.

A related insight Suskind made concerned the assumption that kids like Owen are *context-blind*: incapable of processing their surroundings. Owen, for instance, had a difficult time understanding why his older brother became embarrassed by his public conduct, which often seemed inappropriate given the setting. What Suskind inferred, however, was that Owen was very context-sensitive when it came to the world that he inhabited, one filled with Disney narratives. "Context blind?" asked Suskind. "Suddenly we see him mastering a context that's invisible to us" as a nine-year-old autistic presumed to have no sense of his surroundings. Within the world that he occupied, however, he was able to construct an affective life, becoming "expressive and affectionate with these characters in ways he rarely is with us, or anyone else."

He later elaborated on the context of Owen's experience: "a river of symbols that flow" in his darkened room of cathode illumination. This observation tends to be unavailable to the clinical diagnostician who, in controlled office visits, can only see what happens *outside the contexts of performance that characterize daily life*. The Suskinds, in contrast, were able to study these contexts in detail and over time in the setting of the family home and its portal to the animated world of Disney films, making them, in effect, *loving ethnographers* of their own home life—not just of Owen, the putative object of their attention, but of themselves as central aspects and mediators of his environment.

Parental Conflicts Between Expectations and Actuality

The Suskinds thus found themselves caught between their world of normal expectations and the world of Disney through which Owen found meaning in his emotional development. Suskind admitted that he still fought the stigma of an autism diagnosis, as many parents do when difference is pathologized. Owen presented the common autistic trait of pursuing self-directed, narrow interests in his immersion in the Disney world, a practice cultivated by his parents. At the same time, they wished for him to be more like other kids, to fit in better with the mainstream of society.

The Suskinds faced a conundrum of many such families, and applied commonsense rules to an uncommon situation (see Chap. 9). Children are often discouraged from being narrow. They are often, for instance, required by adults to read a wider range of authors, engage in a broader array of activities, and so on, so as not to limit their life's possibilities. Yet doing so can amplify feelings of anxiety for those on the autism spectrum, such that they are far more fretful when doing "normal" things such as diversifying their interests than when comfortably ensconced in their narrow focuses (see Chap. 3).

The Suskinds at one point, after learning that Owen was defying controls they tried to place on him by watching videos in the middle of the night, took severe measures to limit his Disney obsession, padlocking the TV cabinet so that he could not access the monitor by himself. Their own expectations for normalcy overrode their growing understanding that Owen thrived in the TV room in ways not available to him outside its darkened confines. Later, Suskind found meaning in William Blake's aphorism that one should seek "to see the world in a grain of sand ... and eternity in an hour," a recognition that an intense, narrow focus can produce greater insight than broad vision more widely distributed. Arriving at that insight, however, took a lot of work, and a lot of faith in his own understandings in relation to the pathologizing discourse surrounding autism.

Suskind later described his ambivalence over his tendencies to control matters and fix problems, and his need to follow Owen's lead. "It's a difficult impulse for me to control," he acknowledged: "I want to fix everything make it just so, make it right. But singing 'Hakuna Matata' [from *The Lion King*] with him eases me and my corrective impulses."

The fit that Owen found with Disney productions was at odds with his conduct in school, a place where his differences became his defining characteristic, leading to his removal from school after school. Owen's difficulty in picking up social cues, said one school administrator, was too great a burden for teachers and classmates, and such a disruptive student had to be removed so that the others could proceed with the learning scripts.

Schools require students to adapt to their rules and codes of conduct. In contrast, at home, the family adjusted to Owen (see Chap. 3), an easier task given the more flexible set of goals and expectations and absence of a plan to disrupt. Suskind describes how a whole extended family, top to bottom, gets changed by someone who stops the constant drumbeat of me and mine, who's up, who's down, the irresistible drama of bloodlines, birth orders, and familial politics. Why? Because the ways he's different compels a minute-to-minute search, humanizing and heart-filling, for all the ways he's not different. It's us at our best.

In school, Owen was viewed as disruptive because he could not perform within the expected social scripts played by obedient students. At home, his points of difference, rather than serving as distractions, were adapted to by those who surrounded him, creating a mediating environment in which his assets could emerge and be cultivated. Rather than being pathologized for his differences, he was nurtured in light of them. "Us at our best": It's hard to argue with Suskind's self-appraisal.

Finding a Role Within the Disney Archetypes

Owen's developing obsession eventually began to include drawing Disney characters, an activity through which he began to demonstrate remarkable skill in graphic production. "It freaks me out," confided Suskind: "He can't write his name legibly," but he could reproduce character drawings with remarkable fidelity. These renderings prompted additional wondering about what they might mean to Owen. Superficially, they appeared to serve as graphic echolalia in that they seemed to involve mimicry without meaning. But Suskind, in his role as loving ethnographer, had learned to look behind appearances and wonder if something of greater substance might be behind them. When looking through Owen's drawings, Suskind found the beginnings of an answer in Owen's scrawl at the end of a sketchbook: "I Am The Protekter of Sidekicks.... No Sidekick Gets Left Behind." Owen's identity was distilled in this expression, and his particular orientation to a specific category of Disney characters took on, for his parents, a new meaning. In Disney's world of heroes, villains, princesses, and supporting characters, Owen saw himself in the role of the sidekick, one who, as Owen later said, "helps the hero fulfill his destiny."

Suskind's processing of this role led to new insights about his son, and about the Disney franchise's character formations. Heroes, he noted, tend to be flat and simple. The supporting players, in contrast, are varied and vivid: "The spectrum of complex human emotions is housed with the sidekicks." This identity was not simply a role, but an identity infused with emotion. Suskind invoked the case of autistic agriculturalist Temple Grandin, who developed a machine that squeezed a person to produce a feeling of comfort—something she had learned about through her experiences with cows panicking while being herded to slaughter—leading to the rare revelation about *how it feels to be autistic*, an issue overlooked in the pathologizing field of autism research.

With Owen incapable of meeting the behavioral standards of formal schools, the Suskinds decided that Cornelia would homeschool him. This decision was informed by a realization that they finally accepted as "overwhelming and indisputable: Our son has turned his affinity for animated movies, mostly Disney, into a language to shape his identity and access emotions that are untouchable and unmanageable for most teenagers, and even adults." Such an affiliation was not cultivated in normal schools, and indeed invited derision and discouragement. In the Vygotskian sense, then, the Suskinds constructed a social setting at home that enabled Owen to become involved in valued cultural activity such that his points of difference became less of a perceived handicap and more viewed as assets in his pursuit of meaningful goals.

The Constructive Role of Imitation

Vygotsky (1934/1987) sees a role for imitation in his account of the zone of proximal development, although his view of imitation includes processes of agency and adaptation. Imitation in his conception requires that "there must be some possibility of moving from what I can do to what I cannot" beyond "mechanical activity" (p. 209), which he believes better characterizes the training of animals. Imitation is involved in what Vygotsky calls "instruction" in which one learns something fundamentally new (p. 210). Van der Veer and Valsiner (1991) describe this distinction as being "between insightful learning and trial-and-error learning.... children are capable of intellectual, insightful imitation.... teaching can evoke and promote their cognitive development" (pp. 344–345). This capacity for mindful imitation is illustrated by the role of play as a way of helping to create a zone of proximal development such that upper thresholds are extended through "the active imitation of a model through play" (Vygotsky 1934/1987, p. 345). Both instruction and play can push and extend one's threshold for learning toward something fundamentally new, and ultimately rule-governed, revealing the dynamic, flexible, and teleological nature of the zone of proximal development (ZPD).

Imitation is, thus, in Holzman's (2010) paradox, fundamentally *creative* in that it helps to construct the ZPD that enables learners to grow toward socially valued ways of being. To Holzman,

> environment must be both what is—the specific sociocultural-historical conditions in which child and mother are located—and what is coming into existence—the changed environment being created by their language activity. In other words, this environment is as much activity as it is context.... It is this activity, I suggest, that is and creates the ZPD—and through which the child develops as a speaker, meaning maker and language user. (p. 33)

This constructive view of imitation helps to explain the difference between echolalia and ventriloquation, a distinction that required close observation on the part of the Suskinds to understand in Owen's appropriation of Disney storylines to provide the contours for his own development. At one point, Owen did an Internet search for the script of *Aladdin* and copied it into a Word file, then laboriously rewrote parts of the story as his own, typing with one finger. Suskind described his process as follows:

> What's running through his noggin is now on the page, as though this was the way the movie might have been, maybe should have been.
>
> Even years later, when he told us about this night when he changed this *Aladdin* script, he explained that there was a problem to be solved. He'd long ago turned [the evil sidekick Iago] into someone he could confide in, something I'd discovered from under the bedspread that night many years before. How, though, could a villain's sidekick be Owen's dear friend. At some point, after umpteen viewings, this insight about good and evil, and one's capacity to change, took shape. Did he know when? Not exactly. Did he impute it by observing real people in real situation? He can't say. All he knows is that he secretly changed this plot, so a villain's sidekick could switch sides, free prisoners from a dungeon, and help a hero fulfill his destiny. (pp. 166–167)

Suskind's insight about Owen's appropriation and adaptation of the plot suggest Ricoeur's (1983) notion of how stories may become *emplotted*, that is, situated in dialogue with and in extension of other, previous readings and the evocations: the series of images that they associate with them (Rosenblatt 1978). These evocations serve as *configurational acts* enabling readers to bring together diverse texts into a complex whole (see Smagorinsky 2001). Disney stories in this sense provided source material through which Owen constructed his own narratives, interpreting his characters as he saw them rather than as they were conventionally understood or deliberately composed. In school, these liberties would often suggest that he had comprehension problems, but in the world he constructed in his reconfigured home, his imaginative adaptations to the stories made perfect sense. This narrative ultimately coalesced into Owen's orchestration of the whole of the Disney sidekick archetype into his own grand narrative: "Twelve sidekicks searching for a hero. And in their journey, and in the obstacles they face, each finds the hero within themselves."

THE BENEFITS OF A NARROW FOCUS

One of Owen's therapists noted Owen's obsession and how it both conformed to what he had seen in other autism spectrum cases and departed from them. Disney movies, he inferred, "involve relationships and carry emotional complexity," unlike Pokémon or inanimate objects like cars. Having observed my own daughter's obsession with Pokémon and its gateway to the deeply emotional world of more sophisticated anime films and graphic novels, I would dispute the therapist's dismissal of Pokémon as being absent emotional complexity. But his point on the emotional resonance that Disney enabled in Owen is on target and overlooked in much writing on autism.

The therapist also noted that Suskind had been advised by a number of professionals to discourage Owen's obsession with Disney because, as he wrote in his notes, "it's self stimulatory and avoidant—meaning he would use it to avoid social interaction and instead retreat into fantasy. I understood that that would be the professional consensus, but I remember thinking, and maybe even saying, 'I'm not so sure.'" Rather than seeing obsession as narrow and limiting, the therapist acknowledged that by delving so deeply into the genre, Owen might be mining something far richer than was available on the surface, and thus benefiting in ways that non-obsessives have a difficult time relating to and understanding.

Finally, the therapist concluded that he was "blown away at how good [Ron] Suskind was at acting out the scenes. What struck me was, not only did Owen come alive, but Suskind came alive in a way I hadn't seen before, and the connection between them was electric. I noticed so much joy, intensity, spontaneity, laughter, and they seemed much more organically connected. The room crackled with sparks of delight." I find this observation to illuminate much about what we authors are trying to achieve in this volume. The autistic boy with his narrow interest in a single film genre was engaged in highly social play and performance. First, Disney's stories are drawn from ancient tales, reimagined for the late twentieth century and filled with stock characters, one of which, the sidekick, Owen had identified with and incorporated into his self-image. Watching these films with his family had been a social process, even with Owen's frequent solo expeditions to watch and rewind in ways that only he could find interesting. But the family's willingness to take on characters' roles and engage in either verbatim or reconstructed dialogues produced a setting in which Owen could not only thrive in the moment but grow through the enactments and affirmation he received from his family. As Suskind noted, "he seemed to be using this narrative construct to shape his identity. He was clearly transposing his deepest feelings, his fears and aspirations, on the sidekicks."

This infusion of characters with feelings, in turn working through his own emotions about his place in the world, was fundamental to his performative and playful engagement with Disney sidekicks, an observation made by a therapist who noted with interest: "Autistic kids like Owen are not supposed to [empathize like that]—this is getting weird in a very good way." I would argue that the Suskinds' willingness to play along with Owen and validate his engagement with their participation and support contributed to Owen's development of capabilities that his diagnosticians presumed he could not have. Rather than pathologizing him with the assumption that he could not feel for others, the Suskinds, through patient and supportive play *with* Owen over time, saw what is rarely evident to the disinterested diagnostician who, with the *Diagnostic and Statistical Manual of Mental Disorders* (American Psychiatric Association 2013) guiding the procedures, is looking for disabilities, abnormalities, disorders, and deficiencies, rather than abilities and potential.

Owen's obsession with a celluloid world in part shielded him from society's real cruelties, which he experienced late in his teens through bullies at school: seemingly "good" and charismatic teens who knew how to act when adults are watching and how, when they are not, to destroy the confidence of peers without the full range of resources for resilience, like Owen. Following an extensive period of being bullied, Owen worked through his feelings of fear that led to regressions in his social development. At one point, he took on the role of Merlin from *The Sword in the Stone*, in essence providing himself with a sympathetic, understanding counselor. Remarkably, rather than reciting scripts from the film, Owen adapted Merlin to voice the advice he needed to endure the social obstacles constructed for him by the bullies:

> Listen, my boy, knowledge and wisdom are the real power! Now remember, lad, I turned you into a fish. Well, you have to think of that water like the future. It's unknown until you swim in it. And the more you swim, the more you know. About both the deep waters and about yourself. So swim, boy, swim.

Suskind was left to wonder: "Could it be that a separate speech faculty has been developing within him that was unaffected by autism? Or, maybe, in response to how the autism blocked and rewired the normal neural pathways for speech development?" This development, he believed, was predicated on Disney scripts of the sort discouraged by therapists and psychologists. Yet Owen adapted them to his own situations so that his inner speech—which Suskind learned about through his exposure to Vygotsky (1934–1987)—could rely on social scripts adjusted to represent—to emplot—Owen's experiences in archetypal storylines. As the family's education specialist phrased it: "It's not so much how he's used the movies to help with academics. It's how he's used them to guide emotional growth, which, of course, is the bigger and more complex challenge."

When a therapist suggested that Owen write a book called *The Wisdom of Disney, as Told by Owen Suskind to His Father*, Suskind responded, "I'm not sure if the wisdom is with Disney." He then invoked what might be termed a transactional sense of the role of story (see, e.g., Smagorinsky 2001):

> Owen's chosen affinity clearly opened a window to myth, fable, and legend, that Disney lifted and retooled, just like the Grimm Brothers did, from a vast repository of folklore. Countless cultures have told versions of *Beauty and the Beast*, which dates back three thousand years to the Greek's "Cupid and Psyche," and certainly beyond that: these are stories human beings have always told themselves to make their way in the world. It's how people embrace these archetypal tales, and use them to find their way—that's where the wisdom lies.

As a transactional theory of reading suggests, the meaning is not solely in the text, but emerges through a reader's attribution of meaning to the narrative codes. Reading in this sense involves not just decoding texts but *encoding* them by instantiating meaning based on personal knowledge and experiences.

Deep Engagement and Depth of Insight

Owen's next stages would be difficult for the ordinary family—one, that is, without wealth and connections—to replicate. Owen developed the goal of becoming, as he said, "an animator at the Disney Animation Studios in Burbank, California, and usher in a new golden age of hand-drawn animation [through] a movie about the sidekicks' journey using traditional hand-drawn animation. It touches people and saves the world," a story both fictional and real, with Owen in a central role in both. Many kids might harbor such a goal; few have fathers who can make a few calls to help make it happen.

During a birthday call from Jonathan Freeman, a Disney voiceover actor who spoke the lines of Jafar from *Aladdin* among other roles, Jonathan became curious about which themes Owen resonated with most in the films:

> "Isn't it about the forces of good and evil fighting it out," Jonathan proffers. "And how in the end, good triumphs."
>
> "Umm. Sort of. I think it's about more than that," counters Owen.…"I think it's about finally accepting who you really are. And being okay with that."
>
> The sound of sighs and sniffles comes from the phone. "Oh my. How is it I never saw that."

Owen was then able to visit with a variety of Disney animators on a trip to the Disney Animation Studios in Los Angeles. When asked by an animator how it felt to draw, Owen responded, "I feel what the characters do, if they're happy or sad or scared or lighthearted. When I draw it, I can feel it." This insight mapped well onto Walt Disney's own approach to animation, as Suskind noted:

> [Disney] had taken a crafted image, hand-drawn in a way anyone could on a pad—albeit drafted by professional artists—and turned it into a verisimilitude of life that carried basic human emotions. That was his real innovation—presenting lifelike emotions on the screen to draw forth real emotions: "And that's really why Owen's here—emotions.… What the lifelike emotions presented in these movies drew from him, and still do, are *his* emotions, *his* deepest feelings, from his life as our son. Not Walt Disney's."

This interest in and respect for Owen's Disney obsession led Suskind to begin to see Owen as a source of insight, not a boy perpetually locked into childhood, not someone with a pervasive developmental disorder. Toward the end of the memoir, Suskind relates a time when he asked Owen what it was like to watch *Beauty and the Beast* hundreds of times over a period of nearly two decades. Owen replied:

> The movie doesn't change. That is what I love about it. But I change. And each time, it looks different to me. It was scary when I was small. And then I understood that it was about finding beauty, even in places where it's hard to find. But now I realize it's about something else. A bigger thing. It's about finding beauty in yourself, because only then will you really be able to really see it in others, and everywhere…. And now I can see beauty everywhere.

Play and performance in human development: Owen experienced this process through his transactional engagement with Disney characters, supported by his attentive family and treated with respect and dignity in his home. Unlike in his schools and different from his experiences in his peer world, Owen was provided with a mediational setting that cultivated his assets and constructed his points of difference as contributing factors in his growing insights about himself and his social world.

Group Homes

In thinking about mediational settings for autistic youth, I thought about the function of group homes for autistic youth and adults. Like the son of my college friend who is in his mid-20s without having yet spoken, Owen, at the end of his father's memoir, went off to live in a group home, where his developmental trajectory may unfold in an environment in which he and his fellow autistics comprise the norm.

I had hoped to learn more about group home practices, but was quite surprised to find in my searches that there is little research on what happens in a group home. Perhaps Institutional Review Boards are careful in allowing research to be conducted with such a sensitive population, but it appears as if few have even tried. What is available fits within the pathologizing discourse of much autism research, as illustrated by the following abstract:

> A treatment package consisting of a DRO [Differential Reinforcement of Other behavior] procedure, token fines, and prompted relaxation was used to reduce the agitated-disruptive behavior of a person with autism and

mental retardation living in a community group home. The agitated-disruptive behaviors [included] cursing, hitting, kicking, throwing objects, and verbal threats. (Reese et al. 1998, p. 159)

I know that there are kids who strike back at those around them, and I have no solutions to offer as to how to treat them humanely while also protecting others from their conduct, other than to provide environments that elicit potential, a task easier written than achieved. At the same time, for research on a group setting, I find the emphasis on the individual's offensive and dangerous outbursts to be very limiting in understanding how to construct a social setting—such as a group home—so that social activity serves as a developmental channel. Because group homes are undoubtedly idiosyncratic in terms of their supervision, enrollment numbers, characteristics of residents, and other factors, it's difficult to say what they provide, especially given that research thus far appears to be both limited in volume and focused on badly behaved individuals and how to make them less threatening and disruptive. Given that they often serve as the setting in which people on the autism spectrum conduct their daily lives, surely it's critical to undertake research into how they function to mediate the development of autistics, and to understand the endpoints toward which their lives are encouraged.

Discussion

In this chapter, I have taken a family memoir and treated Suskind's report as a loving autoethnography, amenable to illustrating how a setting may be constructed within families and other social units in which young people of neurological difference may find productive channels of activity in which to immerse themselves and help to construct their social futures. I believe that the Suskinds' emotional attachment to their son provided far greater insight into his state of mind than could any observations from detached observers who are trained and tasked to look for deficits. The Suskinds were ever hopeful about Owen's prospects in life, and thus looked for signs of assets and potential instead of behaviors indicating pathology.

Their care-oriented effort to step inside Owen's world illustrates a rare sort of emotional connection, that of *compathy*. Sympathy refers to having feelings of support for others experiencing problems that are not shared by the observer so as to achieve "fellow feeling" for those in distress. Empathy refers to the capacity to share or recognize emotions experienced by another, taking a step closer to emotional resonance than sympathy allows. Compathy takes empathy one great step further, requiring one to *feel with* another, a state that is so difficult to achieve that compathy is barely even a word. Yet that's what I see in the Suskinds' relationships with Owen. That orientation, I assert, makes them far more reliable than diagnosticians who are purportedly objective, even as their perspective requires diagnosing deficits, a framing standpoint that negates claims to objectivity and inevitably constructs difference as deficit.

This compathy enabled the Suskinds to enter Owen's world and become characters in his drama. They set aside their own tastes in film to see Disney through their son's eyes, and to listen carefully to how he understood this world. Rather than relying on adults looking for evidence of developmental deficiencies in their "pervasively developmentally disordered" and often puzzling son, they played and performed along with him, following his insights and learning to appreciate them. Within his family, he was thus not subject to the secondary disability that afflicts those who are bombarded with deficit language and ideology. Rather, he gained in confidence, authoring his own interpretive narrative through which he orchestrated Disney archetypes, emplotted his own experiences and outlook, and constructed a positive social future for himself. Central to this process was his family's commitment to adapting *their* lives to his, motivated by their love and care and willingness to understand his differences and cultivate his assets through playful engagement.

Notes

1. I will refer to Ron Suskind as Suskind, his wife as Cornelia, and his sons as Walt and Owen. I also depart from Suskind's present-tense narrative style, relating his story using past-tense verbs.
2. As described in the Wikipedia (n. d.) entry on shadow: "In Jungian psychology, the *shadow* or '*shadow aspect*' may refer to (1) an unconscious aspect of the personality which the conscious ego does not identify in itself. Because one tends to reject or remain ignorant of the least desirable aspects of one's personality, the shadow is largely negative, or (2) the entirety of the unconscious, that is, everything of which a person is not fully conscious. There are, however, positive aspects which

may also remain hidden in one's shadow (especially in people with low self-esteem). Contrary to a Freudian definition of shadow, therefore, the Jungian shadow can include everything outside the light of consciousness, and may be positive or negative. 'Everyone carries a shadow,' Jung wrote, 'and the less it is embodied in the individual's conscious life, the blacker and denser it is.' It may be (in part) one's link to more primitive animal instincts, which are superseded during early childhood by the conscious mind. According to Jung, the shadow, in being instinctive and irrational, is prone to psychological projection, in which a perceived personal inferiority is recognized as a perceived moral deficiency in someone else. Jung writes that if these projections remain hidden, 'The projection-making factor (the Shadow archetype) then has a free hand and can realize its object—if it has one—or bring about some other situation characteristic of its power.' These projections insulate and harm individuals by acting as a constantly thickening veil of illusion between the ego and the real world. From one perspective, 'the shadow…is roughly equivalent to the whole of the Freudian unconscious'; and Jung himself asserted that 'the result of the Freudian method of elucidation is a minute elaboration of man's shadow-side unexampled in any previous age'. Jung also believed that 'in spite of its function as a reservoir for human darkness—or perhaps because of this—the shadow is the seat of creativity'; so that for some, it may be, 'the dark side of his being, his sinister shadow…represents the true spirit of life as against the arid scholar.'"
3. In Smagorinsky (2011b), I define inner speech as follows: "Inner speech refers to the cognitive processes that follow from the appropriation of both social speech and its ideological framework such that one adopts cultural means of mediation (particularly that provided by speech) for self-regulation, ideas, and other means of acting in the world in accordance with social standards and practices. The endeavor to name inner speech and understand its workings is entirely inferential and only indirectly supportable through empirical evidence" (p. 12).
4. Gottfried lost much of his voiceover work following repugnant jokes he tweeted in March 2011 after the devastating earthquake disaster in Japan.
5. This event is featured in a brief film at http://www.nytimes.com/video/magazine/100000002755397/animating-owen.html?src=vidm

References

American Psychiatric Association (2013). *Diagnostic and statistical manual of mental disorders* (5th ed.). Arlington: Author.

Bakhtin, M. M. (1981). *The dialogic imagination: Four essays by Mikhail Bakhtin* (trans: Emerson, C. & Holquist, M.). Austin: University of Texas Press.

Cole, M. (1996). *Cultural psychology: A once and future discipline*. Cambridge, MA: Harvard University Press.

Holzman, L. (2010). Without creating ZPDs there is no creativity. In M. C. Connery, V. John-Steiner, & A. Marjanovic-Shane (Eds.), *Vygotsky and creativity: A cultural-historical approach to meaning-making, play, and the arts* (pp. 28–39). New York: Peter Lang.

Reese, R. M., Sherman, J. A., & Sheldon, J. B. (1998). Reducing disruptive behavior of a group-home resident with autism and mental retardation. *Journal of Autism and Developmental Disorders, 28*(2), 159–165.

Ricoeur, P. (1983). *Time and narrative* (Vol. 1; trans: McLaughlin, K. & Pellauer, D.). Chicago: University of Chicago Press.

Rosenblatt, L. M. (1978). *The reader, the text, the poem: The transactional theory of the literary work*. Carbondale: Southern Illinois University Press.

Wikipedia. (n. d.). Shadow. Retrieved September 1, 2016 from (psychology). *Wikipedia*. Available at http://en.wikipedia.org/wiki/Shadow_%28psychology%29

Smagorinsky, P. (2001). If meaning is constructed, what is it made from? Toward a cultural theory of reading. *Review of Educational Research, 71*, 133–169.

Smagorinsky, P. (2011a). Confessions of a mad professor: An autoethnographic consideration of neuroatypicality, extranormativity, and education. *Teachers College Record, 113*, 1701–1732. Available at http://www.petersmagorinsky.net/About/PDF/TCR/TCR2011.pdf

Smagorinsky, P. (2011b). *Vygotsky and literacy research: A methodological framework*. Boston: Sense.

Suskind, R. (1998). *A hope in the unseen: An American odyssey from the inner city to the Ivy League*. New York: Broadway Books.

Suskind, R. (2014a). *Life animated: A story of sidekicks, heroes, and autism*. New York: Kingswell.

Suskind, R. (2014b). Reaching my autistic son through Disney. *The New York Times Magazine*. Available at http://www.nytimes.com/2014/03/09/magazine/reaching-my-autistic-son-through-disney.html?

Van der Veer, R., & Valsiner, J. (1991). *Understanding Vygotsky: A quest for synthesis*. Cambridge, MA: Blackwell.

Vygotsky, L. S. (1934/1987). Thinking and speech. In L. S. Vygotsky, *Collected works* (Vol. 1, pp. 39–285) (R. Rieber & A. Carton, Eds; trans: Minick, N.). New York: Plenum.

Wertsch, J. V. (1991). *Voices of the mind: A sociocultural approach to mediated action*. Cambridge, MA: Harvard University Press.

Contributors

Leslie Susan Cook is associate professor in the English Department at Appalachian State University in Boone, North Carolina, where she is co-director of the English Education program. Her doctoral dissertation research with young women diagnosed with depression and related neurodivergent makeups has been a springboard for further work in ending the stigma around neurodiversity and educating future teachers about diversity across the human spectrum.

Christine Dawson is the Director of Student Teaching at Skidmore College. She was a secondary English teacher for ten years, served as an English department coordinator for a middle/high school, and was a literacy coach. She earned her doctorate in Curriculum, Instruction, and Teacher Education from Michigan State University, and she holds an MA in Curriculum and Teaching from Columbia University Teachers College and a BA from the University of Virginia. Her research interests focus on writing studies and pedagogies, English teacher preparation, curriculum design, and the significance of teachers' own writing in their beliefs and pedagogical practices.

Marcy Epstein teaches in comprehensive studies at the University of Michigan-Ann Arbor and manages a private practice for children and adults in literacy, exceptionality, and academic advocacy. Her books include *Deep: Real Life with Spinal Cord Injury* and *Points of Contact: Disability, Art, and Culture*.

294 CONTRIBUTORS

Aaron Feinstein holds an MFA in theater directing from UCLA's School of Theater, Film, and Television. Previously, he co-directed The Miracle Project with Elaine Hall, which was the subject of the two-time Emmy Award winning HBO documentary: "Autism: The Musical." He is currently the Executive Director and Founder of Actionplay, an NYC-based 501(c)(3) programming, outreach, and education organization dedicated to providing children, teens, and adults on the autism spectrum and related conditions equal access to education, arts, and culture. Aaron is the director of the film Ken and Alex (Big Daddy Autism) about the unconditional love of a father and his non-speaking son on the autism spectrum living in NYC.

Paula Heller (MA Theatrical Directing) has taught theater arts for 25 years at Mehlville High School in St. Louis. She has directed over 70 plays with youth of all ages and abilities, and has worked with Theatre Unlimited, a program for adults of various abilities and the Teen Theatre program at the Jewish Community Center, and currently works with That Uppity Theatre Company's DisAbility Project and the Prison Performing Arts organization. Additionally, she teaches at private schools for autistic youngsters through Stage's St. Louis outreach programs. She is working toward Drama Therapy certification through the North American Drama Therapy Association.

Christine LaCerva, M.Ed. is Director of the Social Therapy Group and of the East Side Institute for Group and Short Term Psychotherapy Therapist Training Program. She leads a large group practice that includes clients aged 4–84 years. With Fred Newman, the late founder of social therapy, Christine has worked over 30 years to advance a philosophically inspired, performatory approach to emotional development, helping clients build environments for their emotional growth. Her multi-family groups explore unexpected ways to support the development of families whose children have been diagnosed on the autism spectrum. She completed her graduate studies at Teachers College, Columbia University, in community psychology and special education (including education of the deaf) and has a performance background in dance.

Joan Lipkin co-founded the DisAbility Project, one of the first and longest theater projects for people with disabilities in the country, with the late occupational therapist Fran Cohen, in St. Louis, MO. As the artistic director of That Uppity Theatre Company, she has worked with people with disabilities for over 20 years, and also consulted with other companies on techniques for teaching playwriting and theater to children and youth with ADD, ADHD, OCD, and other learning disabilities. A nationally recognized expert on community-based theater, she has also worked extensively with numerous populations including people in the LGBTQ community, people with Alzheimer's and early onset dementia, women with cancer, survivors of suicide, supporters of reproductive choice, at risk youth, foster children, university students, women who have been sexually trafficked or exploited, those struggling with substance abuse, among many others.

Robin Post specializes in Acting, Voice, Movement, Devising, and Community Engagement Theater. She recently joined the Department of Theatre at The University of North Carolina Wilmington (UNCW) as an assistant professor of acting after a decade teaching for The Ohio State University's (OSU) Department of Theatre. While at OSU, she was the director of a longitudinal empirical research study, Shakespeare and Autism. She is presently establishing programming at UNCW intended to train students majoring in theater, psychology, social work, education, exercise science, and so on on how to implement the work with those on the spectrum. Robin most recently performed with the Royal Shakespeare Company at The Other Place Theatre in a unique production performed with children on the spectrum.

Nicola Shaughnessy is a professor at the University of Kent (UK). Grounded in feminist studies and theater, she now serves as Director and co-founder of Kent's Research Centre for Cognition, Kinesthetics and Performance. Through this role, she investigates the cognitive and physiological processes involved in making, participating in, and experiencing performance. She has also initiated practice-based projects using applied drama and performance in the workplace as part of Kent's Innovation, Creativity and Enterprise network as well as an interdisciplinary project on drama, performance, and intermediality as interventions for autism (www.imaginingautism.org).

Peter Smagorinsky is Distinguished Research Professor of English Education at The University of Georgia. Primarily a literacy education researcher following a career as a high school English teacher, he has begun investigating Asperger's syndrome following his recognition of his own place on the spectrum in conjunction with his daughter's diagnosis. His writing on this topic has been autoethnographic, theoretical, and empirical.

Index

A
ableist attitudes, 170
Actionplay, 140–2, 147, 148
    action, 145–7
    building community, 142–3
    music's role, 142
    normativity and compliance, 143–5
adaptation, 51–73
alien puppet, 187–8
American Psychiatric Association, 11
applied behavioral analysis (ABA), 143, 144
Arendt, H., 35
Asen, E., 89
Asperger's syndrome spectrum, 8, 35, 38, 52, 53, 113, 188, 220, 222, 234
Attention deficit hyperactivity disorder (ADHD), 129–30
Auslander, P., 154
autism spectrum disorders (ASD), 4
autism-spectrum youth, 142
autistics, 134, 144, 274

autoethnography, 269–90
Axline, V., 90

B
Bailey, S., 164
Bakhtin, M.M., 274
Bakhurst, D., 43
banality of evil, 35
Baron-Cohen, S., 156, 200
behavior emotional and social disorders (BESD), 226
benign neglect, 36
Bernauer, D., 44
Blume, H., 10
Boal, A., 149
Bogdashina, O., 200
Bozalek, V., 34–5, 40
brain disorder, 14
Broomhead, K.E., 226
Bryant, C., 144
building community, 142–3
Burrs, G., 192, 196

C
Chaikin, J., 156
Chloe, 219–22, 239–41, 241n1
   commercial potential, 236–7
   contrast to expectations, 226–7
   creativity, 237–9
   life trajectory, 231–4
   otaku, 222–5
   peer relationships, 227–31
   sexuality, 234–6
Christian Science Monitor, 44
City University of New York (CUNY), 145
Coach E, 132–3, 134–6
co-adaptation, 54–8
Cole, M., 47n4, 62
Cook, L.S., 24, 219–41
Crutchfield, S., 171

D
Daiute, C., 63, 71
Damasio, A.R., 61
Daniels, H., 9
Darwin, C., 21, 54–8
Dawson, C.M., 25, 243–66
defectology, 4, 16, 33, 36–8, 46n1
deficiency, 124
DIRFloortime®, 134, 135
DisAbility Project, 22, 153–85
   autism-inclusive performance, 164–6
   mission, 157–9
   origins, 156–7
   participants, 159–60
   post-performance, 166–7
   pre-performance, 162–3
   scripts, 167–71
   survey, 172–3
Disney archetypes, 280–1
Disney narratives, 277–8
Doyoyoying game, 110
Drama Club, 131
dramaturgical prosthesis, 160
dualism, 34, 47n2
Dynamic Story-Telling by Youth (DSTY), 71

E
employment, 170, 184n3, 180–4
Epstein, M., 153–85
extranormal, 38

F
Facts and Figures, 169, 170, 184n3, 178–80
family play, 79–102
Feinstein, A., 23, 129–49
File Transfer Protocol (FTP), 223
Fortune Magazine, 224

G
Galton, F., 54
Gerrig, R.J., 164
Gindis, B., 53
Graham, S., 113
Grandin, T., 3, 210n1
Grasseni, C., 202
Greenspan, N. T., 157
Greenspan, S. I., 23, 134, 135, 138, 157
guided improvisation, 190

H
Haddon, M., 210
handicap, 37
Happé, F., 205
heartbeat hellos, 119
Heathcote, D., 121, 124
Heller, P., 153–85
Higashida, N., 176, 195

Hjörne, E., 9
Hoffman, D., 15, 271
Hoggett, S., 113
Holzman, L., 10, 20, 22, 80, 81, 282
Hoover, H., 67
Howell, A., 203, 204, 206
human development, 6–8
Hunter Heartbeat Method (HHM), 23, 105–8
  circle as activity boundary, 114–15
  empowerment, 116-18 *In Here Out There*, 126
  play, 122–5
  praise, 120–2
  roles and processes, 115–17
  structure, 112–14
  teacher/learner, 108–12
  The Tempest, 125–6
Hunter, K., 115, 116

I
Immordino-Yang, M.H., 61
inadequacy, 38–41
individual adaptation, 65–7
individualistic orientation, 68
inferiorization, 34
interiorization, 39

J
Jones, W., 192

K
Klin, A., 191, 192
Kozulin, A., 53

L
LaCerva, C., 21, 22, 79–102
Lamarckian principles, 61

Lee, K., 6, 53, 60, 61, 63, 69
Lindley, R.A., 61
Lipkin, J., 153–85
Little Foxy, 199
Lobman, C., 148

M
Markram, H., 207
Markram, K., 207
Marxism, 57, 63–4
Master of Fine Arts (MFA), 126
Matthew Effect, 70
mechanical activity, 281
medical model, 8–10
Meisner technique, 123
mental health, 6, 10–15, 33–47
mental illness, 11, 52
Meshcheryakov, A., 43
meta-experience, 39, 69
Miracle Project, 132–3, 139–40, 141, 148, 149
Mitchell, D.T., 160
moral insanity, 38, 40, 240
Moynihan, D.P., 36
music therapy, 142

N
narrative transportation, 164
National Alliance on Mental Illness (NAMI), 11
National Governors Association, 44
National Institute of Neurological Disorders and Stroke, 4
neurodiverse populations, 14
neurodiversity, 9, 10, 20–1
neurological system, 13
neurotypical, 38, 127n2
  population, 108
  syndrome, 8
Newman, F., 22, 80–2, 88–90, 98

New Soviet Man, 57
Nixon, R.M., 36
Nordoff-Robbins method, 142
normalcy, 124, 125, 279
normality, 8, 93

O
obsessive-compulsiveness, 12, 24, 51, 52, 72, 220
obshcheniya, 43
Ockleford, A., 207
Ohio State University (OSU), 127n1, 127n6, 127n7
online anime community, 219–41
oppositional defiant disorder (ODD), 82
othering, 34, 170
Owen, 272–3, 288–9
   deep engagement and depth of insight, 286–7
   Disney, 277–8, 280–1, 283–6
   echolalia and ventriloquation, 273–6
   expectations and actualit, 278–80
   group homes, 287–8
   imitation, 281–3

P
Padden, C., 43
pathology paradigm, 8, 10, 27n1
Pellicano, E., 192, 196
people of difference, 66
pervasive developmental disorder (PDD), 83, 102n1
Pervasive Developmental Disorder-Not Otherwise Specified (PDD-NOS), 222, 233
Phoebe Caldwell foundation, 211n2
play and performance, 5
Pokémon characters, 135–40

positive social updraft, 5, 16–18, 42, 43, 69
Post, R., 23, 105–28
privileged irresponsibility, 34
Prizant, B., 143
prolepsis, 277
proprioceptive sense, 133

R
Rao, A., 90
Revenge of the Godz, 145, 147
Ricoeur, P., 282
Rippl, G., 197
Rodenburg, P., 119
Roth, I., 209
roundabout, 9, 37, 41, 66, 259
Royal Shakespeare Company, 127n6

S
Sainsbury, C., 113, 117, 127n5
Säljö, R., 9
Salomon, 203
Sandahl, C., 154
Sawyer, R.K., 205
Scharf, R., 173
Scholz, M., 89
Scott, 243–4, 262–3
   advanced student of writing, 251–8
   autism, 258–62
   Poet-Memoirist, 245–51
   Research Method, 264–6
secondary disability, 16
sensory experience, 133–5
Shakespeare and Autism, 106–8
Shaughnessy, N., 24, 187–212, 212n9, 212n12
Siegel, D., 157
Silberman, S., 3, 5
Simon, G., 127n3

Smagorinsky, P., 3–27, 33–47, 51–73, 153–85, 219–41, 269–90, 290n3
Smolit, H., 175
Snyder, S.L., 160
Social Emotional NeuroScience Endocrinology (SENSE), 184n2
social environment, 15–16, 58–60
socially mediated neurodiversity paradigm, 14
social therapy, 79–102
social updraft, 16–18, 42, 43
Spencer, H., 54
Stapleton, M., 212n12
Starkloff, M., 156, 157
Stetsenko, A., 55, 56, 60
stimming, 206, 211n1
Suskind, R., 25, 72, 198, 269, 272, 273, 276, 279–1, 282–5, 289, 289n1

T
Templeton, F., 203, 204, 206
therapeutic process, 83
The Tempest, 127n6
Thomson, R.G., 160
Tobin, J., 53
Toku, M., 235
Tourette's syndrome, 24, 51, 52, 219, 222, 233
Tribble, L., 202, 203
Trimingham, M., 212n7, 212n8
Tronto, J., 34, 39, 40

U
Uppity Theater Company, 154

V
Valsiner, J., 281
Van der Veer, R., 281
vestibular sense, 134
Vygotskian scholar Cole, 277
Vygotsky, L.S., 4, 6, 9–11, 13, 16, 18, 19, 21, 33, 43–6, 47n3, 47n4, 53, 54, 56, 58, 59, 64–6, 68–70, 81, 82, 131, 144, 148, 199, 200, 240, 281
  culture, 41–2
  and defectology, 36–8
  inadequacy, 38–41

W
Walgreens Disability Inclusion, 43–6
Walker, N., 8, 9, 26–7n1, 27n3
Walt Disney studios, 270–2, 286
Ward, D., 212n12
Wertsch, J.V., 4, 13, 251, 274
Whitebox, M., 146–7
Williams, D., 144
Wilson, R., 235
Wittgenstein, L., 81, 93
Woodruff, P., 153

Y
Yaroshevsky, M., 18
Yosemite Still Life, 255–6

Z
zone of proximal development (ZPD), 200, 281, 282